Our Black Fathers:
Brave, Bold and Beautiful!

Joslyn Gaines Vanderpool & Anita Royston

Our Black Fathers: *Brave, Bold and Beautiful!*

The Brave, Bold and Beautiful! series was created to inspire, empower, enlighten and recount the personal histories of the forgotten, unknown and unacknowledged, who live or have lived bravely, boldly and beautifully. As storytellers and keepers of the gate, our role is to unleash our truths and preserve our stories for posterity.

Five Sisters Publishing
PO Box 217
Gretna VA 24557
www.5sisterspublishing.com

First Edition: 2008
Second Edition: June 2017
Published in North America by AR Publishing. For information, please contact Five Sisters Publishing c/o Anita McGee Royston, PO Box 217, Gretna, VA 24557.

Library of Congress Cataloguing-In-Publication Data
Library of Congress Control Number:
Joslyn Gaines Vanderpool and Anita McGee Royston
Our Black Fathers Brave, Bold and Beautiful! Joslyn Gaines Vanderpool and Anita McGee Royston and /– 1st ed
p. cm.

ISBN – 978-0-981-7784-0-2
1. SOCIAL SCIENCE / Ethnic Studies / African American Studies. 2. BIOGRAPHY & AUTOBIOGRAPHY / African American & Black see Cultural Heritage. 3. FAMILY & RELATIONSHIPS / Parenting / Fatherhood. 4. ART / American / African American. 5. HISTORY / United States / 20th Century. 6. SOCIAL SCIENCE / Women's Studies

10   9   8   7   6   5   4   3   2   1

Comments about *Our Black Fathers Brave, Bold and Beautiful!* and requests for additional copies, book club rates and author speaking appearances may be addressed to Joslyn Gaines Vanderpool and Anita McGee Royston and or Five Sisters Publishing c/o Anita Royston, PO Box 217, Gretna VA, 24557, or you can send your comments and requests via e-mail to www.5sisterspublishing.com

Also available as an eBook from Internet retailers and from Five Sisters Publishing

Book Design and layout by Christopher Moebs/Pegasus Books

Printed in the United States of America

Contents

Section Two:
For the Love of Him

Section Three: Transformations

Section Five: One Man Show

Dedication

To our remarkable fathers:
Morris Lee Gaines and Josephus McGee, Sr.
for providing powerful legacies of love,
fortitude and faith.

Morris Lee Gaines   Josephus McGee, Sr.

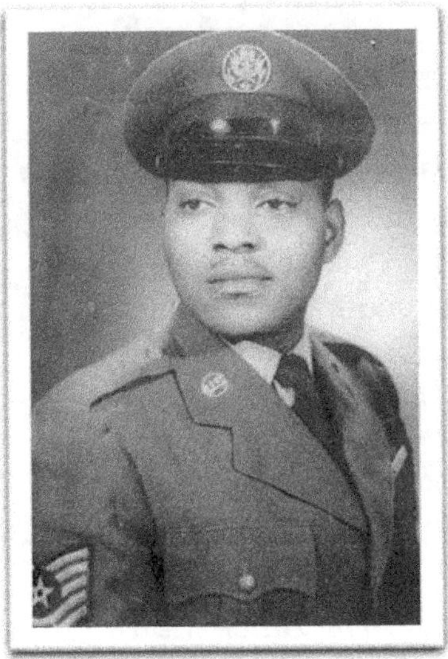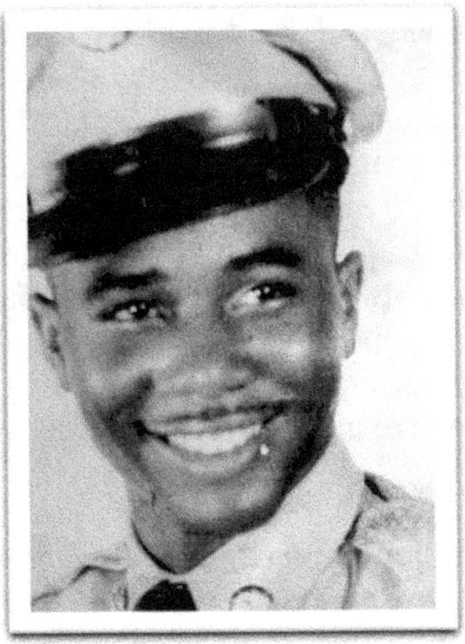

Special Acknowledgements and Thanks...

We'd like to express sincere gratitude to all fathers living or deceased who are/were there for their families. To those committed to raising brave, bold and beautiful children we salute you. Also we'd like to thank the fathers who are in the stories; and the authors for their efforts to shed light on these monumental men in their lives.

Special thanks are extended to Frank Withrow for the use of his powerful poems. We also would like to commend and thank, D'Antoinette, Geisha, Marsha, Sasha, and Vanessa our bright, wonderful, hard-working assistants who have been extremely instrumental in keeping us organized. Many thanks to Clark and Jeremiah of Unison Media who were there when we needed them and willing to pitch into this effort with passion. To our families: you are exceptional. We offer sincere gratitude to our mothers, our husbands, children, grandchildren, siblings, extended families and friends. We appreciate your patience and encouragement and the kind and empowering words of so many others who have entered and stayed, or streamed through our lives at significant times to inspire and support us in this endeavor.

To Alan Govenar, the prolific author of many books about the African American experience and the late Osceola Mays, we offer deep appreciation for allowing us to include, *The Black Man's Plea for Justice* from the beautifully written book, *Osceola: Memories of a Sharecroppers Daughter*.

Most importantly, Anita and I thank God for our collaboration in life, in addition to our partnership in developing this series. And to our late, great fathers, we love and thank you eternally for the lessons you imparted, and the tremendous legacies you've left us.

<h1 style="text-align:center">Extraordinary Praise for
Our Black Fathers: Brave, Bold and Beautiful!</h1>

"Our Black Fathers: Brave, Bold and Beautiful! is simply a magnificent compilation of some of the most absorbing and readable stories of Black fathers on the planet. With each story, the authors have managed to lay before the world the most intimate symbols of what it meant and what it means to be a Black father in America. Moreover, this poignant and impassioned book highlights the quiet strength, the dignified demeanor, the profound courage and the generous spirit that truly defines the essence of Black fatherhood. This is one of the most important books written about the power, genius and dignity of fatherly love. Much, much praise to the storytellers and to the two gifted and incredible authors and creators, for sharing their stories and for letting us know – once and for all – that Black Fathers matter.*" Richard A. Rowe President and Founder, African American Male Leadership Institute*

"I am truly honored to contribute a few words of praise to such a powerful, amazing, rich, and divinely directed project. As it was with Mary, the mother of Jesus, whom God found favor in to bring forth redemption to mankind, his Son, he likewise has once again blessed his family with the possibility of life by giving the creators of this vision an amazing subject, *"Our Black Fathers: Brave, Bold and Beautiful!" RP King Sr., Father, Grandfather, Pastor: Mt Airy Baptist Church- Gretna, VA.*

"Our Black Fathers is one of the most illuminating tributes to African American fatherhood in contemporary popular culture. This compendium of heartfelt memories elucidates the profound love and sense of commitment, Black men feel for their children, and documents the impact of healthy father-child relationships in the African American community." *Jackie Booth, Baltimore FatherHelp*

"Black males and particularly Black fathers, suffer from an image problem. Due to their characterization in the media and the lack of visible evidence of the dedicated and committed relationships so many Black fathers have with their children, has contributed to a less than flattering perception. Any effort that brings balance and celebration to the many unsung Black fathers who have, and continue to do a great job with their children and families warrants our collective support. This timely project, ***Our Black Fathers: Brave, Bold and Beautiful!*** is a prime example of such efforts that are long overdue." -- ***Ronald K. Barrett, Ph.D., F.T., Professor of Psychology, Acting Director, African American Studies Department, Loyola Marymount University***

"Thank you! Finally! A profoundly moving compilation of mesmerizing narratives of the ordinary lives of black fathers as told by their sons and daughters. Some stories are entrancing, others unadorned, however all help to emancipate the all too often, disregarded and mutilated image of the black father. Gaines-Vanderpool and Royston have made all fathers proud. ***Our Black Fathers, Brave, Bold & Beautiful!*** is a must read for anyone who has ever questioned the love, loyalty, strength and commitment of the African-American father." ***David C. Asfall," jBanta Resources & Support for Fathers/Fathers Resource Center Sacramento, CA***

"Our Black Fathers: Brave, Bold and Beautiful! is a true effort to celebrate the rich legacy of African-American fatherhood, which is so necessary at this time. As I read, I went back to days spent side by side with my father, watching the San Francisco 49ers play. These stories mark the rich oral history of our community and give our fathers the inspiration they need to in turn provide rich paternal support to improve the lives of our children, which will ripple through the generations and change the nation!" ***Dr. Ramona Bishop, Superintendent, Del Paso Heights School District***

INTRODUCTION

The saga of Black men on any continent where they've existed is about lives that have been too easily discarded. Tragically, their stories have largely been untold. What makes these men extraordinary is their ability to enlighten those in their charge. Under oppressive circumstances, without any reservoir for their own pain except their faith, they have been there for their children generation-after-generation.

Surviving in a society that has failed to honor their brilliance, our fathers still manage to exhibit love, strength, humility and valor. These amazing Black men cope with racism, discrimination and degradation in their own honorable way while lovingly nurturing and providing for their families. Yes, they are mere mortals with frailties and faults, but they are formidable too, often succeeding despite a myriad of obstacles before them.

These deserving men give so much to their children through lessons of cultural and racial pride, courage, and dignity. The common stereotype of the unaccountable Black father that seems to have permeated our society as the truthful and accurate depiction of Black men, in general, has not been everyone's experience. There are many stories of loving fathers who are very much involved in the upbringing of their children.

Oh we are grateful for our powerful Black patriarchs! Men of promise, king of kings, warriors of the universe. Despite dreams denied, they still rise and conquer the world just by living and refusing to give in, give up, or go away. Hopelessness has no hold on them; but hope, for their children, does.

Beautiful Black men, you are our heroes, and serve as a shining example for others struggling to do the right thing when

they become fathers. In those circumstances where a child needs someone to intervene in their lives with the warm embrace of a father, we thank God for sending other men in the role of father figures as portrayed in some of the stories.

For those men who were ripped from their families in years past, sold into slavery or left to die on the sagging branches of massive trees dotting the American landscape -- you will not be forgotten.

Anita and I were blessed to have fathers who were very much engaged, loving, and accessible to us, and our siblings. Our fathers did all they could for us, and more than likely left this life wanting to do more for their children. Even beyond their physical departures, the powerful, loving spirits of Morris Lee Gaines and Josephus McGee, Sr. remain; and are guiding us in this most important and thrilling journey to bring forth the real life legacies that have been provided by our wonderful authors. The poignant stories that they have graciously shared will **now** live on in the hearts of many who will read about, and embrace these men of perseverance.

Our Black Fathers: Brave, Bold and Beautiful! is a testament of true men and reveals that those acknowledged in the pages to follow, are only a few of many Black men (living and deceased) who have impacted our lives since the advent of time.

Petri Hawkins Byrd (bailiff for the popular Judge Judy program) is truly a loving father who cherishes his role. This was clearly evident when he sent a poignant note explaining his absence when he had to miss a Father's Day event in June 2009 that was hosted by Judge Mabeline Emphraim. We wanted to share it because it personifies the essence, power and true meaning of being one of Our Black Fathers: Brave, Bold and Beautiful!

A Father's Day Promise

Petri Hawkins-Byrd

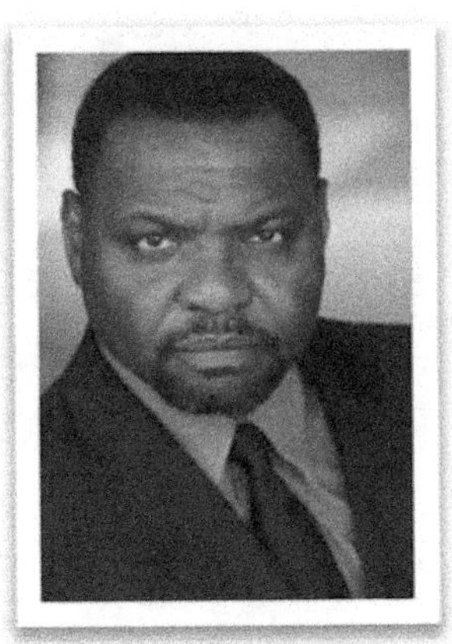

Well folks, as you can tell by now, I didn't make it to this illustrious event this Father's Day. However, I do have a legitimate excuse for my absence. I am busy keeping a promise; to be a good dad.

You see, my youngest daughter, Darcy, was a preemie, born May 28th, 1994 at 28 weeks. She was 1 lb. 14 oz. She fit right in the palm of my hand. Fell in love with her the day I met her. For the next 3 months after she was born, it was touch and go. One June morning we got a call that she might not make it through the day. I began to weep and got down on my knees and made a deal with God. "If you lend her to me," I said "I promise to give You a return on your investment. I promise she will honor You all the days of her life."

Well, yesterday I was back in a hospital room with my baby, bargaining with God again as she battled pneumonia. And again, just like 15 years earlier, I got the best of the bargain. To paraphrase Linus in "A Charlie Brown Christmas," That's what Father's Day is all about, Charlie Brown!"

God bless all the daddies who have bargained with God and upheld their part of the bargain. Happy Father's Day, gentlemen.

Our Black Fathers:
Brave, Bold and Beautiful!

A Tribute to Father

Frank Withrow

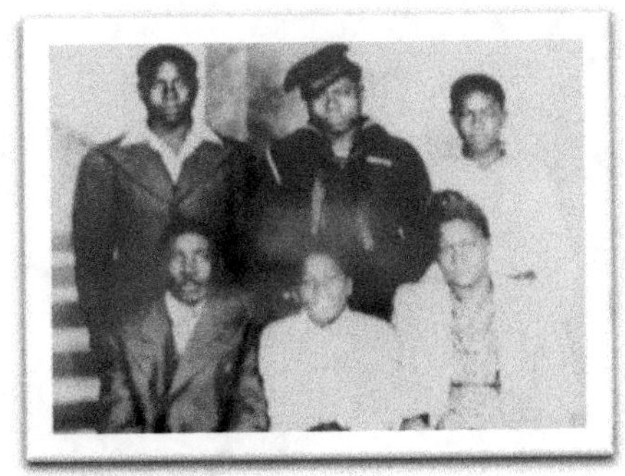

THERE IS A SPECIAL MAN
THAT I LOVE SO DEAR.
HE HAS TAUGHT ME WHAT I KNOW
AND HAS ALWAYS BEEN RIGHT HERE.
HE TREATS ME KIND AND SPECIAL
AND MAKES ME FEEL SO GRAND.
I WOULD NOT BE SUCCESSFUL
IF IT WASN'T FOR THIS MAN.
HE IS ALWAYS THERE WHEN I NEED AN EAR
AND WHEN I AM FEELING LONELY
HE TELLS ME THERE IS NOTHING TO FEAR.
HE HAS SHARED WITH ME HIS WISDOM
AND TOLD ME TO DO MY BEST.
HE HAS HELPED ME TO SEE
THAT I AM BLESSED.
THESE WORDS ARE ABOUT YOU, FATHER.
THEY'RE FROM YOUR NUMBER ONE FAN.
I LOVE, HONOR AND ADORE YOU
AND PROCLAIM YOU
THE BEST FATHER IN THE LAND.

Destiny

Joslyn Gaines Vanderpool

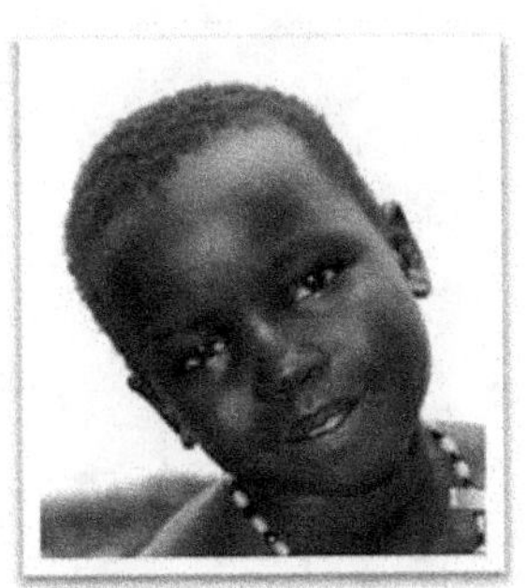

DEAR BELOVED,
AS YOU ASCEND TO YOUR DESTINY
EMBRACE YOUR PROMISE,
GO WITH PRIDE IN THE ACHIEVEMENTS
YOU HAVE ACCOMPLISHED.

REMEMBER THE BRILLIANCE OF YOUR
ANCESTORS FROM WHICH YOU ARE
UNIQUELY WOVEN --

THOSE WHO HAVE GONE BEFORE YOU,
CLEARED A PATH WITH THEIR BLOOD,
SWEAT, TEARS, PROTESTS, PRAYERS AND LIVES–

CONTINUE TO WRITE VIBRANT CHAPTERS
TO OUR STRONG, UNWAVERING LEGACY
THAT BEGAN ON THE SHORES OF AFRICA
WITH YOUR OWN TREMENDOUS STORY.

EMBARK ON YOUR JOURNEY WITH
DIGNITY AND PURPOSE, GIVING BACK
TO THOSE WHO LOOK TO YOU FOR DIRECTION,
FOR WITHIN YOU LIES ALL OF YOUR
MAGNIFICENCE WAITING TO BE REVEALED.

Father Knows Best

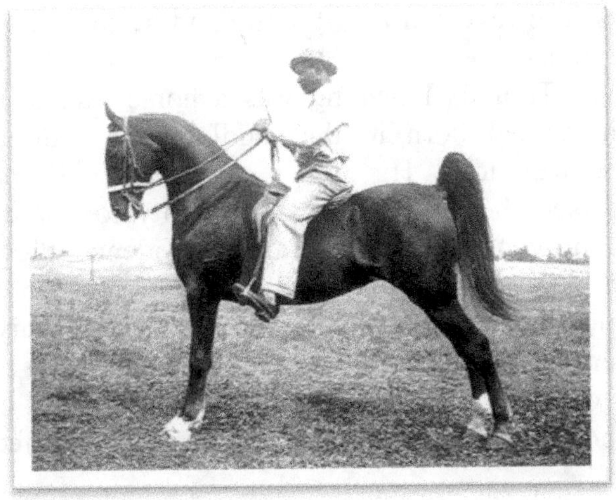

Mr. Thomas Downing astride his horse where he was most comfortable.

A Forgotten Horseman:

A Son's Weekend Memoir
Excerpts from the book, *A Forgotten Horseman: A Son's Weekend Memoir*

Lee Downing
"What is essential is invisible to the eye."- *Antoine de Saint-Exupery*

When I was 16, I held my father's hands while on my knees pleading to God for him not to die.

"Dad! Dad!" and "Dad!" I cried out, as he lay there on his back with his hands and fingers in a firm position, grasping the reins of a five gait mare.

He was in a place of contentment as he spoke, "Whoa mare, that's a girl!" and made those familiar clicking sounds I often heard when I was a little boy watching him ride horses everyday in the summer. Then in a calm moment, with his hands gently relaxed in mine, his face revealed a soft smile and he took his last breath and his last ride.

My father, Thomas Downing was a horse trainer, one of the forgotten horsemen born in the saddlebred kingdom of North Middletown, Kentucky. His was a remarkable gift because my father possessed the natural, uncanny ability to relate to horses, which was proven by the trust and confidence they exhibited toward him. Although my dad was a man of few words, his true voice, a voice that spoke volumes, was revealed in his work and accomplishments with the horses he trained. He often preferred to spend time with the horses over the company of most people; and it was that bond which enabled him to train them so effectively.

My father then told me, "The most difficult things in life are the best things in life for you."

As a ten year old, during a summer weekend in 1959, I had the pleasure of helping my father at an American Saddlebred Horse Show. It was that weekend I learned invaluable lessons of life that underscored the importance of integrity, honor, respect and the significance of principles and fortitude. It was a weekend I came to appreciate the meaning of having a work ethic in life. My father then told me, "the most difficult things in life are the best things in life for you." At the time, I truly didn't fully comprehend the importance of his words, but those words, like a mantra, stayed with me. Then my father imparted words of advice that are so very true. "Through hard work, good things will happen for you."

That summer weekend was a *coming of age* time when a boy began his journey to becoming a man. I worked alongside my father, my uncles and a group of Black horsemen who forever shaped the profession of American Saddlebred horse training. However, because of the social and racial injustices of the time, these men never received recognition for their talents and contributions to the saddlebred horse world.

Although many years have passed since that memorable weekend with my father and his fellow horsemen, I still find myself recalling those days. That is especially true whenever I see a horse trailer traveling down the interstate or when watching horses graze on the soft green grass as I pass by in my car. I smile each time and think how blessed I have been to experience such a moment in life. There is an old adage I once heard, "Memory is the only way home." As I think back to that memorable weekend, going home makes me proud and content. In my comfortable lifestyle, I often wonder in amazement how my father and his fellow horsemen managed to persevere through those times, and still find ways to ensure my smooth journey through life.

The great Jackie Robinson once said, "A life is not important except in the impact it has on other lives." My father and his "forgotten horsemen" friends certainly had an impact, not only on my life, but the lives of many. Their impact was made without substantial amounts of money or materialistic items, but with their teachings of courage, respect, and dignity -- all virtues, unlike money or materialism, which last a lifetime.

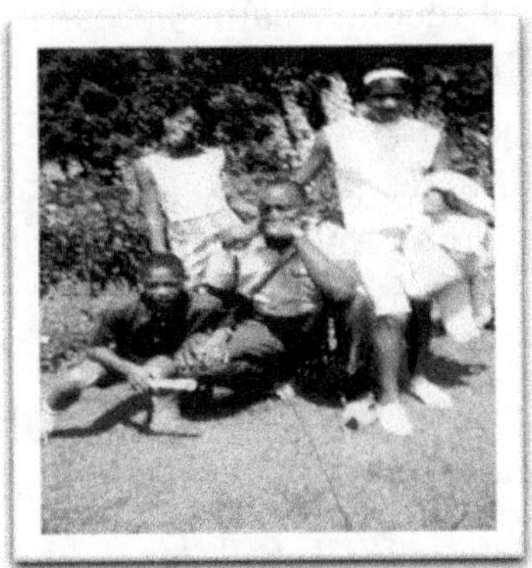

Mr. Laybon Jones Sr. surrounded by his loving children circa in 1964.

Hope for Dad's First Born

Dera R. Williams

A whiff of tobacco, the curling smoke of a pipe, an olive bathed in a martini, a brand new book with pages still stuck together. Those images bring back memories of my dad.

To "Cocoa" Hopes for a Dad's First Born

"Not quite 9 months old are you, my darling -- bordering between a baby's chubbiness and a little girl's nymph-like slimness. The laments, "Mommie" and Da Da" have attained distinctness, but words with more than one syllable are beyond your grasp. I look into your pecan-brown face, with dark eyes so like your mother's, and I think of all the hopes I have for you. Hopes which, if they are to crystallize, must survive a world on the brink of nihilism."

So begins the letter Daddy wrote to me over fifty years ago when I was a toddler. I recently came across this letter while going through some files of documents, birth certificates and diplomas.

My mother had given me the letter a few months after my father's death in 1990. I was just as touched and amazed as the first time when I read the words my father had written to me, his eldest child, and daughter.

Daddy calmly told us, "Look straight and hold up your heads." He refused to acknowledge ignorance at any level.

Laybon Jones Sr. loved to express himself through the written word. Fancying himself a wordsmith as well as a philosopher in the order of Socrates, he was on his college newspaper staff, and at one time thought of journalism as a career. He delighted in fancy writing pens and a well-stocked home office.

"You are happy, my sweet, as only a baby who has had the love and care of devoted parents could be. But what about your chances of happiness when you are 21? Through your formative years, will I be able to shelter you from the ravages of a cruel world? I have no illusions that I will. Yet I trust God that He will imbue me with the strength to impart to you an intrinsic armor of love and beauty that will withstand the adversities of a temporal existence."

Daddy had a proud spirit -- one born of growing up in poverty, learning to cope with the abandonment by his own father at a young age; and having to scuffle and work hard to prove that he was capable of achieving success. However, deep down Daddy had an inferiority complex about being poor in the '30s and '40s as well as being disadvantaged because of his Black skin. He also harbored the feeling of shame because he came to the big city of Little Rock wearing the same ragged coveralls he wore in the small farming community in eastern Arkansas where he was born.

The little country boy tried to fit into his new community in the midst of *Jim Crow laws* of the South, while determined to avail himself of new friendships among the up-and-coming African American middle-class of that city. However, it would be the military that provided a means to an end for my father, who served four years in the segregated Navy during World War II.

When my father was 22 he used his benefits from the GI Education Bill to enroll in Philander Smith, a small Black Methodist college in Little Rock. Four years later, Daddy graduated and married my mother and had three children of whom he was very proud.

We moved to Oakland, California from Little Rock, Arkansas when I was two. Like other Black families, we migrated to California for better employment and economic opportunities. Daddy's first job was in a furniture store as a stock boy.

"I wish I could tell you that you were born into a world of brotherhood and love for all mankind. But to tell you this would only make your awakening more poignant and frustrating. So I must tell you the truth; the unrelenting bitter truth. The world isn't serene and garden-like, it is turbulent and savage. While there is some vestige of brotherly love scattered about the various facets of earth, the core of mankind is hard and replete with hatred, avarice, and prejudice. Nations are against nations; ideologies are clashing, with their ominous voices echoing throughout the world. Men are dying -- some for what they believe -- others for that they don't understand."

My father shielded me, my younger brother, and sister from as much pain and hurt as he could. Raised in multicultural California, we were not prepared for separate public facilities when we went on family summer trips in the 1960s South.

We expressed amazement more than fear when a raggedy truck roared by with a motley crew of bedraggled young adults who began to angrily hoop and holler, and heckle us as we rode down the Texas highway in our brand new Buick.

Daddy calmly told us to, "look straight and hold up your heads." He refused to acknowledge ignorance at any level.

In the hallway of our home, there is a picture of my dad as a young man in a pristine white sailor suit, proudly worn as an enlistee in the United States Navy. He is poised and well-groomed with an air of assurance because that was how he portrayed himself, as a king on a throne. At six feet three inches, with a sinewy lean build that commanded attention, he posed for that picture with one leg propped up, leaning forward, looking directly into the camera, flirting with it. That was my dad.

"But it isn't all dark, my honey. For a ray of hope penetrates the abysmal well of confusion and frustration. That ray of hope springs from the progenitors of this generation. And you of my flesh and blood I fervently hope will fortify yourself to meet the tide. It is my hope that you will possess strength, and dignity without ostentation, and love tempered with understanding. To insure this, I must teach you to revere His word..."Thou shalt love thy neighbor as thy self....." Stand up straight and look the world in the eye. Face the vicissitudes of life with resolute calmness. Never tire of a deep thirst for knowledge and understanding. Never lose a respect for the desires of others. And above all, keep the faith in God and confidences in yourself."

Daddy liked the finer things: a cold martini, a good biography and first class hotels. He appreciated a woman wearing a hat to church on Sundays and a minister that exalted the *word of God* in an old-fashioned but dignified manner. He also loved learning. So he exposed his family to travel, books, and a broader view of the world that was beyond our society's self-imposed limitations. Since books were important to my father, they became significant to his children as well.

My childhood home had built-in book cases that were always filled with all kind of treasures. Censorship was nonexistent in the Jones household; anything in that bookcase was fair game. Although there was a variety of nonfiction titles that far exceeded my comprehension at age ten, we could still read or attempt to read anything on the shelf. So it was there where I discovered James Baldwin, Langston Hughes and William Faulkner.

My father's life varied greatly from his days in the small farming community in eastern Arkansas, to a remarkable career track as a real estate broker, educator, director in a government agency, and a consultant for minority contracts.

When I pass by the newsstand in downtown Oakland, I cannot help but think about Daddy going there every Sunday after church to pick up the *New York Times*. He would come home, light his pipe, prop his feet up on his desk and become immersed in what was going on in the world.

At age 66, Daddy was taken away much too soon, but he lived to see sweeping changes in the country, including the transformation of the South through the Civil Rights movement.

The same luxury hotel in Dallas which refused us entry in 1963, welcomed us with open arms five years later. Daddy not only achieved some of his goals and dreams, he lived to see his children, one of whom was that little chubby girl of 9 months, achieve some of their dreams too.

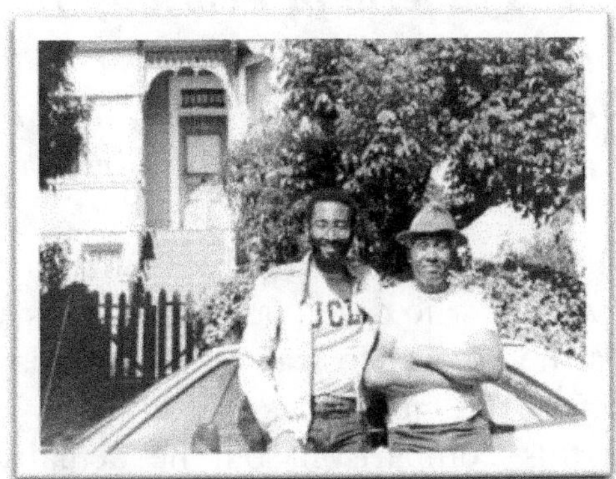

*Author and his father, Mr. Benjamin **Daddy** Royston 1982.*

We Are Professionals!

Steven A. Royston

Like Jesus, Daddy was a Carpenter
And like Jesus, Daddy was a carpenter who would scoff at this comparison, but actually he was a master carpenter and cabinetmaker to boot.

I really miss my daddy, Benjamin Henry Royston. I could talk to him about anything. He was my best friend; and I haven't seen him since Tuesday, February 14, 1995.

I remember the last day Daddy graced my eyes. My older brother, Philip was in an asthma-induced coma at Kaiser Hospital in Richmond, California. My dad was hovering over him. The very next day, as if to spare my brother from his apparent fate, Daddy had a massive heart attack and died before hitting the dining room floor in his home in nearby Berkeley. Philip recovered about nine days later.

At my daddy's funeral in February 1995, I recalled my favorite story about him and me. I was happy that I loved him. He knew it. He loved me, and I knew it. And we enjoyed ourselves for forty years.

What I really miss about Daddy is that he was a smart, muscular, hard worker who doled out lots of hugs and tickles to his five children that he loved. He was a great Sunday school teacher and Bible student. And like Jesus, Daddy was a carpenter who would scoff at this comparison; but he actually was a master carpenter and cabinetmaker to boot.

<u>When Sons were Expected to Do Stuff</u>
Not all daddies were warm and friendly like mine, but the majority of them would not abide boys not being taught how to work, fix things and do stuff.

I came up during a time in the '50s and '60s when fathers were handy and could do a lot, and expected their boys to do the same. Not all daddies were warm and friendly like mine, but the majority of them would not abide boys not being taught how to work, fix things and do stuff.

One vivid lesson is forever etched in my mind. Daddy and I were working in someone's kitchen one weekday night after nine o'clock. This was late for us, but not too unusual because Royston Cabinets' workers went where the work was to be done every day and night, except Sundays.

We were installing a big, heavy electric oven in a new cabinet we built in our shop. It was about seven feet tall and made of ash or birch wood. I was about eight or nine and my daddy was about 43. By then, installing cabinets was *old hat*. I just wanted to hurry up and get *outta* there and go watch TV at our house, which was in front of the backyard cabinet shop.

On this project we were doing something I never experienced before. As the designated *number two helper son,* running hot wires into a metal junction box on the wall behind the oven, and fitting the outlet to receive the three pronged 220 volt plug was new to me. I had seen so many ordinary household 110 volt electrical jobs that it was no longer interesting. But this was different … and I believed, dangerous for us. I was really afraid my daddy was out of his league and was going to get shocked. Surely this was a job for a real electrician.

<u>Hey Daddy, Do We Know How to Do This?</u>
For a minute, I thought I might get in trouble, or at least receive the evil eye.

With all the lack of cool a nine year old could muster, I said loud enough for the family who lived in the house to hear, "Hey Daddy, do we know how to do this?" If my mother had been there she would have knocked *the crap outta me* for embarrassing her like that. Patience with loud, uncool children was, and is not, one of her virtues. But one of the things I loved about my daddy was we could talk. And I didn't have to be anybody but myself when we did.

For a minute, I thought I might get in trouble, or at least receive the evil eye. But instead, Daddy drew me close to him, hugged me hard and said, "Of course we can, Bub because *we are professionals!*" When he said *"professionals,"* he put his thumb and forefinger together as if to indicate that everything was *a-okay*. Then he thrust his right arm forward to signal *success* and laughed that spirited, low tenor Arkansas "Ha! Ha! Ha!" laugh of his to punctuate the point.

Daddy started explaining what he was doing and why. He told me about the ground wire, the hot wires and how to plug in the three pronged big plug in the correct outlet holes. When it was finished, the oven worked like a charm. Daddy showed me how to work the timers, clock, broiler and so forth. That oven was much fancier than the one we had in our kitchen, but my daddy had that *sucker* all figured out.

Confidence is a Wonderful Thing for a Boy
I left that kitchen confident that whatever my daddy set out to do would be right.

I was so proud that my daddy knew how to do complicated work like wiring. I left that kitchen confident that whatever my daddy set out to do, it would be right.

I am a lawyer now. At my daddy's funeral in February 1995, I recalled my favorite story about him and me. I was happy that I loved him. He knew it. He loved me, and I knew it. And we enjoyed ourselves for forty years.

When I think about the things Daddy saw in me, in comparison to what he must have seen in other Black boys like him, who grew up in the dangerous, rural, segregated South of the '20s, and inhospitable wartime California in the '40s, I hope he reveled in how far the Roystons had come in forty short years.

Daddy, who was born in 1919, knew people who had been slaves, and here he lived to see his son become a lawyer. He also witnessed the advent of computers and other crazy technological advances.

Confidence is a wonderful thing for a boy. I'm glad I learned it from my daddy. He taught me how to try to be a good man, and like he was to me, a good daddy too.

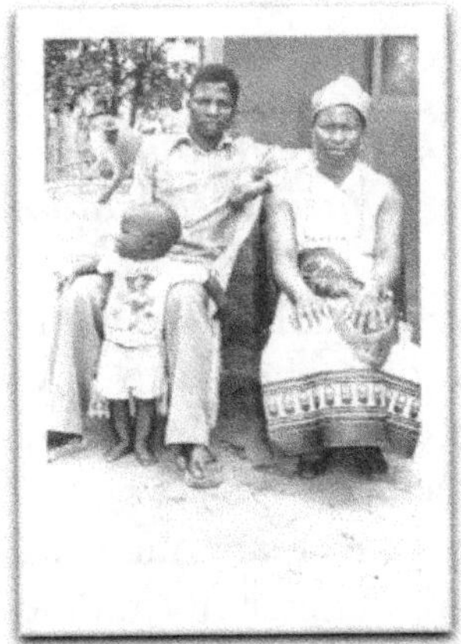

The authors parents, Mr. & Mrs. Thomas T.K. Kalimba and young Sam.

Mtandire's Tinsmith

Sam Kalimba

<u>A Difficult Place to Exist</u>

In the 1980s no member of the community dared mention that they came from Mtandire.

During the reign of President Kamuzu there lived a tinsmith in Lilongwe, the capital of Malawi, in Mtandire to be precise. Banda was his clan. His first name was Thomas; and the family name was Kalimba. He was my father, who I affectionately refer to as TK.

In the 1980s no member of the community dared mention that they came from Mtandire. Many referred to it as Area 47, while others used Area 49 as their place of residence when questioned at the hospital or any other areas of formal interrogations. Due to thugs, gangs, and robbers, the region was so notorious no one wanted to be associated with it.

A Father's Great Struggle
It was not that easy to rear four sons, let alone assure them a formal education.

My man, TK lived in Mtandire with his wife Delia and four sons. Although he didn't choose to have only these sons, nature was a formidable force, despite having our mother go for prenatal services six other times.

It was not that easy to rear four sons, let alone assure them a formal education. I remember my mother cutting my father's old trousers. She gave the upper part of the pants to the eldest son, and sewed the lower part of the pants together with extra fabric to form shorts for my younger brother. All this was done under the auspices of TK to achieve his goal of sending his sons to school.

Oh the land! ...the bicycle, the shorts, the 24 hour business, and all of the sacrifices my father made for his son were not in vain.

I can still see my father coming home early in the morning with pieces of iron sheets on his shoulders ready to make aluminum pots during the day. All the effort was intended to support my brother, Maxwell's pursuit of an education.

At the close of his work day, TK was not at peace after poor sales. Therefore, it forced him to utilize the night hours to work in an area of new development for well-to-do folks, as a watchman. Unfortunately, both sources of income were insufficient for home upkeep as well as school fees for a secondary school education for Maxwell.

My mother had a cousin, who led a softer life that lived at Mchesi in the same city. She owned a plot of land at Mtandire and had two grass thatched houses there. So TK went to Mchesi to meet his in-law to garner funds for Maxwell's fees, to which she provided a donation.

A Bicycle, a Plot of Land, and a Kiss
Without hesitation, my father looked around and found the bicycle he was using for his business.

As had happened before, the fees for my brother's education for the following term troubled TK. Without hesitation, my father looked around and found the bicycle he was using for his business. He kissed it, and said good-bye before relinquishing it. The money from the sale was channeled to Maxwell's fees.

The year of Maxwell's Junior Certificate Examinations brought forth another big problem for TK regarding costs. He tried Delia's brother for support, but could garner none. TK's conscience forced him to sell part of his plot of land too. To his encouragement, Maxwell passed his examinations and got selected to Dzenza Secondary School.

TK's struggles didn't end until good Samaritans relieved him from this panic. Father George, a Polish parish priest came to my father's rescue and extended his hand to the welfare of the whole family. Indeed "God helps he who helps himself."

Death Could not Deter a Dream
Sadly however, there was one most unfortunate thing…

Thomas did not stop working hard for his other sons. Felix, Maxwell's younger brother, dropped out from primary school due to his lack of confidence in his father's ability to manage paying for both sons to attend school. So TK sent him to a certain garage in town to learn about motor vehicle mechanics. The other two sons were very young and had not yet started their primary school education. My father advised Maxwell to work hard to support his younger brothers, Samson and Godfrey.

Oh the land! the beloved bicycle, the shorts, the 24 hour business, and all of the sacrifices my father made for his son were not in vain. In 2001, Maxell became Airport Manager for the then Union Transport Freight Company. Sadly however, there was one most unfortunate thing…Maxwell did not see his father's grave as he was the first to succumb to death; may the souls of father and son rest in peace. Both accomplished a dream that death could not deter.

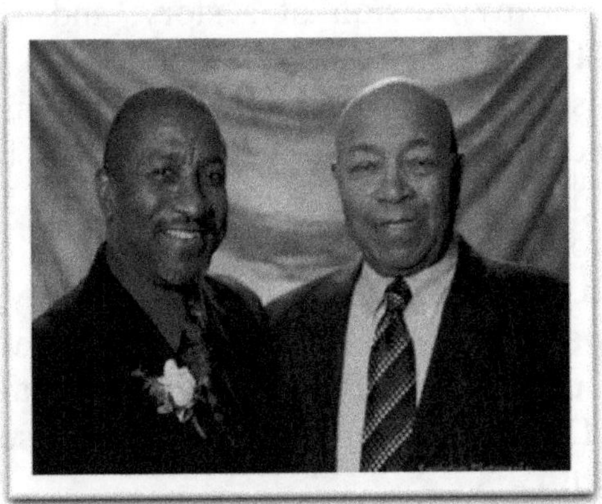

Author and his father (right), Mr. Joseph Marshall, Sr.

The Tallest Man

Jeri Marshall

I kept my eyes set for a tall, slender figure with bowed legs. He walked like a cowboy, and was to me, the biggest, strongest, toughest man in the world.

<ins>Raise the Window Down!!!</ins>
"You cannot raise a window down. Raise means to go up. So say, let the window down."

How does one capture the life of his father in words that will express love, appreciation and gratitude? I guess the best way is to simply tell my story about Joseph Earl Marshall Sr.

My father raised nine children and has entered into his 64th year of marriage to the same woman, which means that this is only one-tenth of my father's story. I know the others in my family all have their favorite remembrances and recollections about life with Dad. What follows is my version of a story, and a memory that the entire family still relives.

When I was five or six years old we were on one of our many car rides. I had no idea where we were going, but one of the car windows was down. "Raise the window down!" I implored.

A voice from the driver's side replied, "You cannot raise a window down. Raise means to go up. So say, let the window down." This was my first vivid memory of my father correcting me in the proper use of the English language. Although he is not a perfectionist, Dad believes that the standard use of language has been clearly set.

Even today at age 84, my father has a passion for language. Just last week as we discussed the writings of Omary Khayyam, I referred to something as "enormously huge." Even though I'm 54, Dad promptly interjected, "Jeri-boy, if it's enormous, it's already huge."

An Ungodly Hour
Each morning Dad would wake us up at some ungodly hour.

Dad was in the military and served in World War II. My brothers, sisters and I were a part of Buck Sergeant Marshall's squad, which is one of the common stories that several of us share about our father.

In the late '50s, we were living in a two-bedroom house on 62nd and Western Avenue in Los Angeles, California. Each morning Dad would wake us up at some ungodly hour. I say ungodly because it was still dark as we huddled around the floor heater to keep warm. We dressed before the crack of dawn as the sun began to rise and prepared to go to nearby Harvard Park for our daily exercises.

My dad thought our morning ritual was a great family activity because we had the whole park to ourselves for push-ups, jumping jacks and other assorted exercises. Six skinny little children marching across the street in the wee hours of the morning was a sight to see. Perhaps my reference to marching may have been overstated. Actually we sort of huddled together and ran across the street in a desperate attempt to keep warm.

My Brother's Keeper
In order to keep the family together, Dad expected the older kids to watch over the younger ones, and everyone was responsible for watching over the babies.

Whether we have fond or not so fond memories of our morning routine, it was one of many activities that kept us together which was important to my dad. To him, family was everything. Displaying no favoritism for one child over another Dad loved raising us. All of us have been accepted based on each of our individual personalities.

In order to keep the family together, Dad expected the older kids to watch over the younger ones, and everyone was responsible for watching over the babies. In our family, we were grouped mainly by ages. The older kids were Joe Jr., Debra and James. John, Jeri and Denise formed the middle group, while Diane, Donna and Doris rounded out *Team Marshall* as the youngest children. When he left for work after our morning exercise sessions and breakfast, Dad knew we would be there for each other.

Tell The Boss Man, I'm Going to the Doctor
Except for the love from his family, there was no real exit from the stress and demands put on my father.

While growing up everything wasn't a *crystal stair*. My father moved our family from St. Louis, Missouri to California to give us a better life. Although we lived in a tiny house, I had no idea we were poor. What I distinctly remember is that our father sacrificed much, and went through *hell and high water* to give his kids the best he could.

My father's work life wasn't easy. Except for the love from his family, there was no real exit from the stress and demands put on him. Nor was there any level of respect given to a talented Black man with an inventive mind.

Dad was a consistent provider, but when he needed a day off, he told us to tell the boss, "He was gone to the doctor," at least that way his employer couldn't tell him to come in when he was really feeling sick, and of course, tired. For those rare moments away from the daily grind, Dad could escape the racism and other difficulties on the job.

Since we couldn't afford a lot as a family, we made the best of our lives by doing creative things and enjoying what we had. We always played baseball in the park or made home movies with an 8mm projector which became a highlight at family gatherings. Dad even taught us how to make toys.

I remember one particular family excursion to Disneyland. I desperately wanted a pair of Mickey Mouse ears, but my father said, "Those are too expensive, Jeri-boy."

I walked away dejected, so my father decided to make a pair of ears for me. The version Dad crafted were huge! I didn't want to wear them back then; but now I appreciate my father's love in trying to make me happy. When we did receive store bought items like bicycles, model planes and skates, we were elated.

Dad's the Man!
You're the name that we claim.

There was no doubt that Dad was the man. My sisters, brothers and I honored him in different ways. Sometimes we would conduct plays for our parents in the large dirt yard behind the house to show them how much they meant to us. My late brother John, and my sisters Denise and Diane set up a cardboard stage with flood lights, boxes and odds and ends. I ran electrical wires from the house to the stage, and we used string that stretched from the trees for the curtains.

I can't recall what the plays were about, but they were quite a production. So much went into designing costumes, making popcorn, setting up chairs from the kitchen and hustling between acts before preparing for the grand finale, which always ended with the *Thank You* song honoring our father:

We thank you for the education you provide
and the love you hold inside
And we want you to know what we think of you
You're the name that we claim
Never ever – be forgotten
So father we love you….

Daddy's Home! Daddy's Home!
Once I saw Dad coming down our street, I began running towards him.

Much like our mornings which began with Dad, our evenings ended the same way. We eagerly awaited his return from a long, hard day of work with the Southern California Gas Company. Each evening I could be found in the front yard looking westward into the setting sun for Dad, who caught the bus and walked the rest of the way to our house. He was distinguishable. I kept my eyes set for a tall, slender figure with bowed legs. He walked like a cowboy, and was to me, the biggest, strongest, toughest man in the world.

Once I saw Dad coming down our street, I began running towards him. He would catch me and any one of my siblings and swing us in the air in a spectacular feat of strength. We would jump on him and he would carry all of us at one time. We hung onto his arms, legs, back, and even rode on his shoulders. Then he would stop and wrestle all of the boys. It wasn't until we were grown men that all of us could wrestle our father to the ground.

Even though my brothers and I eventually managed to hold Dad down, what we can never do is wrestle his incredible spirit and the love he has for his family. And for that, we thank you father.

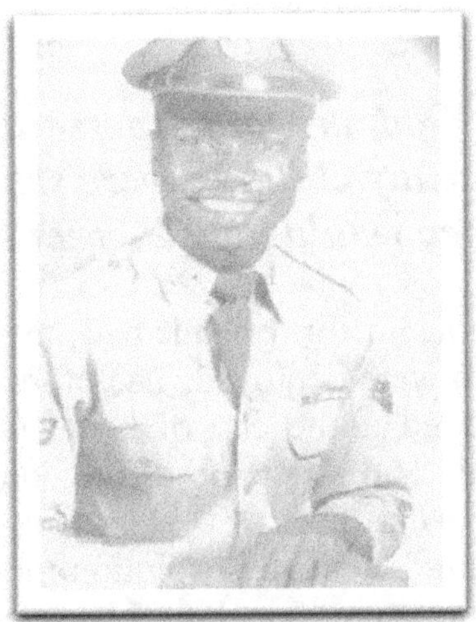

Master Sergeant Henry McNair, Jr.

Peace in the Midst of the Storm

Dedicated to my father, Henry McNair Jr., my peace in the midst of the storm

Jona McNair Brown

.

Who Would Care for our Children?
"Trust and have faith in God and he will see you through."

During the 1990s we were a military family who found ourselves in the beginning stages of war -- Operation Desert Shield/Storm. That August, my husband, children and I were stationed in Frankfurt, Germany. Shortly after I gave birth to my third child, Dominique, my husband received deployment orders to South West Asia (Kuwait). A series of discussions ensued concerning the welfare of our children, finances, soldiering, the fear of the unknown, and death.

As a man of God, my father personifies greatness. So I knew that once my children were settled at my father's house they would have a great experience.

A married couple in my brigade had no one to care for their children when both were deployed. Therefore, the Army forced the mother out which led to the end of her career. My husband and I knew that we only had a few months to come up with a plan for our family in the event that I was also deployed. I was confident that my parents would be the best solution for our situation.

Before I had to leave for duty I boarded a plane with my children to spend the Christmas holidays with my parents and other family members. Saying goodbye was hard to do but I was steadied by my family's support and my father's sense of *peace*. As a Viet Nam veteran he understood what my husband and I were going through as we prepared for war.

"The just man walketh in his integrity and his children are blessed, after him."
-Proverbs 20:7

As a man of God, my father personifies greatness. So I knew that once my children were settled at my father's house they would have a great experience. In our absence, my father was essentially in charge of the two older children, and my mother focused on the newborn baby.

In the care of my father, my children attended public school for the first time. They were never latch key kids because my dad dropped them off and picked them up from school every day. For the first time our children were living a normal family life. Their grandparents were instrumental in instilling integrity, building strong family values as well as shaping and molding their character. With my mother and father's guidance, they were experiencing new activities like Sunday school and choir rehearsal on a regular basis.

I don't know how my parents found the strength and energy to step in and raise my children, but they did. In July 1991, they flew to Germany with the children and stayed until they became attuned to us again.

<u>A Soldier's Poignant Words</u>
My father used the most poignant words when reminding us of the road ahead.

Although my husband and I had been in the military for several years, my father related to our plight and gave us powerful advice that was critical not only to the mission at hand, but would be invaluable in our daily lives.

My father used the most poignant words when reminding us of the road ahead. "War is what, and why we train and when it all transpires fear will step aside and your survival skills will take over. Trust and have faith in God and he will see you through." With his wisdom, words and the value he's added to our lives, Henry McNair, Jr. will always be my peace in the midst of the storm.

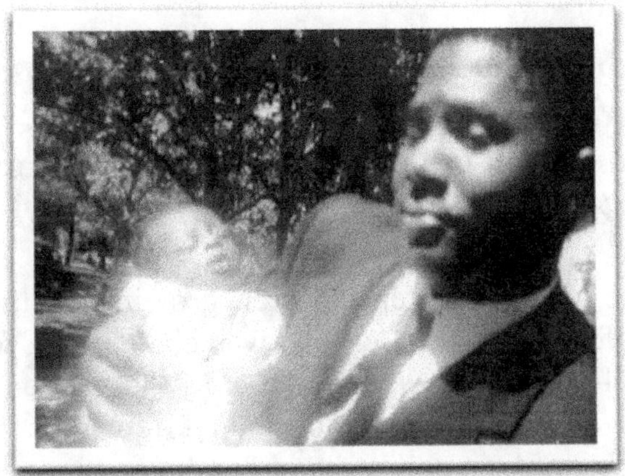

The author and his Superhero, Dr. Josephus McGee, Sr.

A Real Superhero

Dr. Jerome McGee

<u>Who Is Your Hero?</u>
***To my surprise some of my peers laughed when I
identified my hero.***

In December 1986, we were assigned to Langley Air Force
Base in Virginia, and were several weeks from my wife giving
birth to our third child. Upon recommendation, I was attending the
U.S. Air Force Non-Commissioned Officers Leadership School.
During a presentation on *Morals and Needs,* the instructor asked a
question that for the first time in my life, generated sincere
introspection.

"Who is Your Hero?" was the question, to which everyone was
required to respond. As I listened to some of what I considered to

be the most ridiculous responses, I immediately began to search my past to find my hero.

While my peers identified Bat Man, Superman and other fictitious characters as their heroes, it was now my turn to name my hero and tell why. So when asked, "Who is your hero?" I said, "My dad."

I was the seventh of ten children growing up in the '60s and '70s in California's capital city. It was challenging for the McGee family who lived on Strawberry Lane. My father had to be at work before 7:00 a.m. On some mornings I remembered waking up before sunrise to the smell of breakfast being prepared for my dad and the sound of his conversation with my mother.

When Dad returned from work, he'd join me, my brother Donald, and some of our friends from time-to-time in the school parking lot, which was next to our house. Dad would kick, hit, catch the ball or sometimes even run the bases. We played until it was time to eat.

Dinner was always a time for family togetherness but there were some occasions when Mom and Dad watched the news while the children ate. In those days, Dad came into the kitchen and asked if we had enough. If we weren't sated, he'd say, "Get some more."

Now I realize that those were the days that there wasn't enough food for everyone. So my parents made sure their children never went to bed hungry. Looking back, I see that we would have probably been categorized as poor, but we younger children never knew it.

My dad worked two jobs to take care of his wife and children. I remembered him walking me to my Cub Scout meetings, taking my little brother and me to a *big time* wrestling match, attending parent teacher conferences and little league baseball games.

While my peers identified *Bat Man, Superman* and other fictitious characters as their heroes, it was now my turn to name my hero and tell why. So when asked, "Who is your hero?" I said, "My dad."

"Your dad?" the instructor asked, perplexed.

Yes I thought, certain and firm in my response. My reflections regarding my father were now from an adult perspective. I was a man with my own family who was viewing my father's past with a different understanding and appreciation.

To my surprise, some of my peers laughed when I identified my dad as my hero. Then I told them the following: "My dad was always there for us. He taught me by example how to love my wife and children."

A Broad Compassion
He took care of his family, fed hungry people, and welcomed homeless families into our home...

Despite the fact that they were often financially challenged, my father and mother protected their children from the cares that confronted our family. I recounted that I didn't even know we were poor until I grew up because all of my needs were always met.

My father's compassion was broad. He took care of his family, fed hungry people and welcomed homeless families into our home until they were able to get on their feet, without ever taking away from his own family. As a pastor of a Baptist church in Sacramento, my dad was the first to license and ordain women. He embraced everyone and encouraged young ministers by providing a platform to develop and launch their gift.

The memories of my father continued to flow. Before my dad became a pastor, he was a traveling evangelist who took his choir (that would be his children) with him. Before there was a Partridge family, there were the McGee's.

In the late '60s my dad bought a small yellow school bus, which had a white stripe painted around it, and chrome letters written behind the passengers' door. He told us it was a sports van. Almost every summer we spent five weeks on the road traveling from the cotton fields of Mississippi to the Cathedrals in the suburbs of Pittsburg and Canada.

The Total Package
It was as though we were the only people in the room. My hero was proud of me. Wow!

To me my dad was the total package -- my natural and spiritual father and my mentor. I wonder how many pastors have a father like my dad, a man who trained and mentored pastors and ministry leaders? A man who just a few years before his transition into the presence of the Lord, chose me to pastor him and my mom.

I'll never forget the Sunday my father was asked to make a special presentation to me, as it was my 42nd birthday. Dr. Josephus McGee Sr. walked to the front of the church, stood before the congregation and began to speak.

"Since I've been here at Jubilee, every time I hear somebody say Pastor McGee, I turn around. You see I've been Pastor McGee for many years, then I remember they're not talking to me, but to my pastor -- my son, Pastor Jerome Justin McGee, Sr. I'm proud of you Son."

It was as though we were the only people in the room. My hero was proud of me. *Wow!*

Always there, my father gave me an advantage in life. I could talk to him about anything. He was instrumental in helping me avoid many of the pitfalls of pasturing, and he counseled me in ways I could better serve my community. My dad, Josephus McGee Sr. will always have the love of his wife and children; the admiration and respect of a community of church and civic leaders; and he will always be my hero.

God used my dad's life to teach me how to honor my wife and be a good provider for my family. For me to have the same degree of admiration, love, and respect from my wife, children and grandchildren that my father so deservedly enjoyed, would be the greatest gift, not including salvation, that any man could receive.

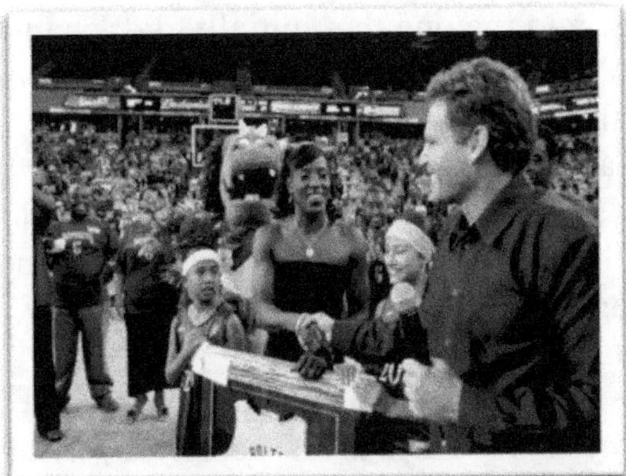

Retiring author's jersey with WNBA, Sacramento Monarchs.

Thanks for the Incredible Ride Dad!

Ruthie Bolton

Breaking My Fall
Thank you for believing in me when I didn't believe in myself.

There are not enough words to describe the impact my dad made on my life. My father was my friend, mentor, pastor, and leader, but most of all he was an ambassador for Christ.

Oh how I miss you, Dad. And I thank you so much for giving me and my other 19 siblings such a solid foundation to stand on. Thank you for believing in me when I didn't believe in myself.

From the college ranks, to not being invited to try out for the U.S. Women's National Basketball team, to working hard, making the team, and winning Olympic gold medals, your presence was felt.

Even when the other colleges didn't recruit me for their basketball teams, and the one that initially did, changed their mind, you still said, "You'll be alright, just keep the P.M.A.," which was a positive mental attitude.

I remember saying, "Is that all?"

And you said, "Yes daughter," because you couldn't remember my name. You helped break my fall through all my struggles by not only inspiring me, but empowering me.

A Well Taught Lesson
Daddy always said, "Life is ten percent of what happens to you and 90 percent of how you respond."

When I was younger, I didn't' realize as much as I do now about how keeping a positive mental attitude would play a major role in every aspect of my life. Daddy, you preached this over and over!

I can remember how you made sure that the paper outlining those principles stayed taped to one of the doors in the hallway of our house. At times I wondered what the big deal was concerning those words. We had read it already.

I soon understood what you were trying to accomplish. You were just trying to get the P.M.A embedded in our heads, our hearts, and our souls. You wanted it to become a part of who we are, and often said that there are three things that make up an individual, whether they believe it or not: *"attitude, motive, and character."*

Sharing Your Lessons to Enlighten a New Generation
Throughout my life my character has been shaped by the adversity, rejection, and disappointments I've encountered.

According to your teachings we all have an attitude about what we do, whether positive or negative. We also have a motive or purpose for what we do. And last, our character is what defines and shapes us. It is our portfolio. How you live your life and how you respond to life's adversities will determine the DNA makeup of our character.

Throughout my life, my character has been shaped by the adversity, rejection, and disappointments I've encountered in every facet of my journey. From the college ranks, to not being invited to try out for the U.S. Women's National Basketball team, to working hard, making the team and winning Olympic gold medals, your presence was felt. During a storied career in the *WNBA with the Sacramento Monarchs and beyond, you were there, guiding me with your lessons of empowerment and faith.

Due to your wisdom Dad, I have chosen to share what I've learned. As a matter of fact, I'm involved in *Aim High,* a character building after school program. I share with the kids everything that I have lived and experienced in my lifetime. We talk about attitude, peer pressure, discipline, respect, accountability, challenges, perseverance and self- image.

In order to help youth deal with who they are, and who they could become, my goal is to give them some of the principles you gave me. I wish to convey to them, as clearly and distinctly as you did for me, that *character is the core of who they are.*

"If you carry with you in life a few principles, you won't need a suitcase full of rules."

One of my dad's many sayings was, "If you carry with you in life a few principles, you won't need a suitcase full of rules." I heard this repeatedly, but didn't understand it like I do today.

There is so much to thank you for Daddy: the late night family devotions, the teachings about being *Born Again* and your role as our spiritual eyes and ears. But most of all thank you for being persistent and constant in my life.

<u>Well Done Dad!!!</u>
I want to share that in spite of all my ups and downs I hung in there because I had my role model, friend and my loving daddy by my side.

Besides my community activities to empower youth, I am also writing a book called *The Ride of a Lifetime.* Through my book I hope to reveal how incredible our ride was. I sincerely want the readers to get a glimpse of my experience with you Daddy and how formidable we were together. I want to share with others that in spite of all my ups and downs I hung in there because I had my role model, friend, and my loving daddy by my side. What's so sweet is that I have learned more about you since you've passed on. I can just sit and reminisce about some of our conversations and be inspired. I try to hold on to every word because you were truly amazing!

What made my daddy so incredible was that he had an unbelievable woman by his side. The saying goes something like this, "Behind every great man, is an even greater woman." That's why since 1998, (after my dad's death) I sign all my autographs M/D for Mom and Dad, just behind my name in recognition and gratitude for the impact my parents made in my life.

Well done Dad. Rest in peace!!!

*Women's National Basketball Association

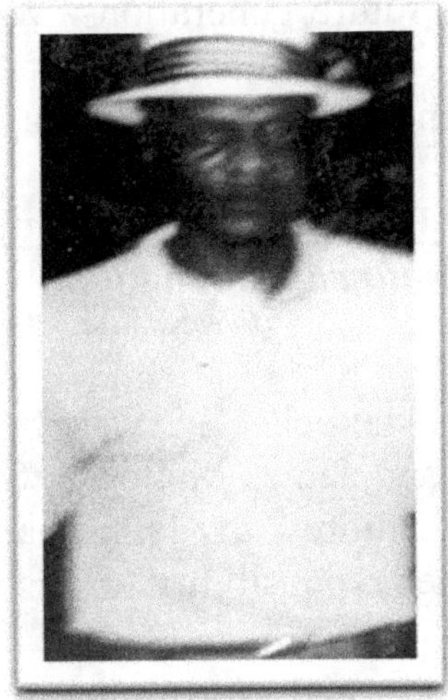

One of the great leaders of his time, Mr. Gerald Mattocks, Sr.

A Well Lit Path to Wisdom

In Remembrance of my Father

Carolyn Mattocks

<u>Great Men Think Alike</u>

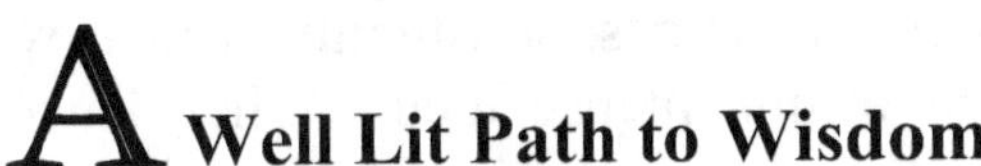

I have often thought my father's passing in February 2002 during Black History Month was significant.

My father was not Frederick Douglass, Booker T. Washington, W.E.B. DuBois, Marcus Garvey, the Honorable Elijah Muhammad, Dr. Martin Luther King Jr. or Malcolm X, but he possessed the wisdom of them all. Thus I have often thought my father's passing in February 2002 during Black History Month was significant.

Like the aforementioned great men of African descent, my father also saw the need for unity among our people as well as a need to prepare for future generations. While their greatness was defined by various historical movements, my father's greatness was his role as our mentor and most importantly, our father.

<u>An Educator without an Education</u>
"It is not about education all the time, but wisdom."
-- Carolyn Mattocks

Gerald Bernard Mattocks Sr. was born in Florence, North Carolina to Lenora and James Mattocks, Sr. on October 20, 1930. The oldest of seven children, my father had to forego an education of his own to assume responsibility for his siblings when his father suffered a stroke.

Even without a formal education, my father was wise and always tried to see a lesson in everything. So I believe that it is not about education all the time, but wisdom.

Despite many challenges, spirituality, which was central to my father's life, gave him intense focus. When I was a young child, my father gathered my brothers, sisters and I around the kitchen table after he came home from work. He discussed things that he observed on a daily basis, such as the racism he and other Black men encountered.

> ***Even without a formal education, my father was wise and always tried to see a lesson in everything. So I believe that it is not about education all the time, but wisdom.***

My father shared his stories about his struggles because he wanted for us to work and be respected. Due to the racially hostile times, personal circumstances, and the lack of opportunities afforded him, my father never wanted us to experience what he had, which was to work, as it was termed in those days, *like a nigger* – a degrading position of no respect.

My father toiled doing back-breaking work for 33 years at the Coca-Cola Bottling Company in New Bern, North Carolina. The heavy lifting and physical exertion required for the job is what ultimately led to a decline in his health. So he strongly emphasized the importance of education to garner better opportunities for his children.

In regard to making better choices about men, my father's lessons about what to look for were very insightful. He'd say, "Focus on a man who uses his head first, not a man focused only on what's in his pants." But his most important lesson was to "Use your own head" and "Stay focused," in order to make the appropriate decision.

Once Upon a Time When Men were Raised
While men struggle today to raise their Generation X sons, my father raised men that understood that manhood is not defined by the number of children that you produce.

Even though he could not read or write, my father possessed common sense, intelligence, and enough insight to realize that there were great difficulties ahead. Today when society is debating about how to prepare the next generation, my father was explaining to my siblings and me the importance of establishing a foundation for those whom would follow.

My father had every reason to give up in frustration; however, he never relinquished his responsibilities; and never gave up on us. Instead, he stretched limited resources to maintain his family. And he expected the same of us.

"Children do not ask to come here, but once they are here, you must take care of them," my father said. So when my brother's son was born, he reiterated his point, "Start saving for the baby now."

While men struggle to raise their Generation "X" sons, my father raised men that understood that manhood is not defined by the number of children that you produce. To him, accepting responsibility was the key.

<u>A Lasting Legacy</u>
African American people have always been taught that
"knowledge is power," but I have learned that knowledge is only
potential power.

It was on the backs of my parents that I received a good education. More importantly, my father enriched us and taught us to seek knowledge. African American people have always been taught that *knowledge is power,* but I have learned that knowledge is only potential power. It only becomes power when one acquires wisdom from that knowledge, then acts accordingly.

Sometimes in my quiet space, I think about how my father impacted my siblings and me in our decisions today. There is an old saying, "You can tell a tree by the fruit it bears." As a result, my father's well-lit path to wisdom has bore many wise children, grandchildren and future generations to come.

Father to Son

Frank Withrow

You might pull your pants down when you're in the street
but you're not leaving this house embarrassing me

You say I'm talking like a fool
Well, this is my house and I make the rules

Don't let your mouth get you in trouble
First I'll check you and then tell your mother

If I get a call from school I better be told
that you just made the honor roll

And if you go out and make a baby
you'll take care of the child and the young lady

We will help you go to college or learn a trade
But I'm not your banker and your mother isn't your maid

Go look around and find some real men
They're not living off their family or staying with friends

Sometimes you struggle and need a little help
But a real man can take care of his family and himself

Son, I love you but you must understand
I'm just trying to teach you how to be a man

Author and her father, Dr. Sheldon Duruisseau, the man who dared to dream.

The Audacity to Dream

Shelia Duruisseau-Sidqe

When I think of my father, I think humble, courageous, determined, visionary, leader, educator, humanitarian, and role model. These are just a few words that describe Shelton James Duruisseau, my father – a man who dared to dream.

As the youngest son of six children, my father was born in the small town of Labeau, Louisiana to Joseph and Victoria Duruisseau. He spent many hot and tireless days picking cotton and farming land but realized early in his life that although this way of living was one that many endured, it was not for him. So at the age of 16 my father left Labeau and his family in search of a different life. A life without cotton fields, hard labor, and little returns.

I thank my father for having the courage to leave his family and the cotton fields at such a young age, and having the wherewithal to know that he wanted a different existence for himself and for the next generation of Duruisseaus.'

In his future, my father envisioned books and using his mind rather than his hands. He saw himself as an educator, rather than a farmer. This audacious move ultimately changed not only his future, but those for generations to come. He knew that he could create a different reality for himself. And it would be education, determination and discipline that would transport him to where he wanted to go.

As a father, he has passed on his vision and determination to succeed. He has shown me by example, the importance of being an educated person and just how far it can take you when teamed with courage and discipline. What I have learned from him is that you can do anything in life that you put your mind to. He is a role model who has provided a strong foundation that provides our family with security, strength, and wisdom.

I thank my father for having the courage to leave his family and the cotton fields at such a young age, and having the wherewithal to know that he wanted a different existence for himself and for the next generation of Duruisseaus.' I thank him for having the determination and discipline to pursue an education and for being the pillar that holds our family together by setting such a good example of what being a real man, a real husband, and a real father truly means.

From audacity to excellence, Shelton Duruisseau, Ph.D. has attained numerous academic and career achievements. With a strong record of public service and an extensive background in health care, he was appointed to the Medical Board of California by Governor Arnold Schwarzenegger in 2004. Currently he is the executive associate director of External Affairs for University of California Health System.

The young man from Labeau is a long way from his earnest beginnings. He used his mind, worked hard and netted bountiful returns by not only having a dream, but audaciously pursuing it until it was fully realized.

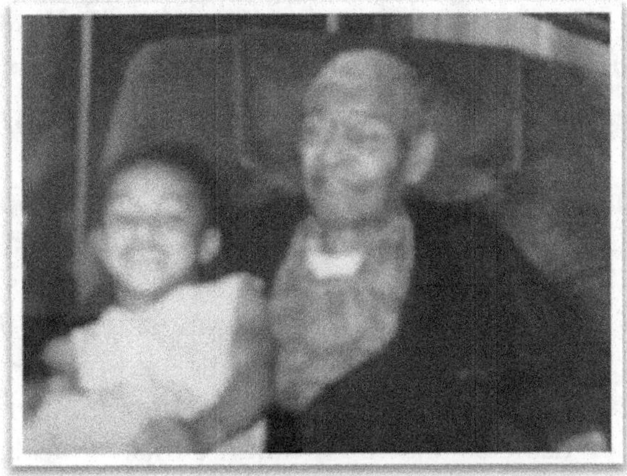

JT Whitaker, A Good Man

Alfreda Abdul-Ahad

John Thomas Whitaker, my maternal grandfather, was a rare breed, a black man who never worked for a white man in his entire adult life. Born in 1908, he ran a successful grocery business selling goods of all types from his own store that he built. He had a successful fish house, which sold all types of seafood on ice, and had an ice delivery business that had a fleet of trucks, all of this while living in the segregated town of Belhaven, North Carolina.

As a boy, young John witnessed his parents, who were sharecroppers without a formal education, repeatedly being cheated by the white folks whose land they worked, and decided early on, that he was going to work for himself.

In my entire life, I never heard my grandfather complain, except when watching the Watergate

***hearings. Now, as an adult in America in this
21st century, the enormity of what he did, owning his
own business, for all that time, is awe-inspiring.***

Like many Black and Native American families of that time, and that region, they saw the importance of education as a means for their children to better themselves. This was very true in my grandfather's case. He told us, his grandchildren, the story of how when he was 10 or 11 years old and had broken his leg, his grandmother, a full-blooded Cherokee Indian, carried him to school on her back so that he wouldn't miss time learning. He did finish school, and before setting out on his destined path, attended one year of college at Elizabeth City State Colored Normal School, known today as Elizabeth City State University, a Historically Black College

Along the way to becoming the man that many blacks in Belhaven still remember so well, my grandfather had to suffer many injustices at the hands of white folks, in order to remain in business. Growing up, I never realized all that he must have gone through, so that his family could live comfortably and his grandchildren could work summers for him, "for fun", dipping ice cream, selling candy, cookies, and pickles, learning to count money, and to deal respectfully with people of all ages.

In my entire life, I never heard my grandfather complain, except when watching the Watergate hearings. Now, as an adult in America in this 21st century, the enormity of what he did, owning his own business, for all that time, is awe inspiring. The very thought, takes me back to an event that I witnessed as a child of about 8 or 9 years old, around 1968 or '69.

A Day of Reckoning

One day while we were sitting in the "shop" (grandfather's store), a very old and decrepit white man who was assisted by some other young white men, walked in. Naturally everyone became very quiet, wondering what was going on. He asked to speak to "nigger John", referring to my grandfather. Someone went out back to get him.

What I do remember, is that little old white man asking my grandfather, the one he still referred to as "nigger John", to forgive him for the wrong he had done to him.

When grandfather came in, he went up to the white men, and the old white man began to speak. I don't remember all what was said, but evidently, he'd done some evil things to my grandfather over the course of some time in his business dealings with him to procure some of the goods he needed to sell in his store. What I do remember, is that little old white man asking my grandfather, the one he still referred to as "nigger John", to forgive him for the wrong he had done to him. When he was done, the other young white men gathered him up, and assisted him out, in the same manner in which he'd come in.

We were later told that the old man was about to die and wanted to clear his conscience, and my grandfather allowed that, in a dignified way. As a result, my grandfather, who also helped two of his brothers become successful store owners, was a well-loved and well respected man in his home town because of the way that he treated everyone; something he also instilled in us, his grandchildren.

Many in the town came to grandfather's homegoing celebration when he went on to meet the Lord in 1986. Afterwards, while cleaning out his office, my mom found an old journal, that went back for decades, with names, dates, and large and small sums of money written in it. At that time, and in that place, black people could not just go to the bank and get a loan when in need, but my grandfather, in his compassion, lent to most of the black people in town, to pay on homes, doctor bills, rent, or just to buy food, most of which was never paid off; but that was the kind of man he was, a good man.

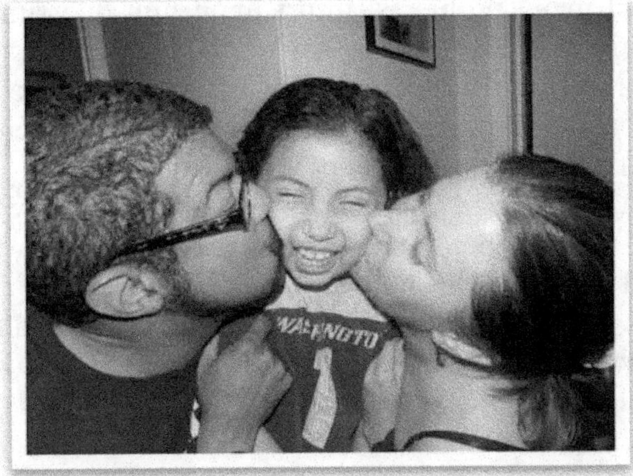

The Million Dollar Man

Audrey Booth

There are a million wonderful things that I could say about my dad. He's brilliant, kind, and strong. He's passionate, and somehow always seems to find a creative solution to any problem (no matter how frustrating the problem may be). Maybe his problem solving skills are a result of his doctorate in environmental engineering, or maybe he was just born that way. I don't know (after all, he's my dad, and I wasn't around when he was a kid).

"Everything I have done is because someone told me I couldn't do it." D. Booth

My dad, Derrick Booth, was born on June 9, 1968, in Los Angeles, California. From a young age, he learned that life is not fair, and he had to persevere in order to achieve his goals. He experienced many problems, thrust upon him due simply to the color of his skin. He was a smart child, which some of his teachers gracefully accepted, while his other teachers tried to hold him back because he is black. Throughout his school years, he endured some classes where his teachers held him to a different standard than the other (predominantly white) students. He talked to me about many instances where he was treated poorly and unfairly. But he learned valuable lessons from those incidences. He gives a lot of credit to his mom and dad for raising him in a way that taught him to move forward and learn from those challenges.

Doubts, Denials, Degradation Didn't Deter My Dad

My dad experienced many unjust situations in life, and many people who doubted his ability to succeed. However, through it all, he managed to persevere. One day, when we were driving home, he said to me, "Everything I have done is because someone told me I couldn't do it." There are two types of anger—blind anger, that can lead you to make unwise decisions, and productive anger, in which the emotion is channeled to produce a better outcome than was otherwise possible. My dad was angry at the people who told him he couldn't follow his dreams, so he used those feelings as motivation to achieve his goals.

> *My dad has also always been a leader, which is another thing he was told he was incapable of becoming. Yet, despite people's doubt, my dad became a leader of countless organizations...*

Once, my dad and his cousin went to visit a university they wanted to attend, and went to talk to the man in charge of recruitment and scholarships for the physics department. The man mentioned how he needed to find a person of a minority group to whom he could give a scholarship, because someone had just turned one down. At this, my dad mentioned that he was very interested in studying physics, and was in need of a scholarship. Then, without even asking about my dad's academic history or qualifications, the man in charge of the scholarships got annoyed and started ranting about how he was *tired of minorities,* and told my dad he had no chance of going there. Now, as I mentioned before, my dad doesn't give up easily. So, frustrated by the physics department, he walked across the street to the engineering department, where he presented his qualifications and was immediately welcomed and later offered major scholarship money. He went on to receive his doctorate in environmental *engineering* at this same school.

My dad has also always been a leader, which is another thing he was told he was incapable of becoming. Yet, despite people's doubt, my dad became a leader of countless organizations, several of which he founded, and has even been the dean of several different departments at American River College.

Lifting Us to a Place where Angels Soar

Aside from achieving so much in his education and career, he also has been an amazing father at home. My dad always tries hard to make things fun for me and my siblings; every year, he makes it a priority to do everything he can to make holidays exciting and special. At Christmas time, we spend hours as a family decorating the Christmas tree. We have a crazy amount of ornaments, and each year my dad insists on buying each of us a new, special ornament. He quite frequently buys a Spiderman ornament, because he loves Spiderman more than any other fictional character. (If you were to walk around our house, you would find countless different Spiderman toys, trinkets, and comics. Even his car has Spiderman stickers, and a Spiderman steering wheel cover.)

My dad also makes it a tradition that every year, a different child gets to put the Christmas angel on top

***of the tree; we have two black angels, one wearing a
red Christmas dress, and the other wearing a white
dress that lights up and changes color. Each year we
alternate between siblings, and my dad lifts one of us
up high to place the angel on top.***

So, our collection of Christmas ornaments gradually gets
bigger and bigger. When we decorate the tree, he lets my siblings
and me pick a theme for the tree and choose what color bulbs and
lights we use. It used to drive my dad crazy when we hung the
ornaments too close together and crowded the tree, but eventually
we got the hang of it, and decorating the tree became easier as we
got older. My dad also makes it a tradition that every year, a
different child gets to put the Christmas angel on top of the tree;
we have two black angels, one wearing a red Christmas dress,
and the other wearing a white dress that lights up and changes
color. Each year we alternate between siblings, and my dad lifts
one of us up high to place the angel on top.

But the inside is not the extent to which my dad works—he
also spends hours outside, setting up many different inflatable
decorations, and setting up lights in the trees and lights on the
fence. We are always the most decorated house on the street—no
one can match my dad's eagerness to make the most wonderful,
fun Christmas every year.

Once, when my brother was young, my dad and my uncle
schemed to make him believe in Santa Claus. I wasn't a
witness—my mother was pregnant with me at the time. But
nevertheless, the story shows how much my dad always cares
about making stuff exciting for kids. My dad took my brother
across the street to his friend's house, with my uncle dressed up
in a Santa Claus outfit. While my brother was with his friend, my
Dad managed to climb up on the roof and walked around, acting
like he was Santa delivering gifts. My brother and his friend
could hear him on the roof, and were immediately convinced of
his existence.

The Holidays are Not Just for Kids – How My Dad Holds on to Hope

He also likes to make holidays fun for adults. One year, my dad anonymously hooked up one of our inflatable Mickey Mouse Christmas decorations on our neighbor's lawn. They were an elderly couple, and the husband was very ill – my dad thought they needed a bit of cheer to help them out. So late one night, my dad went out and hooked up the inflatable decoration. Unfortunately, that same night, the husband passed away. Eventually we found out that they really appreciated the inflatable decoration; it was a blessing to them, and helped brighten that very sad time.

My dad also spends hours decorating for Halloween. As with Christmas, we have boxes and boxes of Halloween decorations, for both the inside of the house and the outside. Every year we go out and buy new decorations, from plastic skeleton parts to dry ice and fog machines. He always covers the house in candles and ghosts, and goes outside and covers the yard in gravestones, skeletons, and cotton spider webs.

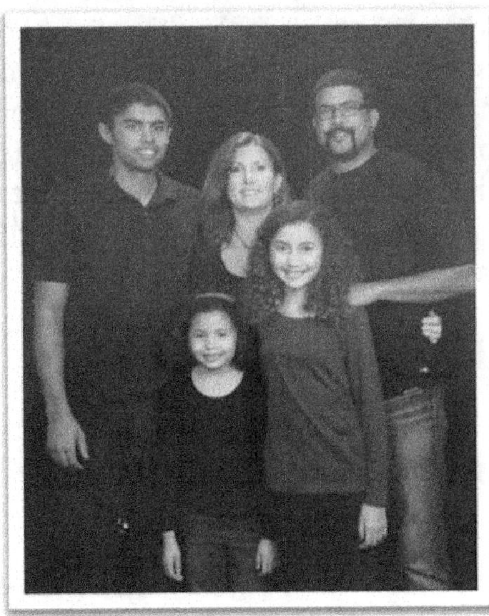

My dad does things daily to make life interesting, and he makes the most of any given situation. He never gives up, and always finds a way through any problem, whether it is a major situation or a small issue.

My dad sometimes even spends hours carving pumpkins, creating intricate designs of characters, including Ariel and Snow White for my sister and me. When we were younger and had Halloween parties, he would make a Puking Pumpkin. This entailed carving the usual Jack-O-Lantern face onto a pumpkin, then pouring in some weird combination of kitchen ingredients that would foam and pour out of the pumpkin's mouth, as if it was puking. It was gross, but incredibly funny, and all the kids at the parties went crazy over it.

He even dressed up with us. My dad has never really been one to wear anything extravagant, but he would still make an effort to wear some form of a costume. One year, he dressed up as a Cereal Killer. Yes, that's right, a *Cereal Killer*, not a *Serial killer*. We had the miniature boxes of cereal for my sister, who at the time was just a toddler. He took one and jabbed a steak knife into it, leaving it halfway in, with the knife handle sticking out. Then, he took red wax from one of the Halloween candles and poured it around the "wound", as if the cereal was bleeding. He then connected the cereal box to a string, and wore it around his neck as his costume. It was so funny, and everyone loved it.

My dad does things daily to make life interesting, and he makes the most of any given situation. He never gives up, and always finds a way through any problem, whether it is a major situation or a small issue. Not only does he find solutions, but he somehow manages to make even the most arduous tasks bearable. That's what I love about my dad—he is ingenious, fun, and full of love. He always holds on to hope, and never gives up.

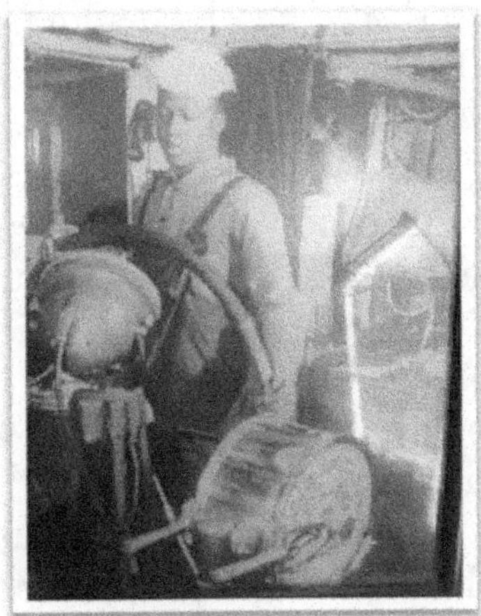

One Day I'm Gonna' Get Out of Here!

In tribute to Alfred Stephens, Jr.

Alfreda Abdul-Ahad

<u>Not a Stay in Your Place Kind of Guy</u>

Alfred Stephens Jr., was a dreamer, but not just a dreamer. He was a doer too and a great storyteller. One of the earliest stories I remember him telling me and my brothers was how as a child he'd sit by the side of the road and watch trucks go by, and say to himself, "One day I'm gonna' get out of here!"

Blacks were supposed to know their place and remain in it to avoid any trouble. By nature, my dad wasn't a "stay in your place kind of guy," so he found himself in trouble at times from both blacks and whites.

Born in 1929, my dad was the third child of a lumber tallyman by day, and preacher by calling, and a homemaker mother. In his early life, he saw a lot of disparity in his segregated hometown of Belhaven, North Carolina. Blacks lived on one side of town, and whites lived in the nicer homes on Main Street, and the other side of town. Blacks were supposed to know their place and remain in it to avoid any trouble. By nature, my dad wasn't a "stay in your place kind of guy," so he found himself in trouble at times from both blacks and whites. Needless to say, Hattie, his mother kept him in prayer, and he loved her dearly.

Since his father was a preacher, my dad often told stories about church, and church folk, particularly preachers. One story he told us was about some of the roaming preachers that would not only come to town, but often to dinner. Mind you, this is not very long after the Great Depression when things were tight for all, especially black people. According to my dad, these roaming preachers were treated like royalty, and given the best of the food and drink from poor folks, who could barely feed their families.

My dad told of a time when his mother had gotten a chicken, plucked, and fried it. Oh, how the aroma filled his head with visions of the glorious meal to be eaten that day, when this one particular roaming preacher showed up. As the preacher and grown folks sat down to eat, (children often ate after the guests), my dad watched as the preacher ate the best of the pieces of chicken, one-by-one.

Finally, he couldn't stand it any longer, and blurted out, "Momma he's gonna' eat all the chicken!" Of course, he suffered the consequences for his action, but the things he saw and experienced from organized religion kept him away from church, except holidays, until much later in his life.

Blazing a Path: From Disparity to a Dream

At 17, bored with school, and weary of the disparity he saw in his hometown, my dad dropped out of high school for the second time and joined the newly integrated U. S. Coast Guard. When asked, "Why the Coast Guard?" he said that he really liked the uniform. Though he ended up having to go back and get his father's signature to enlist, his dream of leaving Belhaven was becoming a reality.

In 1947, my dad went to basic training in Mayport, Florida. He said that Mayport was one of the most prejudiced places he'd ever been, but he made it through. At that time, most blacks in the Coast Guard had to become a steward's mate where they essentially served the white officers. One thing for sure was that my dad did not want to be a steward's mate.

Though later in life, my dad was to spend 27 years in a wheelchair, he didn't let that stop him from living fully.

Fortunately, the Coast Guard was expanding and there was another rate option, commissary man, and my father chose that rate. Commissary men cooked, supervised cooks, ordered the supplies that stocked the ships and bases, and kept records. In that rate, my dad traveled the world, literally. He served on several icebreakers, the big ships that travelled the world delivering supplies to Coast Guard outposts like in Antarctica, where those special ships were needed to cut through the ice. He was also stationed in Japan on his first tour of duty.

In the Name of My Father: A Tree and a Powerful Legacy Live On
I am named after my father, something that I am very proud of.

After retiring from the Coast Guard, my father moved our family to the Bay Area of Northern California, where he later worked as a U. S. Postal Carrier. Naturally a "people person", others gravitated toward him on that job. Between my mom and dad, our house was always full of people, especially around the holidays, and my dad always had a good story or two to tell. Those were some of the happiest times of my life.

Looking back, Little Alfred did indeed 'get out of there', as one of those proud, strong, post-World War I born African American military men…

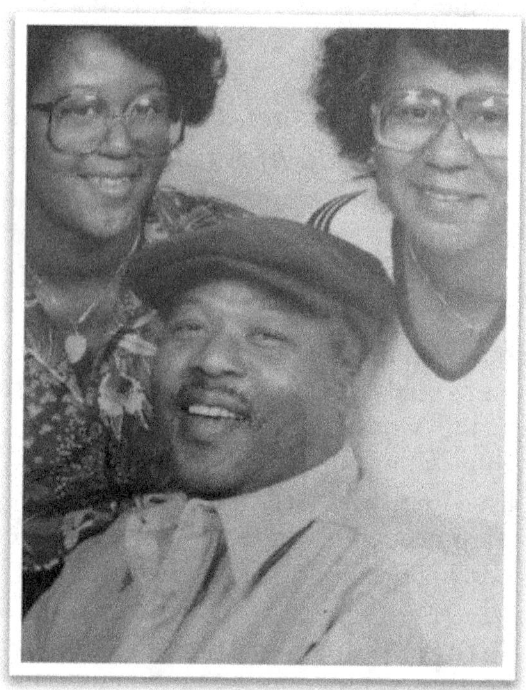

In later life, my dad was to spend 27 years in a wheelchair, but he didn't let that stop him from living fully. Initially a quadriplegic, my dad was unable to use his arms and legs. However, through physical therapy, and the support of his wife, friends, and family, he regained the use of his arms, and was eventually able to drive again, traveling across country visiting friends and family throughout the United States, and going to Europe, as well. Even when I was in college, living in the dorms, my father would come by to take me and my friends to run errands sometimes, and one of my friends said to me, "You wouldn't even know your dad was in a wheelchair, if you didn't see it." That was how he lived his life, with my mom right there by his side.

My dad became active in the California Association of the Physically Handicapped (CAPH), known today as Californians for Disability Rights, and was a founding member of Retired Armed Services Personnel (RASP), a non-profit organization that brought primarily, retired African American military men together, and provided scholarships to students pursuing higher education.

In remembrance, there is a tree planted, and plaque dedicated to my dad in Memorial Park on the campus of the California State University Maritime Academy in Vallejo, California. He provided an exciting life for his family, moving from coast-to-coast in the United States, amassing a plethora of friends. As a proud merchant marine, he kept his identification card updated and on him at all times.

Looking back, Little Alfred did indeed 'get out of there', as one of those proud, strong, post-World War I born African American military men, whose numbers, though dwindling, left a proud legacy within their families, and communities throughout the United States.

When I was asked, if I was named after my father, I said, "Yes. I am named after my father, something I am very proud of."

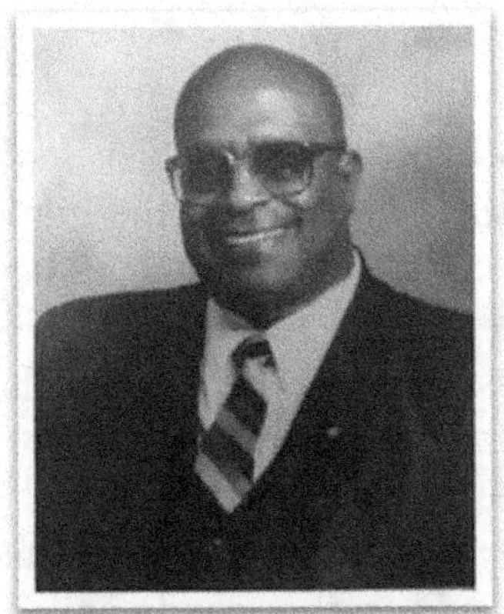

The Art of Loving, The Satterfield Way

Katha Redmon and Karen Satterfield

Sidelined a Lesson Learned

Arthur Satterfield was born June 22, 1940 in Memphis, Tennessee; and attended Booker T. Washington High School where he met and later married his high school sweetheart, Josie Brown. The oldest of four children, with two brothers and one sister, Art played high school football where the field would become the foundation and source of many life lessons including the art of humility. Due to his great athletic prowess and natural instincts, he was one of the best players on the team and one of the most popular students among his peers.

"They're calling your name," the coach said. Art replied excitedly, "Yes Sir, they are." The coach then turned to Art and said, "Well it sounds like they want you up there with them, so why don't you go join your

friends and watch the rest of the game from the stands.

During one football game in his Senior year, the coach surprised Art by pulling him out of the game early in the fourth quarter. Not realizing that the coach had pulled him from the game because he was not performing up to his normal standards and abilities, Art assumed that the coach had sidelined him so that he could rest up and have stamina remaining for the final minutes of the game. He repeatedly asked the coach, "Put me back in the game," and the coach ignored his requests. You see, his girlfriend, Josie, was in the stands and he wanted to impress her with his football talent.

Since the coach was ignoring his requests, Art decided to capitalize on his popularity and evoke support from the crowd in the stands. He thought that if he could get them to call his name, the coach would relent and return him to the game. At his urging, the crowd began to yell "Satterfield, Satterfield, Satterfield." After growing tired of hearing this chant, the coach called Art over. As he walked toward the coach with a big smile on his face, Art knew the coach was about to put him back in the game.

"They're calling your name," the coach said. Art replied excitedly, "Yes Sir, they are." The coach then turned to Art and said, "Well it sounds like they want you up there with them, so why don't you go join your friends and watch the rest of the game from the stands."

Art's team ultimately lost the game without him. The lesson that Art learned that night was that in life, there is a lesson to be learned in all things that happen and by trying to manipulate the outcome, you may miss that intended lesson. The football lesson was that no one individual is bigger than the team and we are all on the same playing field. The life lesson was that no one is bigger than God. He learned that you must pay attention and evaluate the circumstances when setbacks occur because there is usually a larger message being conveyed to help us through each stage as we navigate the journey of life.

The Art of Preparation, Persistence and Performance

Art worked as a sales manager for Montgomery Ward and was also a car and insurance salesman. He was a big guy with a big personality. He had an infectious and gregarious way about him that made him appeal to almost everyone. He was extremely intelligent and meticulous in his preparation and the performance of any job he had. He did not believe in doing things halfway and always gave his best effort, whether it was proofreading a document or running an automotive store. He imparted this wisdom to his daughters and his grandchildren by encouraging them to go to college and completely maximize their potential to achieve their ultimate goals.

Education above all else was important to Art because he recognized its importance and encouraged his loved ones to remove the limits to their lives by furthering their education and giving their best effort. His words and deeds served as an example to his daughters and grandchildren in that they have all attended and graduated from college, with his granddaughter recently earning her Master's degree. No matter how large or small the accomplishment, Art was always encouraging. He was always interested in learning about and discussing our future plans and always reminded us that we were smart enough to be anything we wanted to be.

"It's not the mistakes you make, it's what you do after the mistake that makes the difference. Don't sweat the small stuff because most things are small."

An avid golfer, Art utilized the sport of golf to impart wisdom on life. He used to say that in golf you're not competing with anyone but yourself and he believed the same was true in life. He believed that we should be competing with ourselves to be the best version of ourselves we can be. Not to measure ourselves based upon the accomplishments or positions of others, but to dig deep within ourselves and strive to be the absolute best at whatever we chose to do. He would practice for hours on the golf course to improve his swing and his putting skills. This persistence was the source of another metaphor he used to apply to life. Get prepared by reading, studying and focusing on goals and aspirations and once you're fully prepared, you'll be able to swing with confidence at your goal and ultimately achieve them at the highest levels.

Art instilled in his children and grandchildren that there is no such thing as arbitrarily being lucky to attain success. He strongly believed that you generate your own luck by being prepared. He consistently preached to us that success is the result of persistent and relentless preparation and that true success occurs when that preparation meets opportunity and you maximize and capitalize on those opportunities. Art was a positive person and a realist in many ways. He did not shy away from talking about the mistakes or bad decisions he made in his life. He summed it up by saying "God looks after children and fools," recognizing his shortcomings when they occurred and knowing that God had intervened throughout his life.

The Art of Being a Better Version of Yourself

Always looking forward, Art found ways and opportunities to improve and become a better version of himself and regularly reflected on the mistakes he made in life and provided insight on how he could have done things differently to produce a better outcome. He once said, "It's not the mistakes you make, it's what you do after the mistake that makes the difference. Don't sweat the small stuff because most things are small." Art believed that you should always focus on the bigger picture by keeping your "eyes on the prize". He stated that small mistakes will occur along the way, but the key is to not continually repeat those small mistakes as you make the journey to the bigger goal. His children and grandchildren are so grateful to have had Art in our lives to love us and to instill this type of work ethic in each of us. We have all accomplished our goals due to the many life lessons that he taught us and we will pass these lessons along to future generations.

Later in his life, Art not only inspired his children and grandchildren, he passed on his years of wisdom and learning to other young people while he worked for the Sacramento school system where he had the opportunity to stress the importance of how to present ones' self to the world. His passion for mentoring to youth, especially young boys, was reignited in his role; and he took pride and joy in seeing those young boys begin to focus on the positive aspects of life and blossom into proud and successful young men.

Artfully Said and Done

One last story that still makes us smile to this day is the recollection of Art desperately wanting to attend a sold-out baseball game. At the last minute, he was finally able to obtain a set of tickets to this game. When he got home, he relayed to us that "those seats were so high up in the stands that I could see Jesus!" It gives his loved ones great comfort to know that he is with the Lord and now really "sees Jesus" every day.

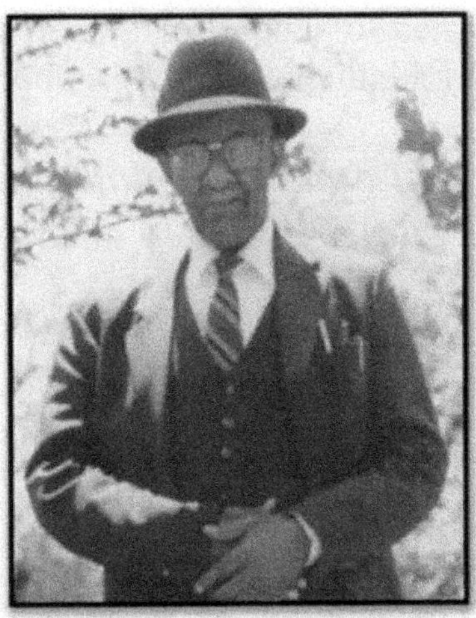

Deacon Roy "Banks" Breedlove—
A Man of Extraordinary Vision

Everlena Ross

Meet a Blessed and True Miracle!

Mr. Roy Banks Breedlove was born on July 22, 1905 to the parents of Booker and Emma Davis Breedlove. He had four brothers, Willie, Jim, Richard, and Joe Davis, and one sister, Everlena Breedlove Hairston. At an early age he was accidentally shot in his left eye which totally destroyed the vision in that eye, and nearly his life as his parents were told that he would not live 30 days. He stayed in a coma for 25 days and in the hospital for three months. The next five years were spent recovering and gaining sight in his right eye. During this healing time, his mom and dad read scriptures to him, and read to him as much as they could because he wanted to attend school like his siblings. When he was 16, he returned to school for a short period of time, but had to quit, and work on the farm to help support his family.

Voting is my right and if folk don't vote, they might just get something they don't want."

To help the family, Breedlove's public work history began at the age of 17 at the Hooker Furniture Factory in Martinsville. While still working on the farm, he maintained a second public job at the Stowe's Sawmill in Whitmell, Virginia where he worked 30 years full time in the winter and part-time during farming season. In April 1938, Mr. Breedlove met and married the beautiful Lucy Inez Inge, and together they lived with his parents, continued farming, continued public work and raised two daughters, Lillie Kate Breedlove Isler and Everlena Breedlove Ross.

If You Can't Attain an Education, Give One

Mr. Breedlove never completed high school due to a lifetime of working to support his family. Although he had to sacrifice an education that he so desired as a child, he never forgot its importance and always recognized its value. In fact, he learned and could recite every state, the state capitals, and the presidents and he wanted more or his daughters, than he could ever achieve.

Realizing the importance of a good education, Mr. Breedlove insisted that his daughters finish high school and get a college education. He also encouraged and helped his nieces, nephews, and children of families in the community to strive for the highest level of education they could get. When Deacon Breedlove celebrated his 100th Birthday, his nephews announced the establishment of the ROY BANKS BREEDLOVE QUEST FOR EXCELLENCE SCHOLARSHIP to honor him and his commitment to education. The first scholarship was presented in 2006 and a scholarship in the amount of $1000.00 has been presented to a graduating senior enrolling in a school of higher learning yearly since then. Another graduating senior will be the recipient of a $1000.00 scholarship in July of 2017 in celebration and memory of Deacon Roy Banks Breedlove.

One Hundred Years of Clear Vision

A devoted believer in the Lord, Mr. Breedlove confessed his faith openly and was baptized and became a leader at the Union Hall Baptist Church serving as Sunday school teacher, Sunday school superintendent, church treasurer and a deacon. In addition, he was active in the community and always wanted to help others. Serving as a Mason, he also was a life member of the Pittsylvania County Branch of the NAACP; and in 2006 became a fully paid lifetime Golden Heritage Member of the National Association for the Advancement of Colored People, granted for voting in every election. He always said, "Voting is my right and if folk don't vote, they might just get something they don't want."

Participation in the voting process had never been easy for African Americans, particularly before the 1965 Voting Rights Act. Many African Americans who tried to vote, often faced harassment, discrimination and even death. Breedlove always realized the importance of exercising his right and once he became of age, voted in every election. When he could no longer physically go to the polls, he cast his absenteeism ballot.

Mr. Breedlove had more than sight vision that he had once lost, he had foresight. Although he was shot in the eye with a gun as youth, he could still see that there was a path for him; even though it would entail hard work and an end to his personal education dream, he still learned, was a teacher in many respects and used his true vision in service to God, family and the community.

Note: Individuals or organizations that share the Roy Banks Breedlove philosophy of *a quality education for all children*

are entitled to receive are encouraged to make a donation to the Roy Banks Breedlove Quest for Excellence Fund. Checks and Money Orders can be made payable to The Roy "Banks" Breedlove Scholarship Fund, Attention: Mrs. Everlena Ross, 1265 F. C. Beverly Road, Dry Fork, Virginia. This scholarship program was established to honor Deacon Ray "Banks" Breedlove's dedication to education.

For The Love Of Him

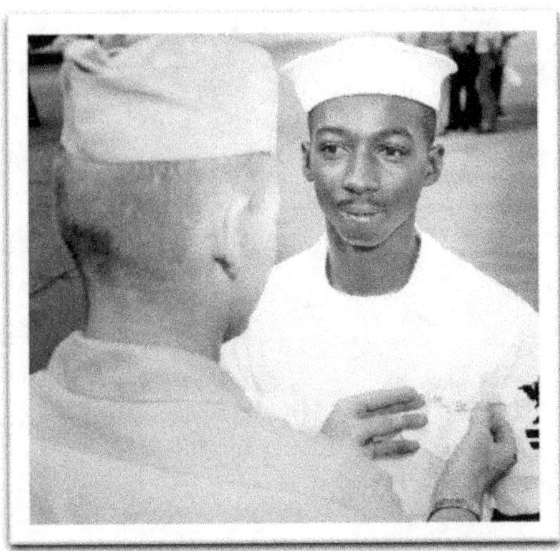

Young Don Bailey getting his wings.

Men of Excellence

Frank Withrow

Men of Excellence understand
the true reality of being a man
Being responsible and working to succeed
Standing tall and not working for greed
They meet challenges in trying times
Men of Excellence won't be denied
They work for the betterment of all mankind
Men of Excellence are never left behind
Look for them in leadership roles
They are born to be in full control
Men of Excellence are truly strong
They make sure right overcomes wrong
Nothing and no one can stand in their way
Men of Excellence do their best every day

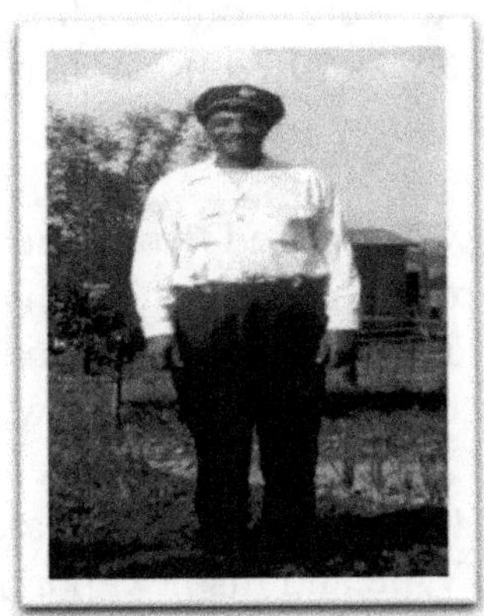

The author's father "Mr. Big Wheel."

Mr. Big Wheel

Beatrice M. Hogg

<u>A Coal Miner's Diversion</u>
***Even though he was retired from the coal mine, he wasn't
retired from life.***

As a little girl growing up in a coal-mining town in western
Pennsylvania, I thought my father was a giant. Daddy was only
five foot ten, but he was thin with big feet and big strong hands.
When he wore sleeveless undershirts in the summer, his dark
brown arms bulged with sinewy muscles sculpted by years of
mining coal. His round, regal head was almost bald, with only a
thin crown of gray curly hair. He had a big, pointed nose and high
cheekbones. He didn't have any wrinkles other than the fine lines
around his dark, direct eyes. To me, Daddy looked like a brave
Indian chief or a noble Masai warrior.

Daddy never raised his voice, even if he was excited or upset.
His voice was soft, but firm, with a hint of a Kentucky twang. A

twist at the end of some words sounded like a steel guitar. When he smiled, his entire face was lifted up. When he laughed, he made a snuffling sound, like the swish of the coal sliding down the chute at the mine.

Even though he was retired from the coal mine, he wasn't retired from life. From the time he finished his breakfast and morning coffee, Daddy was busy. His main diversion was his car. Right before he retired, he got the first of what would be a series of Cadillacs. The first Cadillac was a classic: a big, white Coupe de Ville with enormous tail fins. Two years later, he traded the Coupe for a white Sedan de Ville and his next purchase, a silver Eldorado, was the most elegant car I'd ever seen.

In the Driver's Seat
***Momma and I knew not to bother Daddy when he
was washing the car.***

Daddy never had a car payment. He paid cash for each of his three status cars and he was proud he could afford them. Every spring and summer morning, Daddy would pull the car out of the garage, which was a separate concrete structure behind our house. The garage was Daddy's space. The walls were lined with handmade shelves holding a lifetime's accumulation of tools and maps. It smelled of oil and old wood.

Once Daddy's car was out of the garage, he circled it, looking for any changes from the previous day's inspection. Then he checked the tires and looked under the hood. If he hadn't washed the car the day before, he would put out his buckets and hoses and give his chariot a morning bath. The local Black radio station would be blaring from the speakers because he loved to listen to music.

***When Daddy drove his Cadillac, he was no longer an
illiterate retired coal miner. He was a "Big Wheel," the***

nickname that Pete Jones gave him, a man to be respected and admired.

Momma and I knew not to bother Daddy when he was washing the car. Maybe it was his time to think, to plan his day, or just meditate in his own way.

When the car was spotless, it was time for Daddy's morning drive around the neighborhood. He opened up the green wooden gate, got back in the car, adjusted his mirrors and headed up the street. Even though Momma and I were rarely invited to accompany him, we knew where he was going.

Hills Station only had four streets, so his choices were limited. First, he would go to the post office to pick up the mail. At the post office, he would meet many of his fellow retirees, stopping to talk to them in the front office or one of the benches in front of Babe's Bar, which was next to the post office on Main Street. The latest exploits of the Pittsburgh Pirates, the operation of the local mine and the most recent United Mine Workers of America news were topics of discussion.

After conversing, it was back in the car and a drive up the street to the only store in town: Pete's Dairy Bar, which wasn't a bar or a dairy but a tiny store that sold sundries on credit to the town's citizens. There he would pick up groceries for Momma, candy for me, and cigars for himself. If his groceries weren't perishable, he might stop by the fire hall to see if any other volunteer firemen were there, or go over to Third Street to visit his best friend, Mr. Pete Jones, if he missed seeing him at the post office.

Around noon, Daddy would return home. If he planned to go out later in the day, he would park in front of the house or driveway. I was always excited at the sight of the car in the front of the house. It meant that an adventure could be in store for the rest of the day.

Our Chariot Awaits!
Sometimes after lunch Daddy would pick up his car keys and say, "Let's go for a ride."

In the summer, I lived for Daddy's impromptu adventures. Sometimes after lunch Daddy would pick up his car keys and say, "Let's go for a ride." Momma would get in the passenger seat and I would stretch out in the spacious back seat. We never asked about our destination, because with Daddy, the ride was the real fun.

Our excursions could be to Canonsburg, the nearest town, or to Pittsburgh, the closest city, or all the way to the West Virginia panhandle or north to the New York border. Momma and Daddy had lived in western Pennsylvania for more than thirty years and they had friends everywhere.

A drive down dusty, unpaved roads could lead us to the home of an old buddy who still made his own moonshine. A cruise on the new interstate highway could take us to the banks of Lake Erie. Once, we took the Pennsylvania Turnpike to visit Momma's relatives in Harrisburg for a few hours, and then drove all the way back home in the same day.

Besides short trips every other year, we would go to visit relatives in North Carolina, Kentucky and Indiana. That trip took about a week, with a night or two spent at each destination. I loved to watch the scenery speed by the rear window.

Daddy had always been a car fanatic. In Momma's photo album of old black and white pictures, there is a picture of Daddy and Momma sitting on a car in the middle of a dirt road. By the style of the car and the clothes they have on, this picture looks like it is from the forties. Leaning on the enormous hood of the car, they stare at the camera with contented smiles. Daddy has on light colored pants, a short-sleeved shirt with big pockets and a jaunty hat cocked to one side. Momma has on light colored slacks, a matching blouse and a big, wide brimmed straw hat.

As I look through the album, I discover that there is a car in almost all of the pictures of Daddy – pictures of Daddy standing by the door of what looked like an old Packard and other pictures with him posing near other cars.

A Man Should Never be without a Cherished Possession
On the day that Daddy sold his beloved Eldorado, a spark died in his heart, leaving ashes that were never rekindled.

As the years passed, both Daddy and Momma developed health problems. Since I was adopted as an infant when they were in their late fifties, I was not even a teenager when the mortality of my parents became clear to me.

Momma died of diabetes in 1970, when I was thirteen. After her death, Daddy seemed to shrink. Grief had stolen his once proud stature. He was no longer the fun, adventurous Daddy of my youth. Illness encroached –stealing our time together.

Black Lung Disease took Daddy's breath away and an old mining injury eventually took away his mobility. After a few years, he was confined to a wheelchair. When Daddy lost his ability to drive, he lost a lot more than transportation. He lost his independence, his individuality and his pride.

Daddy was no longer an illiterate retired coal miner when he drove his Cadillac. He was a *"Big Wheel,"* the nickname that Pete Jones gave him, a man to be respected and admired. On the day that Daddy sold his beloved Eldorado, a spark died in his heart, leaving ashes that were never rekindled.

Daddy has been gone over thirty years now, but I can still see him behind the wheel of a car. I think of him whenever I see a Cadillac. Whenever I find myself in the driver's seat of a car, the spirit of *Mr. Big Wheel* is always beside me. Let's go for a ride today, Daddy!

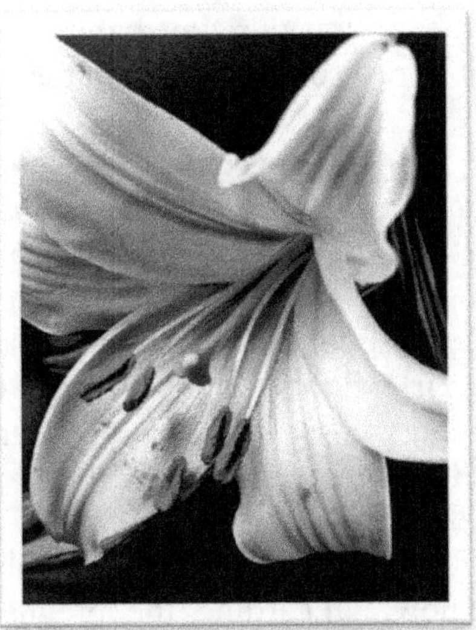

A Father with No Child to Love

Joslyn Gaines Vanderpool

Sometimes Dreams Don't Always Come True
Everything seemed surreal when my husband appeared at the hospital looking bewildered, his jeans stained with blood.

Our first attempt at parenthood never materialized. For me, it was the greatest tragedy I'd ever experienced. As for my husband, he had lost his beloved sister when she was only in her twenties. So death wasn't foreign, but I was wrong about how the loss of our child would level him.

Everything seemed surreal when my husband appeared at the hospital looking bewildered, his jeans stained with blood. I felt a quiet sorrow for him that I've never revealed. Not long before his arrival, the ambulance whisked our daughter and me to the emergency ward of a nearby hospital. A team of anxious paramedics ran ahead with our tiny baby dangling in their arms, desperately trying to resuscitate her along the way.

An Appreciated Presence
"I don't feel right," I distinctly remember saying to Peter.
"Could you call the doctor?"

As I lay on the hospital bed, I wondered about the fate of our beautiful Kiara, a girl whose eyelashes laid like long silken strands against her face, and whose little finger tenaciously gripped mine. We weren't expecting her to emerge nearly three months before her due date, but she did.

The week before Kiara's passing, our obstetrician talked of "Smooth sailing now," regarding the pregnancy. Several days after that promising visit, I felt strange. So I decided to leave a conference I was attending to get some rest. Unexpectedly, when I walked through the door, my husband was home. His presence was appreciated because without him, there would be no other witness to the tragedy that would unfold. It was definitely an experience that no one should go through alone.

"I don't feel right," I distinctly remember saying to Peter. "Could you call the doctor?"

The physician on-call referred us to the pharmacy, but before my husband had a chance to pick up the prescription, a ferocious pain shot through my back. Contraction or not, prepared or not, there she was, my first-born landing in my outstretched hands.

Tears pooled in his eyes – the unvarnished, raw and bitter truth, finally, painfully acknowledged.

"You're not supposed to be here. Not now!" I screamed, looking helplessly down at my baby.

In those confusing moments there was no time to spare. My husband was about to call my doctor after hearing my screams.

"No! 9-1-1!" I shouted from the other room.

The operator instructed us to wrap the baby in a towel to keep her warm. Within minutes, seven paramedics sprinted inside our bedroom. They all looked shocked and ashen. It was a *"What do we do now?"* moment. *"Do we attend to the mother or handle the baby first?"* I didn't fault them. For some reason the circumstances they faced seemed new, like they had never seen it before. Or perhaps they knew this case wasn't going to turn out well.

After the initial shock and confusion, the paramedics severed the umbilical cord, the last connection that Kiara and I shared before we were both rushed to the awaiting ambulance. Racing through the dry New Mexico desert, I watched in stunned silence as a paramedic relentlessly tried to breathe life into the baby's lungs. From the corner of my eye I could see a few tumbleweeds ambling across the road through the back window, but I couldn't hear the siren. My husband followed behind, dealing with his own emotions.

<u>Hoping Against Hope</u>
Before he could slip further into a deep abyss of denial, I shook my head, and turned to the wall, murmuring, "She died honey."

The medical team that attended to me went about their tasks mechanically as if it was just another day. They seemed unaware that my baby wasn't in with the other newborns that were healthy, vibrant and waiting to see their parents' excited faces. Kiara was on life support, and I was dying emotionally, not knowing if I would ever see my child again. After the medical team was done working on me, I was left alone to meet the doctors who were monitoring the baby.

As my mother would later explain, I was hoping-against-hope for a miracle. Before Peter arrived, I was told matter-of-factly of Kiara's fate by a towering physician with a stethoscope anchored around her neck. "If she would have arrived a week later, her chances of survival would have been better. These things happen."

"Her lungs were underdeveloped and she would have most likely suffered from brain damage," another physician added, his tone as cursory as his female colleague's. Translation: it was not to be. After living almost an hour on her own, Kiara passed away.

A chaplain-in-training came to pray with me, and suggested that I hold my deceased baby, which I thought would send me over the edge. When Kiara was brought in the room to be cradled and blessed, I was certain that she had already ascended to Heaven. With her high cheekbones and those amazing eyelashes, she looked tranquil, like an angel. Nestled in an ultra small knit cap and warm blankets, she was carefully wrapped like a precious gift.

After nearly getting into a wreck, Peter finally got to the hospital. Seeing the baby lying peacefully in my arms gave him hope. Although he thought she was just sleeping, my red, blurry eyes contradicted the peaceful portrait of bliss that he had imagined. It was all so unfair to him, because at least I got to see the baby alive all the way to the hospital.

I knew the hurt that lay within me, steadily rising to the surface would explode. I had been living, although briefly, with the knowledge that our child was dead without the presence of my confidant and best friend nearby to buffer the heart-wrenching blow.

I blurted out the devastating news, "She gone!"

Peter desperately wanted to hold his daughter and prove me wrong. So he delicately lifted Kiara into his arms and gently rocked her in an attempt to awaken her. Again, my heart sank when he seemed to deny the reality.

"She's not dead! She's warm," he said repeatedly, continuing to try to spur Kiara to life, and convince me to understand. His handsome face was a distorted composition of anxiety, angst, and fear when he looked at me.

Before he could slip further into a deep abyss of denial, I shook my head and turned to the wall, murmuring, "She died honey. They wrapped her in warm blankets. That's why she feels alive."

Tears pooled in his eyes – the unvarnished, raw and bitter truth, finally, painfully acknowledged.

<u>A Lonelier Journey to Recovery</u>

In one instant Peter was on cloud nine anticipating being a father, to being inconsolable at Kiara's memorial service.

There was nothing for us in that darkened, sterile room but stale air and the smell of death. Looking out on the plains, a spattering of lights dotted the pitch black Southwestern night. There were no stars to wish upon. No debonair television host to slyly announce, "You are in the twilight zone."

It was apparent to everyone that we needed to check out early and go home to grieve. Before we left the hospital, one of the nurses told us that the paramedics who had tried to save our little girl were very upset and emotional about her death. One even sent us a card a week later on behalf of the crew expressing their sympathies about the loss of our daughter.

Painful reminders of the baby lingered throughout our empty townhouse. Music boxes, stuffed bunnies, baby blankets, and unwrapped toys and gifts were in her nursery. We had to dismantle Kiara's crib and return it to the store. That's when Peter's pain really hit me. I allowed my own grief to subside momentarily because he looked defeated as he took the railings down and packed the mattress to load in the car. When asked by the sales people if there was anything wrong with the crib, my husband divulged, nearly inaudibly, "The baby didn't make it."

Imagining each word he spoke, and the agony seeping from his wounded heart as he explained, was extremely sad. Numbed by the sudden turn of events, Peter and I didn't have the wherewithal to arrange a funeral because it never entered our minds that we would face an ending before we had a chance for a beginning. Fortunately for us, my sister flew in from California the next day and handled everything, including around the clock care for me. She even beautifully sang, *Jesus Loves Me* at the service for Kiara. In one instant Peter was on cloud nine anticipating being a father, to being inconsolable at Kiara's memorial service.

Twelve years have passed since our baby's death. I never asked Peter about his frantic drive to the hospital until recently. Not knowing if our daughter was going to live or die flooded his senses. He couldn't even focus on the road.

"I didn't know where I was going, or what I was doing," he quietly offered.

As devastating as the baby's death was for me, I had friends who called, and sent cards and flowers to uplift me. One girlfriend at work visited my office daily to help me get through the tragedy. I even had a dream about Kiara, who seemed to be about eight years old. She had thick, black, curly hair and an infectious smile; and she lived in a little blue house where she was waving to me from a wheat field.

"It's okay Mommy. You can go now," I heard her sweetly say, releasing me from my worries about how she was. Those words, and clearly seeing her in my mind, gave me some closure and a small semblance of peace that she was in a better place.

Unfortunately, Peter didn't have as many outlets to expunge his heartache. His was a lonelier journey to recovery. Each of us struggled to cope in our own way. Our love for our daughter was already established from the day we knew she existed, to her unexpected arrival. She was so real to us. We had dreams, hopes and plans for her.

Even though Peter had no child to love, everything he breathed, believed and had done signified that he was a loving father, if only for a brief moment. If anyone wanted to be a father it was him because he had so much love to give.

Today my husband's love is being put to good use because at last he is a father with a child to love! However, the memory of Kiara will never leave us. She will always be to us, the littlest angel that Heaven has known.

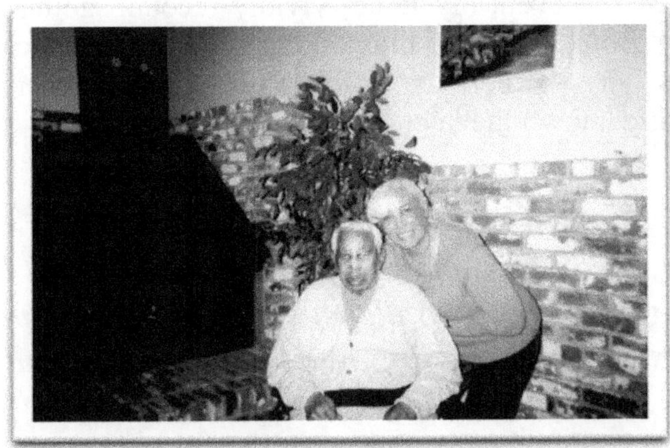

*Mr. George Rene Francis, The Oldest Man
in America, and the author.*

A Man of Three Centuries

The Oldest Male in America

Shirley Francis Wade

<u>Living History Through Papa's Eyes</u>
*As a young boy of seven, my father vividly recounts going to
hear a speech by Booker T. Washington...*

At the age of 112, my father, George Rene Francis is a man
whose life has spanned the nineteenth, twentieth and twenty-first
centuries. Born in New Orleans, Louisiana on June 6, 1896, he has
been deemed and honored by the Guinness Book of Records as the
Oldest Male in America. His birth precedes many inventions and
historical events.

My father has lived through many moments of history and
witnessed first hand, what many only have read about. As

a young boy of seven, my father vividly recounts going to hear a speech by Booker T. Washington, the legendary educator. And *Papa,* as my father is affectionately known, reminisces about having known the late, great Louis Armstrong.

Always self-employed, my father variously was a barber, mechanic, chauffer and a lightweight boxer. A caring provider who dispensed love and support, his efforts aided in keeping our family strong and very closely connected.

Throughout the years, many articles have been written about my father in newspapers and newsletters. Commendations from the California State Assembly and Senate, and the County of Sacramento have been awarded him. Recently, he was featured in *Soul Corner* in the *Wee Pals* newspaper comic strip by Morrie Turner.

<u>Will You Give Me Justice Now?</u>
Since I was a child, my father has brilliantly recited a poem titled, The Black Man's Plea for Justice to his children and thereafter, to each successive generation.

Raised in the 7th Ward, a mostly Creole area of New Orleans, my father married Josephine Alcidia Johnson in 1918 as World War I raged. They had four children. In the 1940s the family relocated to California. Always self-employed, my father variously was a barber, mechanic, chauffer and a lightweight boxer. A caring provider who dispensed love and support, his efforts aided in keeping our family strong and very closely connected.

Since I was a child my father has brilliantly recited a poem titled, *The Black Man's Plea for Justice* to his children and thereafter, to each successive generation.

The stories Papa relays, his memories of times long ago are shared with, and treasured by loved ones.

<u>A Strong, Religious Man</u>
After 45 years of marriage Papa became a widower in 1964.

My father continues to live very happily with his children, grandchildren, great grandchildren and great-great grandchildren who love him dearly. After 45 years of marriage, Papa became a widower in 1964. However, being a very strong religious man, he managed to move on from the sadness in his life.

Besides family, Papa's joys have been catching crabs and crawdads, and fishing. He loved to cook and would always invite family and friends over to feast on the seafood he caught.

<u>Papa Could Do the Splits!</u>
In his eighties, Papa was still dancing.

Being a *people person*, Papa's friendliness and outgoing personality has gained the affection of many people, including friends and acquaintances. They have stayed by his side for years and years and are still with him.

In his eighties, Papa was still dancing. The ladies were happy when he asked them to ballroom dance with him where he would surprisingly do the splits!

<u>An Inspiration for All</u>
The stories he relays, his memories of times long ago are
shared with and treasured by loved ones.

Papa is an inspiration to all. With his positive attitude he has always been about life. At one point he asked, "When will I be 150?"

It is apparent that my father is not planning on going anywhere other than where he lives now -- an Eskaton Care Center, visiting with his family when they take him to their homes and gatherings.

Editor's Note

In order to grasp the magnitude of what has transpired from 1896 to present, which is the lifespan of George Rene Francis, we wanted to list a few of the significant historical events that have occurred in the 112 remarkable years he has graced this earth.

Nineteenth Century 1800-1899

In the nineteenth century, the century of George Rene Francis' birth, Thomas Jefferson was president in the beginning of the 1800s. Slavery existed until 1863. In May 1896, a month before George Rene Francis was born, the U.S. Supreme Court ruled in favor of maintaining separate facilities for *Negroes*, provided they were equal in *Plessy vs. Ferguson*. The first modern day Olympics were held in Athens, Greece in 1896, and in the same year, Utah was admitted as the 46th state to the Union.

Known as the Industrial Age, horse drawn carriages and trains were the major mode of transportation, gas lanterns were used to illuminate homes, and much of the American landscape was still being transformed. Lynching of Black Americans was prevalent. Although the 15th Amendment gave Black men the right to vote in 1870, Black Americans were constantly thwarted and denied the right to exercise their voice until the Civil Rights movement of the 1950s and '60s.

Twentieth Century 1900-1999

By the Twentieth century, the National Association for the Advancement of Colored People (NAACP) was established in 1909. Two World Wars were fought; the Armed Services were integrated in 1948; a man landed on the moon; and the advent of modern technology from cars and airplanes to television and computers, changed the world. However, there was no change more significant to African Americans than *Brown vs. the Board of Education*, the landmark 1954 case which overturned *Plessy vs.*

Ferguson. A year later, in December 1955, Rosa Parks refused to give up her bus seat to a White passenger in Montgomery, Alabama. Her actions ignited a movement that would place the plight of African Americans at the epicenter of America's conscience in regard to the inhumanity of racial hatred and inequality that would consequently ignite the long fight to gain Civil Rights.

<u>Twenty First Century 2000-present</u>

Today in the Twenty-first century, a Black man is a major contender for the presidency of the United States…all this, and so much more has happened in the years of George Rene Francis' lifetime. Not only has he lived through numerous historical events, he has made history, and is a most extraordinary American treasure.

The Black Man's Plea for Justice

Osceola Mays
Excerpted from Osceola: Memories of a Sharecropper's Daughter

Hear me, statesman,
I am pleading to defend
the black man's cause.
Will you give me the protection
to outline your laws?
Will your lawyers plead my cases
in your courts?
Am I not a citizen?
Will you recognize my votes?
I pay dear for transportation
over all your railroad track.
I come up to every requirement
and I always pay my tax.

And when I don't fill in blanks correctly,
will you kindly teach me how?
Ruling power of this nation,
will you give me justice now?
I prepared your wedding supper
and I dug your father's grave.
I did everything you asked me
just because I was your slave.
I helped build your great bridges
and I laid your railroad steel.
Oh, I been a mighty power
in your great financial wheel.
And when I don't do jobs correctly
will you kindly teach me how?
Ruling power of this nation

will you give me justice now?
I plowed your mules
I kept your rules
I fed and milked your cows
I kept my every vow.
I scraped the dirty mud from your shoes
I walked in snow to carry your news;
though I was not allowed to pray
because you guarded me every day.
I worked your fields
I prepared your meals—

And when I don't feed dogs and cats correctly,
will you kindly teach me how?
Ruling power of this nation
will you give me justice now?

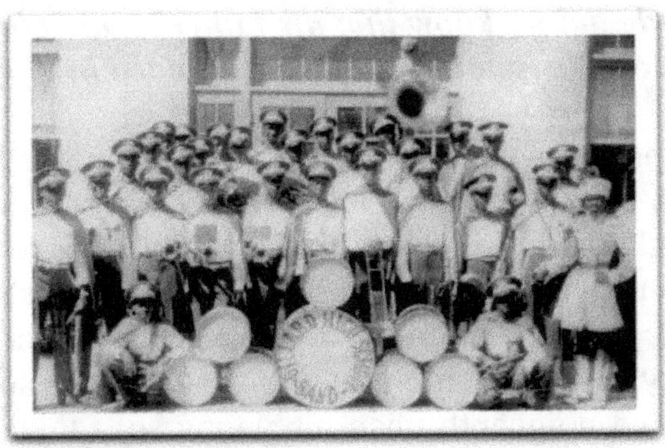

*Young Henry Mc Nair, Jr. on the left with Dillard high school
marching band, circa 1948.*

No Barriers Could Stop Henry's Cadence

Jona McNair

Putting the Rattle in the Rattlers' Step
***To this day, the FAMU Rattlers marching band starts each
performance with a series of rapid steps…***

Nicknamed, *Dude,* my father was a drummer when he was a
student at Dillard high school. While there, he developed an
innovative, unique cadence that was introduced by some of his
band mates attending Florida A&M University. To this day, the
FAMU Rattlers marching band starts each performance with a
series of rapid steps like the swift steps of a rattle snake – *that's
Henry's cadence.*

Little Did We Know
Little did we know that my father would play an
indirect role in the events that unfolded in July 1999.

When the plane of John F. Kennedy Jr. disappeared in the dark, murky waters of the Atlantic Ocean nearly ten summers ago, the world watched anxiously hoping that his, and the lives of his wife and sister-in-law would not be cut short like his father's.

In November 1963, the funeral of President John F. Kennedy brought many poignant moments, but none was etched more prominently and poignantly than his young son, John saluting his father's flag draped casket. Little did we know that my father would play an indirect role in the events that unfolded in July 1999.

My father is a part of American history. Although he wasn't involved in the rescue mission of John F. Kennedy Jr., he did have an indirect role. He is also immortalized as a part of Florida A&M University lore.

Uncle Henry Can Fix Anything!
My mother remembers a little girl who lived next door named Fran excitedly exclaiming, "Uncle Henry can fix anything!"

Only a few years before JFK, Jr. was born, my father was stationed at Greenville Air Force Base in Mississippi. My mother remembers a little girl who lived next door named Fran excitedly exclaiming, "Uncle Henry can fix anything!"

Even a small child recognized that there was something special about my father, who is a mathematical genius, ace jet mechanic, and highly decorated for meritorious service to his country.

Little Fran was right. My dad could do many things and fix anything!

More than Capable -- He's Exceptional
Consequently, there would be times when a man with my father's capabilities was needed.

A man of faith, and a great father, Henry McNair, Jr. is blessed with brilliance, integrity and other exceptional talents. After graduating from Dillard High School in 1951, he knew that the nation was drafting Black men for the United States Army. However, my dad had a passion for planes; so he enlisted in the Air Force in 1952 where he developed many skills. Consequently, there would be times when a man with my father's capabilities was needed.

Although my father was not a part of the actual rescue mission of John Jr., he built the prototype that the U.S. Coast Guard used for training, which was the same type of helicopter that was eventually utilized. Tragically, JFK Jr. and his family didn't survive that fateful day, but the image of the young boy honoring his father will live on in the annals of American history.

Today I honor the many efforts and accomplishments of my father, who is a Viet Nam veteran, member of the Miami chapter of the *Tuskegee Airmen*, and an active member of his church, Mount Hermon. He's happily married to Katherine Edwards of Fort Valley, Georgia and is the father of two boys, two girls, six grandchildren and four great grandchildren. Not only is my father the illustrator of my children's book, *The Shade Tree*, he is a masterpiece of love, dignity, honor and faith.

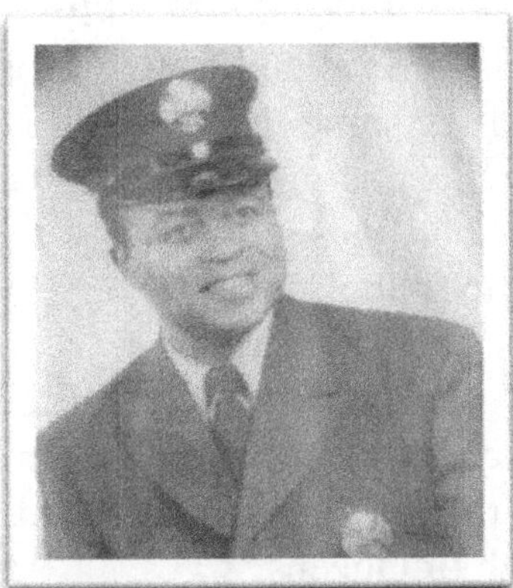

Author's father in uniform as a member of the NYFD.

The Necessity to Nurture

Theodore R. White

My child, help your father in his old age, and do not grieve him as long as he lives; even if his mind fails, be patient with him; because you have all your faculties, do not despise him. For kindness to a father will not be forgotten, and will be credited to you against your sins; in the day of your distress it will be remembered in your favor; like frost in fair weather, your sins will melt away.
from the 1989 revised Bible on Wisdom of Jesus on Son of Sirach

<u>Educate the Children and They Shall Teach the Father</u>
Great Grandfather Reuben knew how to work that land, but he didn't know how to read until his loving children, whom he made sure attended school taught him.

I regret that I never met my great grandparents, Reuben and Cora who raised ten fine children. Fortunately, the family provided oral as well as some written history for us to appreciate. We also had our parents and grandparents who played a prominent role in helping shape our lives.

Six years after the abolition of slavery, my paternal great grandfather, Reuben White was born on August 22, 1869 in Georgia. He was a successful father and farmer whose legacy of nurturance and hard work lived on through my dad, who at age 82, is a retired New York City firefighter and an active real estate broker in the borough of Queens.

Great Grandfather Reuben knew how to work that land, but he didn't know how to read until his loving children, whom he made sure attended school taught him. From time-to-time he kept some of them home from school to perform crucial tasks on the farm but education remained a priority in the family. The children taught Reuben so well that he rose to become a deacon at his church.

<u>We Were Robbed but not Deterred</u>
Just as I mounted my bike two boys about my age, which was around 12, ran by and snatched my brother's bag and ripped the side of mine, then disappeared around the corner.

My mother and father, like our great grandparents and grandparents, shared the same philosophy about the positive aspects of honest work and the necessity to nurture the family. For as long as I can remember, my father always projected those principles.

Our father patiently listened to our sad urban tale and basically tried to assure us that the incident was not our fault.

One bright summer afternoon when Dad was off-duty for several days, he gave me money to share with my younger brother.

So we took off on our bikes to White Castle, the favorite hamburger place back then.

The White Castle we went to was on Hollis Avenue, a *tough* neighborhood. I got the take-out orders perfect, and gave one of the two large bags to my brother who was waiting outside guarding our bicycles. Just as I mounted my bike two boys about my age, which was around 12, ran by and snatched my brother's bag and ripped the side of mine, then disappeared around the corner. Shocked, I ordered my brother to *stay put, watch both bikes*, and *guard* the one surviving soda!

I took off at full speed and ran down the nearest side street as I followed the two kids. They ran into someone's driveway and cut through the backyard. I lost them. They must have jumped over a backyard fence. So I rejoined my brother, and we went home upset.

A Father's Calming Assurance
My father's calm, intuitive reaction to our crisis served as a life lesson.

Our father patiently listened to our sad urban tale and basically tried to assure us that the incident was not our fault.

Dad said it was a situation completely out of our control. Kids in that area could be rough. Had I caught them I would have been lucky to survive because I didn't really know how to fight then.

My father drove us back to White Castle, not to protect us, but so that we could possibly spot the *little thugs*. As stoic as my father can be, I know he would have cursed them out had we found them. His quiet demeanor belies his militaristic core. My father's calm, intuitive reaction to our crisis served as a life lesson that has endured. Dad knew I was upset because I routinely protected my brother. I joked from time-to-time that I was his other father. But I failed him that day.

Cheeseburgers, Fries and Smiles!
On that afternoon more than forty years ago, Dad put smiles on our faces as we sat in our kitchen enjoying plenty of cheeseburgers and fries!

With five children and four grandchildren of my own, I tend to emulate my father's reserve by not *going off* in times of difficulty. On that afternoon more than forty years ago, Dad put smiles on our faces as we sat in our kitchen enjoying plenty of cheeseburgers and fries!

Ironically some years later, my brother retired as a professional full-contact kick boxer, and I am a third degree black belt. Both of us have nurtured and coached many children and adults in self-defense classes throughout the years, but our greatest sense of accomplishment stems from knowing it was more than karate we were teaching. We were fostering self-esteem and self-respect in others' lives, just as our father had done for us. As for that former neighborhood, it evolved into a respectable middle class haven.

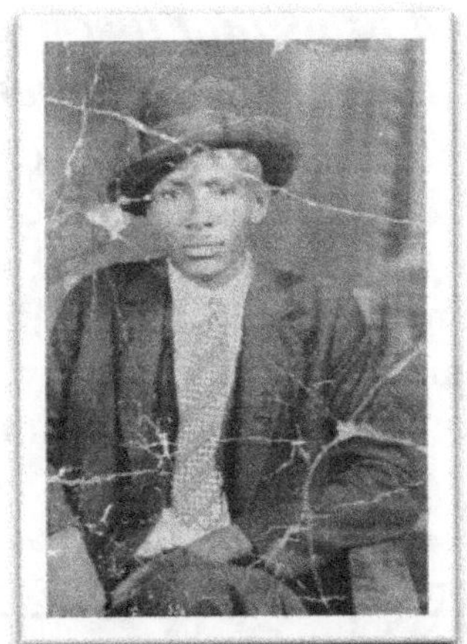

Mr. Jesse Mitchell, circa 1920s.

What's in a Name?

Hortense Mitchell-Brown

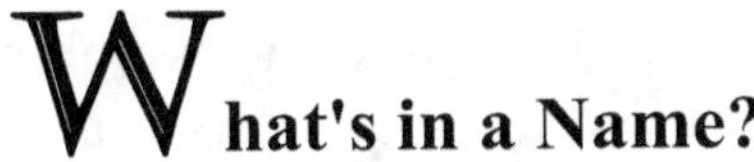

<u>Supreme Provider</u>
As did other Black men of that era, my father farmed and worked hard in the fields....

The Census Bureau incorrectly recorded my father's name as "Jessie." He never changed the spelling though. He didn't have to. Mr. Jesse Mitchell knew who he was. To his family he was a principled, patient, proud provider. Born in Sicily Islands, Louisiana to Henry Mitchell and Ollie Blackmon in 1906, he was one of 12 children -- nine boys and three girls. As did other Black men of that era, my father farmed and worked hard in the fields. He grew a variety of vegetables, raised pigs and chickens, and picked a lot of cotton to earn a living for his family.

***Daddy instilled in us that just because somebody
had more than us or may have been smarter than us,
didn't mean they were better than us.***

Our parents raised my six brothers and sisters and I in a three room shotgun house on a gravelly street. Although we subsisted on little money and few material things, we never went to bed hungry. Our clothes were clean and our home was infused with lots of love and laughter.

<u>Black Men Worked There, They Couldn't Play There</u>
***Under the unforgiving Louisiana sun, my father's light
complexion was toasted a deep brown hue.***

Standing six feet three inches and weighing between 195-200 pounds, my father toiled as a laborer six and a half days a week during the summers at an exclusive *White Members Only* country club. Seven, if there was a tournament. Along with other Black men, including his two brothers, my father mowed the *greens* for the professional and not so professional golfers.

Under the unforgiving Louisiana sun, my father's light complexion was toasted a deep brown hue. For protection against the elements, he donned what we children called a *jungle hat* that resembled what the White hunters wore in the old *Tarzan* movies and a long sleeved shirt as protection from tanning. Unfortunately, all of his precautions did little to ward off the heat and humidity.

The other Black men who worked at the country club looked toward my father as somewhat of a leader because he kept up with everyone's time and took calls if anyone had to miss work.

There were men who did their jobs well, but a few who didn't. So when my mother asked my father why he didn't take the higher paying foreman job that was offered him, my father respectfully said, "No thanks. If the men aren't going to work for the White man, they sure aren't going to work for me."

To my father, the little extra money wasn't worth his peace of mind.

<u>There are Some Things a Man Won't Sell</u>
***Whatever my father went through on the job, he did what he
had to in order to provide for his family.***

Our family continued to survive on what my parents could
eke out for a living. My mother worked hard as a maid earning
meager wages. Whatever my father went through on the job, he did
what he had to in order to provide for his family.

Despite turning down the additional pay and unbearable
pressures that would be sure to accompany the foreman position,
my father found other ways to honestly earn extra money. He cut
neighbors' and friends' hair, sold rabbits and squirrels he hunted,
as well as golf balls he found at his job. Daddy fished too, but he
didn't sell any of it. What he reeled in was sacred because the
catch was our dinner!

<u>My Father the Spoiler</u>
***In the evening Daddy waited on the porch for my mother
to return from work.***

I remember how my father brought breakfast to *Muddear* (our
mother) every morning. After a long day, Daddy had dinner
simmering on the stove. He could cook! Even the owner of the
corner grocery store would send food for Daddy to prepare for her.
It was just that good! Mustard greens and cornbread were some of
his best delicacies.

In the evening, Daddy waited on the porch for my mother to
return from work. There he would greet her with coffee and they
sat and ruminated about the events of the day.

My mother, who I loved dearly, was so spoiled by my
father that she had the nerve to get angry one day when he wasn't
feeling well enough to make breakfast and fix the coffee. When my
father asked her if she could take care of it, she did so with
resignation. However, she would have been the first to admit that
she was truly spoiled through the years by Daddy.

My parents union was strong. They were married forty-seven years before my father passed away to be with the Lord.

<u>Right is Right, Wrong is Wrong</u>
To Daddy, right was right and wrong was wrong.

My father was a very strong, proud Black man but he never was too proud to apologize, which was a principle that he passed on to my siblings and I. To Daddy, *right was right and wrong was wrong.*

Daddy instilled in us that just because somebody had more than us or may have been smarter than us, didn't mean they were better than us. Compassionate and caring, he won respect of friends who sought his advice. Children without fathers even referred to him as *Daddy.* He willingly gave love and taught us to work for what we wanted.

Our father never allowed us to bring home anything that he and my mother didn't give us, or anything that they didn't know where it came from. This was clearly demonstrated when my brothers found a bicycle in a ditch and brought it home one afternoon. Without hesitation, my father made them promptly take it back.

<u>An "i" in His Name, No "I" in His Vocabulary</u>
More importantly, the man we knew as Jesse without the "i" in his name or an "I" in his vocabulary, was a family man who never changed his name, principles or priorities.

A man of God, Daddy memorized and checked off Bible scriptures he read, which I follow today, reading what he highlighted.

When Daddy's father became ill and too old to care for himself, he brought him to our home after an aunt and uncle had been caring for him.

"I want to take care of Papa," was Daddy's simple request, which he did until his father died at the age of 93.

On January 9, 1979 my father passed away. He was a good husband, friend, son, and father. More importantly, the man we knew as Jesse without the "i" in his name or an "I" in his vocabulary, was a family man who never changed his name, principles, or priorities.

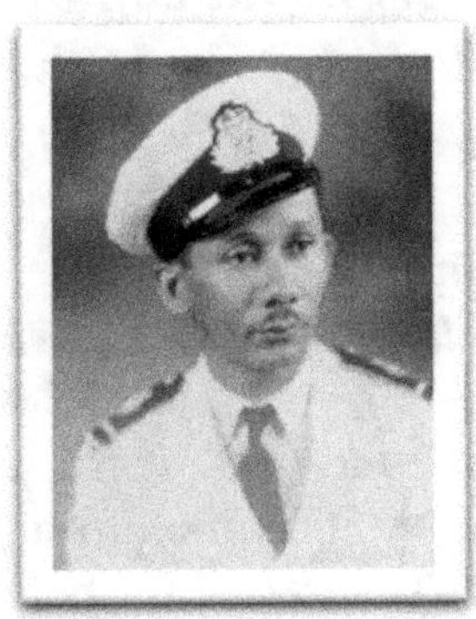 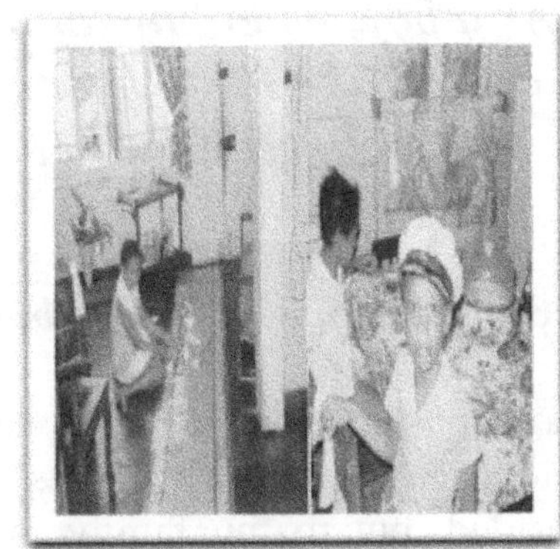

Mr. Barrington Vanderpool and author (right) as
a young boy in Guyana, South America with his sisters.

Man of the Sea, was Simply Dad to Me!

Peter S. Vanderpool

<u>Finding My Way Through My Father's Example</u>
***Reviewing my dad's legacy of love has inspired me to gain
direction…***

Following in my father's footsteps is no easy task. I realize that
I still have a lot of things to accomplish in comparison to what my
father has done.

For many years I lost my way. Reviewing my dad's legacy of
love has inspired me to gain direction as a Black man with the
capability to make a difference in the world, and in the lives of
those I love.

__As a boy, when my father put his naval cap on my head, I felt like I had been anointed captain of the sea; and thus believed that I could be or achieve anything.__

<u>Simple Pleasures, a Simpler Life</u>
Our existence had been about small and simple pleasures.

Our small nation was known all around the world for the Jonestown Massacre, which was more than 100 miles from where we resided, but to my family, who left several years before the tragedy, Guyana was home.

We lived in a one story house on stilts in the city of Georgetown. With no screens on our windows due to humid conditions, every insect imaginable flew through the house, but my mother kept our home immaculate. We were well taken care of because of the sacrifices of our parents. Our existence had been about small and simple pleasures.

In Georgetown, fruit trees of all kinds were abundant. Walking to the market to buy fresh bread fruit, vegetables and spices was an almost daily ritual for my mother. Family drives were a luxury. Although we had no car, my father would borrow a little Mini-Cooper. Then all of us piled into the *licky car,* which is how I pronounced little, and tooled around the countryside or town visiting exotic places of interest.

Our little house seemed to always be infused with the sweet, pungent smells of curried chicken and other delicious delicacies that my mother prepared. The family table was definitely the center of joy. Since televisions weren't available in Guyana, we listened to the BBC and local radio for entertainment and played hop-scotch and cricket to occupy the time.

Life in Guyana was quiet for the most part. Mimicking some of the British traditions, we wore a uniform of sorts to school and had tea and biscuits in the late afternoons. However, when it became apparent that everything would be different with a shift in political power, America, we believed, was where our lives and fortunes could possibly change for the better.

An Uncertain Future
Being poor definitely was a deficit for inspiring youth.

Unfortunately, life in our native Guyana was changing, and not for the better. It was becoming increasingly difficult because of the installation of a new, corrupt government. Consequently, it became a case of *who you knew, not what you knew.* Unless one had a friend in the ruling party, the future could be uncertain, to say the least.

Since there was no university in Guyana at the time, parents whom wanted their children to attain a higher education had to go overseas to accomplish their goals. Being poor definitely was a deficit for inspiring youth.

Due to the dire reality that pervaded our lives, my parents hoped and prayed for an opportunity to get our family of seven to the United States. In 1968 the door began to open when my father had the opportunity to visit his brother in the United States. While there, he applied to the U.S. Department of Labor for a Visa. Based on his experience and skills as a ship's engineer, his application went through.

Little did we know that the country where we were determined to build our hopes and dreams was engaged in a raging war in a country not much bigger than Guyana. That place, I later learned, was Viet Nam. At that time, my oldest brother was a few years away from being eligible for the draft, a reality that we would face sooner than later.

Coming to America
I asked my mom daily, "When is Dad coming home?" Crying myself to sleep was the only thing I knew to do when I was missing my father.

I remember that Dad would be the first to leave for the United States. Although I had been accustomed to him leaving for a week or two at a time to work on ships as a member of the Guyanese

Navy in the '60s, I wasn't at age six, prepared for his absence in America.

Upon returning from the sea, Dad brought adventures to our ordinary lives. When he came home on weekends he was loaded down with armloads of gifts and a broad smile. He shared lively stories about all the ports-of-call he visited, which was like having a mirror to the world. When Dad spoke about far away places, it was as if I was there too. As a boy, when my father put his naval cap on my head, I felt like I had been anointed by the captain of the sea; and thus believed that I could be or achieve anything.

No matter what America had to offer, I still missed Dad.

Life was uncertain knowing my hero and pillar of strength was gone and living in a strange country that I knew nothing about. All I heard about America was that life would be better. It was described as if it was the *Land of Promises,* but no matter what America had to offer, I still missed Dad. I asked my mom daily, "When is Dad coming home?" Crying myself to sleep, was the only thing I knew to do when I was missing my father.

I didn't know that my father was working two jobs in the United States to save enough money to get my Mom and eldest brother and sister, Keith and Pamela, across the Atlantic. But he did, and they soon joined my father while my grandmother looked after me and my other siblings, Patrick and Patricia.

My parents worked diligently to secure the younger children's passage. So my mom worked as a maid at a luxury hotel, and my father was an assistant chief engineer. By August 1971, my mom came back for us and we boarded a Pan American 747 to New York's Kennedy airport. It was the first time I wore long trousers. Thankfully, my fear of flying subsided knowing that I would reunite with the rest of my family, particularly with my father, because he had been away the longest.

Triumphs, Tragedy and a Bully

Our family settled in Washington, D.C., a virtual Mecca of Black culture and racial pride. For almost seven years we lived in a small two bedroom apartment that had a "no children policy," which was waived by management because my father was a valued employee. So we all crammed into our little abode. All five of us children shared one room, and my parents had the other bedroom.

Life in America was filled with triumphs, tragedy, and even a bully. I fell in love with hamburgers, cartoons and the amazing buildings throughout the city. But I wasn't so crazy about a girl who chased me because of my accent. When I said, *I tink,* instead of *I think*, she threatened to attack me. So I learned not to say too much around her and ran whenever she was in sight.

My mother advised that I stay away from my tormentor, but she was in my class!!! I saw her during every recess and she always laid in wait for me after school. Fortunately, the bullying finally subsided.

Our family eventually purchased a large row house that my parents still reside in. No one had to go to war, but my brother Patrick did enlist in the United States Navy and served honorably for 20 years. All of my siblings and I attended high schools in D.C. and entered college. Sadly, however, our beloved sister, Pam died in her twenties of renal failure. A true fighter and inspiration, she is missed more than words can describe.

My father continued to work two jobs to support us until he was in his late sixties, retiring from the U.S. Postal Service after 17 years. Now he enjoys his retirement and extra time with my mom, his children, grandchildren and a few friends from Guyana who also immigrated to the States. The better life my parents had hoped and prayed for came to fruition.

<u>Pete Me Boy!</u>
***As if I were as light as a small boy, my dad has picked me up
when I was a child, and as a grown man, both literally and
figuratively.***

With my dad's positive attitude and unconditional love there
was always an excitement to life. To this day, he religiously sends
cards, letters and emails on special occasions, and for no particular
reason at all. Being that I was a shy boy, Dad was the one who
made me laugh, taught me how to fly kites at the seawalls and gave
me the freedom to dream.

Even though I am in my forties, my father still calls, me, "Pete
me boy!" with his thick West Indian accent that hasn't faded. As if
I were as light as a small boy, my dad has picked me up when I
was a child, and as a grown man, literally and figuratively.
Spinning me around, he then hugs me intensely with no intention
of letting me go. He has encouraged me to get back into the game,
as if I am the captain of my own life.

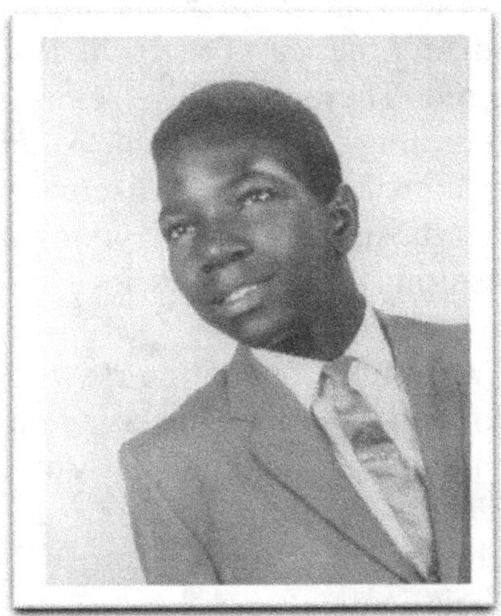

The born leader, Mr. Alfred Walker, Jr.

Born Leader

Trinicia Woodley

<u>Willing to Walk to Learn</u>
He expressed his tenacity for fulfilling his dream by ignoring the impossibilities that were placed before him.

Primed for the events that would clearly define his generation and their greatness in challenging the status quo, my father, Alfred S. Walker, Jr. was attuned to the times. He was born in 1947 and attended public schools in Baton Rogue, Louisiana. When he was a teenager he moved to Sacramento, California where he completed his high school and much of his college education.

Nineteen sixty four was the year that my father turned 17. It was a time when there were a number of major events occurring in the

United States – events that would penetrate the core of the racial divide that existed in America. The Civil Rights movement was scarcely a decade old. There would be setbacks, come backs, but there would be no turning back for Black Americans set to change the legacy of institutional racism and discrimination that pervaded their lives. Not even the deaths of three young men from the North, committed to registering Black voters in Mississippi, could deter the dream outlined by Dr. King.

The 1964 Democratic Convention saw Fannie Lou Hamer become the first African American to serve as a delegate in a major convention from the Deep South. The Voting Rights Act was signed. Young Black Americans seeking an education, pushed institutions of higher learning that were off limits to them to the brink of opening their doors.

The activities of the Civil Rights movement spread as far as California and to Alfred S. Walker, Jr. My father also was determined to obtain the education he so desired.

When then governor, George C. Wallace waged a battle to keep segregation alive by standing defiantly at the entrance of the University of Alabama, America learned that we, as a people, weren't going *to let nobody turn us around.* Under pressure from the federal government, Black students were eventually admitted. And in 1964, James Meredith was the first Black person to graduate from the University of Mississippi.

The activities of the Civil Rights movement spread as far as California and to Alfred S. Walker, Jr. My father also was determined to obtain the education he so desired. He expressed his tenacity for fulfilling his dream by ignoring the impossibilities that were placed before him.

As a student at American River Jr. College in Sacramento, California, my father waged his own movement to gain educational opportunities, not only for himself, but also for the people in his community. Being that there was not a bus route from Del Paso Heights (a mainly African American enclave) to the college, he had no other alternative but to walk in order to learn. This prompted my father to conduct a march so that people on his side of town would also get the opportunity to gain a college education.

My father didn't stop at organizing a march. While in community college he established the Black Student Union and College Awareness & Tutorial Programs. He was the first BSU president at the college. Majoring in human services, he was a member of that department's first graduating class. Afterward, he continued his education at California State University at Sacramento where he earned his B.A. in sociology.

From Learner to Leader
"Enter to learn. Depart to serve."
--Mary McCleod Bethune

My father has the unique ability to serve people, and was honored in 1982 in the ***Outstanding Young Men in America*** publication. Where there is a need, Alfred S. Walker Jr. is there to meet it. He embarked on a career with the Louisiana state government serving in several positions in the social welfare field.

Through the years, my father has ministered in prisons, jails, and youth facilities in Northern California. Never slowing his pace or his concern or compassion for others, Alfred S. Walker Evangelism, Enrichment, Empowerment Ministries will reach billions of people through the China Project during the 2008 Summer Olympics.

From learning to leading, my father's faithfulness is a great inspiration to me. His giving is an illumination expressed through the smiles of all those who have been blessed by his willingness to serve people. My father imparts wisdom, knowledge & understanding using Biblical Principles of the *Word of God*, with simplicity, clarity and motivation. He desires and delights in assisting people reach their full potential.

<u>Still Leading</u>
***My father has impacted the lives of many people who have
shared their testimony of how he has touched them.***

Forty plus years have elapsed, but my father is still leading and touching lives. It elates me to know that I am blessed with a father that not only imparts wisdom and compassion, but others are also being blessed with his gifts.

Many people have shared their testimony of how my father has touched and impacted their lives. I too, am proudly honored to be his daughter. All of his achievements and honors would not mean anything without the loving, faithful compassion he has for people.

On his sixtieth birthday, my husband and I gave my father a party to show our appreciation and gratitude to Alfred S. Walker, Jr. -- licensed and ordained minister, loving husband of his beautiful wife, Latrece and the Godly father of eight children.

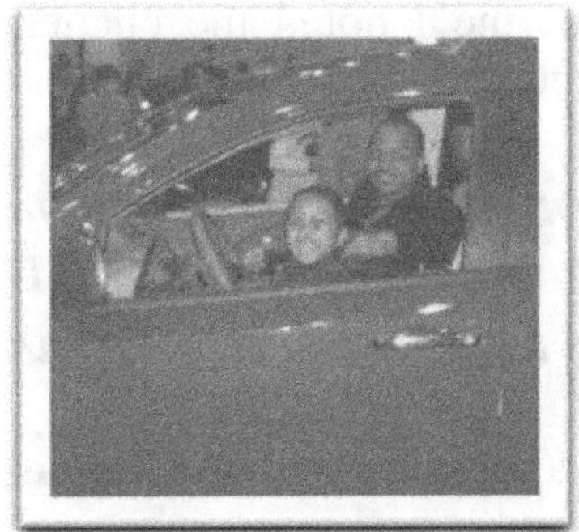

Devin testing out some wheels with Dad and author, Keith by his side.

Same Place, Same Face

Keith D. Morton

<u>The Things People Say</u>
The observant often comment on how similar our features are.

The jagged boardwalk made me nervous. *What if the boy started running (as three-year-olds are inclined to do), crashing to the unwelcoming wood below him, splinters invading his knees and palms?* Thoughts like that had become a common part of my life from the moment I found out my wife was pregnant. That beautiful summer day was no exception as the three of us walked in the shadow of Wonder Wheel trying to find a little peace near the ocean in an otherwise bustling city.

We eventually found a concrete path which took us to one of the most famous hot dog establishments in the world: Nathan's. Devin and I stood outside as my wife went to place an order. People walked back and forth, some sporting a variety of tattoos that were displayed on backs and arms. As always, I was ever vigilant. In front of me I noted the chatter of busy people, and realized it was directed toward me.

Before Devin came along I was poorly defined, but now I see so much of myself in him. It is as if his simple existence has helped to give me definition.

A woman with a lazy eye provided an assessment, "You can't deny that boy is yours!"

"Oh no, you couldn't fight that in court. Look at that boy," her male companion said in agreement.

I smiled not wanting to seem rude. The problem with smiling is that it makes people want to keep on talking when you'd rather not. So I suffered through the standard interrogation that most new parents must endure from strangers, hoping for my wife to emerge and save me. When she came out of the restaurant with cheese covered fries, the conversation and focus shifted toward her.

"Look at you! It's like you didn't have anything to do with making that little boy. You did all the work and get none of the credit."

We laughed at the friendly lady's words and continued on in that fashion for a few more minutes -- then they were gone. It was just another day out in the world with my family.

For as long as my son Devin has been on this earth, and I can count the years on one hand, we have shared both a home and an identical face. The observant often comment on how similar our features are. They talk loud enough for me to hear, because they want to be heard. They want me to know that we have been noticed. The friendly ones, and there are quite a few of those, waltz right up to Devin and I, and say things like "You don't need a DNA test to prove you're the father."

We've heard them all.

<u>Denial is not an Option</u>

I try to imagine myself in a state of daddy denial and I can't.

The attention my son and I get sometimes is fine with me. I like the spotlight as much as anyone that grew from a boy to a man during the ongoing media craze that seems to have engulfed the entire world. It can actually be amusing on the right day, under the right circumstances.

What bothers me is how even the nicest folks inadvertently imply through their wording, that I would ever consider denying that Devin is my son. I'm sure that their comments are not intended to sound negative, but occasionally they do.

I can't even imagine myself in a state of *daddy denial*. The thought of not seeing Devin's face first thing in the morning would be as if I were not seeing my own face. My mother and grandmother have shown me pictures proving that he bears the same countenance as me when I was his age. So how could I deny him?

Before Devin came along I was poorly defined, but now I see so much of myself in him. It is as if his simple existence has helped to give me definition. He's starting to see himself in me too. Not too long ago, and out of nowhere, my son told me, "I want to be good Daddy when I grow up, just like you." After getting over the initial dread of being a grandfather before my time, I understood what he meant. It was his way of telling me that he thought I was doing a good job -- that he loved me.

On a perfect spring day I was thrust into fatherhood, and I'm allowing that momentum to carry me into the future without even the slightest hint of denial.

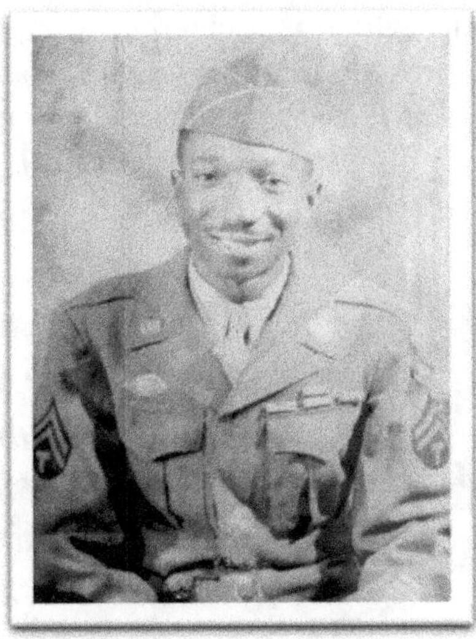

The co-pilot and father.

The Man Who Propelled Me to Soar

In Memory of My Co-Pilot

Don Bailey

<u>If the Front Door is Closed There's Always a Back Door</u>
*As I grew older, my father constantly instilled in me
that I could be whatever I wanted to be.*

A formal education couldn't compete with my father's expansive mind and his large trove of wisdom. The sixth grade was as far as his classroom experience went; however, what he missed in school was richly replaced with other invaluable assets. My father had a warm and generous heart and an outgoing personality. His many powerful lessons and sage advice were instrumental to propelling me to my dreams and passions.

Harry Bailey was born in 1914 in a rural farming community in Accomack, Virginia, which is located on the peninsula, east of the Chesapeake Bay. I was always amazed at his ability to fix anything with a wire hanger, a roll of tar tape and a can of *3-in-1 Oil*. A true family man, he strongly emphasized that a *man must take care of his family, no matter what.*

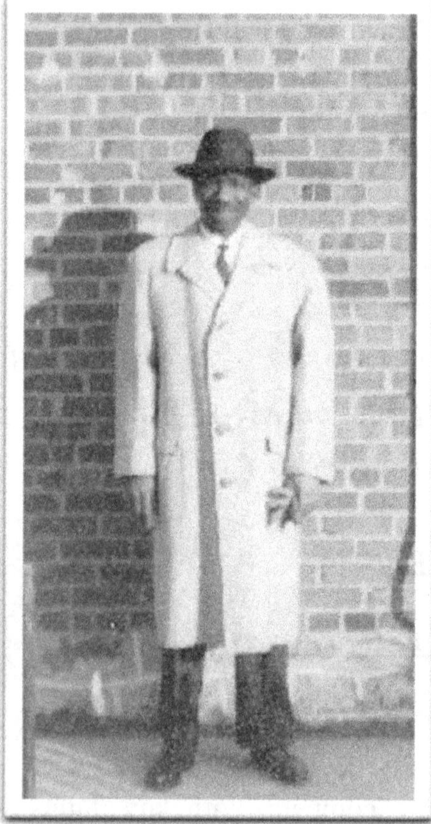

Author's father, Harry Bailey.

My two loves in life were airplanes and television; not watching television, per se, but working behind the scenes. In 1955, those dreams were all but impossible for a Black man to achieve.

I contracted tuberculosis when I was ten. Since we lived in a third floor apartment in Baltimore, my father would come. home for lunch and carry me down stairs to sit on the steps so we could play with paper airplanes. After lunch he would carry me back up the long flight of stairs to the apartment and repeat the process when he got off from work.

As I grew older, my father constantly instilled in me that I could be whatever I wanted to be. Our adopted philosophy was that *if the front door is closed there's always a back door and sometimes it's smarter to open the door slowly rather than try to kick it open.*

<u>A Black Man's Impossible Dreams</u>
"Clean the oil pans, and clean em good."

My two loves in life were airplanes and television; not watching television per se, but working behind the scenes. In 1955, those dreams were all but impossible for a Black man to achieve. However, I would pursue them anyway. First I joined the Navy in 1958 and they immediately wanted to make me a cook. I talked to my father who urged me to continue to let them know what my plan was. It must have worked because I wound up in a Helicopter Squadron, but there was one proviso: they wanted me to clean oil pans.

When I shared what my duties were with my dad, he said "Clean the oil pans, and clean em good." My father's words were in my heart when I later found myself flying as the co-pilot on sea air rescue missions in Sicily or on patrol in the Caribbean.

As the foundation of our family, my father was a source of encouragement for us all. We have all met people in our lives that make us think, "If you

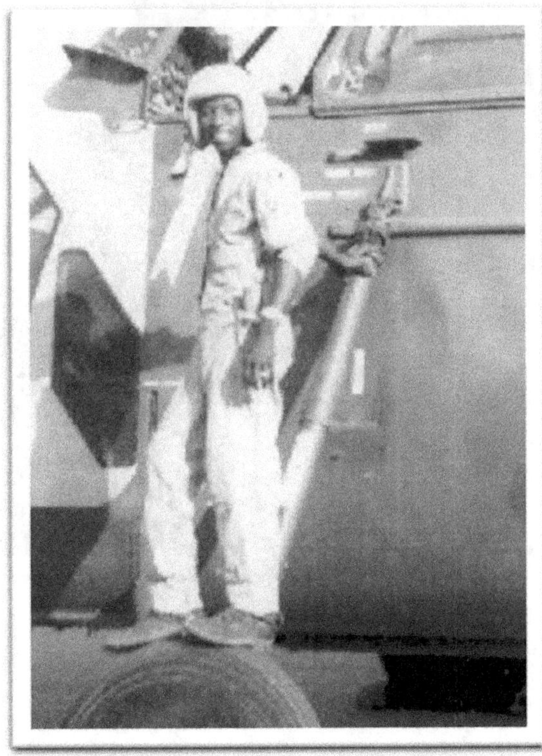

don't like him or her…you have a problem." Well that's how I felt about my father. He was liked by everyone he touched.

Today as I am directing a show, covering a sports event or producing a special for *The Montel Williams Show*, I know it's because my father was there pushing me to be all that I wanted to be. When times get tough I can still hear him say, "Donald, the only way that you can lose your principles is to abandon them," but I won't because my father was my co-pilot – *the wind beneath my wings*. By remembering his words, deeds and the example he set, he continues to guide me as I soar.

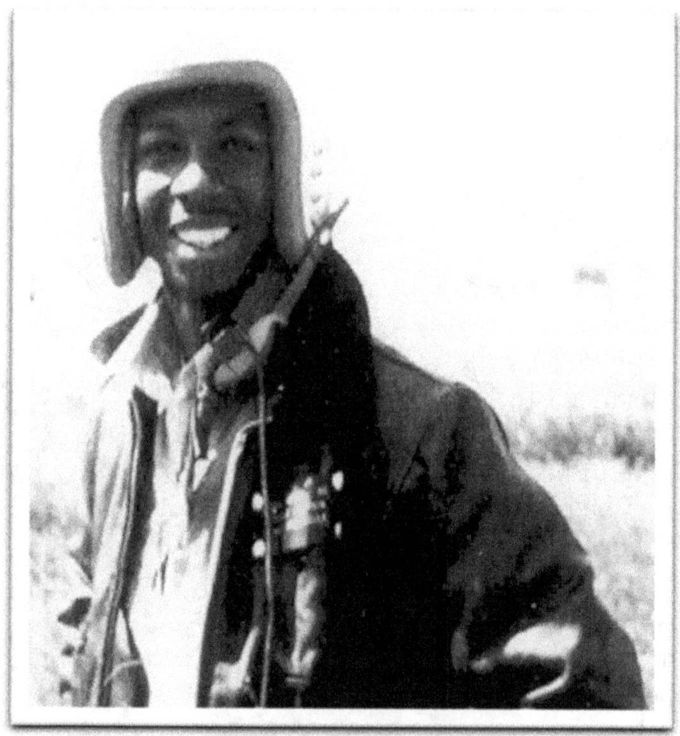

Author set to pilot his helicopter.

Black Fathers

Joslyn Gaines Vanderpool

Black fathers frame
the center of our lives—
giving us assurances
with God we will survive
Black fathers know
pain from what
they've been denied,
but they keep pressing
on, they have families
to raise…
Black fathers are
strong, despite difficult lives.
They've
envisioned for us,
what they never
envisioned for themselves.
They keep pressing on…with
their lessons of love.
Black fathers are symbols of
racial pride,
dignity, eloquence,
brave souls magnified…

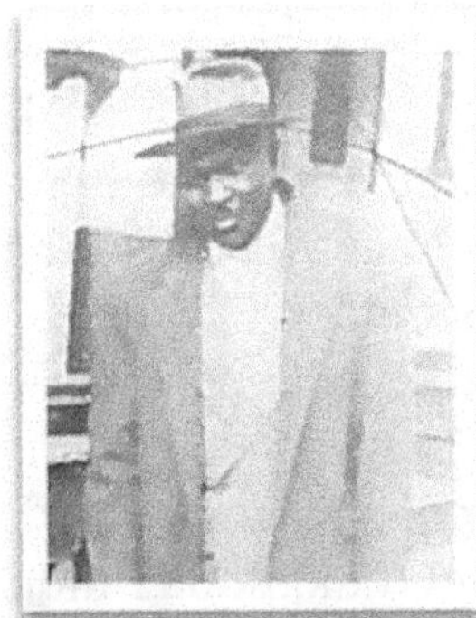 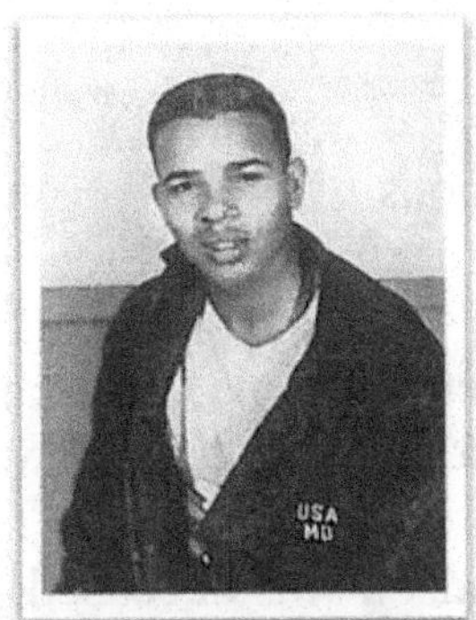

Long Lost, But Not Forgotten – The Tale of Three Uncles

Joslyn Gaines Vanderpool

Purple Heart for a Man with a Heart of Gold

I treasure the fact that my Granduncle Robert "Buddy" Sullivan was a decent, kind man who fought for this country during World War II, despite living in a Jim Crow reality of being treated as a second-class citizen. My mother loved and adored her favorite uncle who was not much older than she. He was a "handsome devil", as Mom states and was a good son to his mother, Adela. Soon after leaving his small town of Albany, Georgia, to join the war effort he was pronounced dead on September 15, 1944 — killed in action in Italy.

"Don't you stop here!" Instinctively, everyone knew that when the postman came to your house in those days of war, it was with a telegram notifying loved

ones that their sons, fathers, brothers, uncles or in this case, grandson was gone.

As if it was yesterday, my mother who was 16 at the time, still envisions when the postman rode up on his bike to my Great Grandmother Frances' tiny house on Mercer Street. She pointed her finger at him and said, "Don't you stop here!"

Instinctively, everyone knew that when the postman came to your house in those days of war, it was with a telegram notifying loved ones that their sons, fathers, brothers, uncles and in this case, grandson was deceased. So, Great Grandmother didn't want anything to do with the postman or what was in his brown mail satchel.

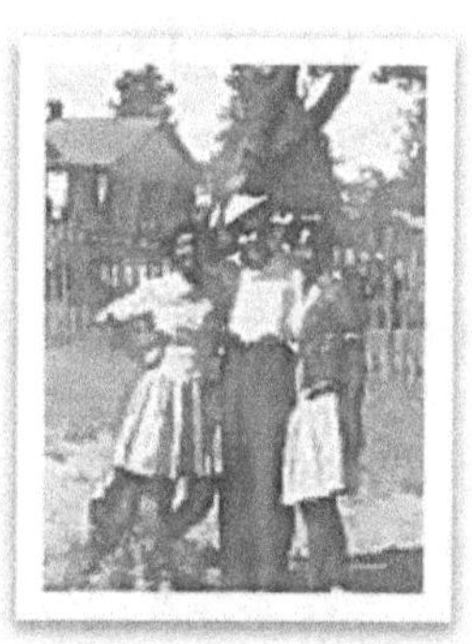

What remains of Uncle Buddy's memory is a well preserved Purple Heart medal, a certificate signed by the Secretary of War, during the administration of President Franklin Delano Roosevelt and a few tattered pictures of him smiling, hat cocked to the side and forever youthful. Although he was physically gone 15 years before my birth, I know of him because my mom always kept his legacy in place as a man with a heart of gold. She had always longed for a large family but was an only child, whose biological father was murdered when she was under the age of ten. That's why Uncle Buddy was a respected father figure who would live on.

The Dreamiest – A Life of Service

Today I am fortunate to write about what my mother has shared through stories and gathering Census Bureau records, pictures, anything she could scrape together to piecemeal her family's story to pass on to us. It was an arduous feat and I can still hear her saying, "These people don't tell you nothing!" when she asked her relatives questions about the past. In those days, such things were no one's business. However, I commend Mom, who is nearly 90, for keeping Uncle Buddy's and everyone's memories alive.

Even though I didn't meet Uncle Buddy, I met his nephew, Jesse Williams, Jr. as our paths crossed through the decades. Like his late Uncle who he emulated and admired, Uncle Jesse, who was affectionately called, Uncle Junior, served his country with valor, intentionally following in his uncle's footsteps. He, himself would do three tours of duty, one in Korea and two in Vietnam. By serving 30 plus years in the Army, every ounce of him was ingrained in military life and service to his country.

My older sister thought he was so handsome in uniform. After my daddy, who my sister planned to marry when she was five or so, Uncle Jr. was the dreamiest man she'd ever seen because of his movie star looks (part Greek and African American).

Born in 1936, Uncle Junior's mother who was Buddy's younger sister, was vibrant and full of life, but she died at 18 shortly after giving birth to her beautiful baby boy. Reportedly she showered, washed her hair, donned a pretty dress and went out for the evening, then came home to sleep and never woke up. The family suspects it was pneumonia. The absence of Uncle Junior's mother drew him close to my mom, because his grandmother and my mom's mother were sisters.

Not long after becoming a teenager Uncle Jr. decided that the military would be his path. Although underage he found a way to enlist. My older sister thought he was so handsome in uniform. After my daddy, who my sister planned to marry when she was five or so, Uncle Jr. was the dreamiest man she'd ever seen because of his movie star looks. He was part Greek and African American.

My father was nine years older than Uncle Jr., but they were very close. When Dad was arrested in 1950 for flooring a state trooper who had called him the "N word" at the Georgia Department of Motor Vehicles, Uncle Jr. was there. Both were in uniform, waiting patiently to get a license for Uncle Jr. However, the trooper refused to serve them and continued to assist white patrons who had arrived well after they had. It was a young and panicked Uncle Jr. who flagged down a cab from the DMV to my mother's house where he nervously exclaimed, "Sis, Sis, Brother's in jail!" Gratefully, Daddy was released and the trooper was transferred to a different field office.

Coming Together in the Worst Way

My introduction to Uncle Jr. occurred when his wife and three children visited us in California when my father was stationed at McClellan Air Force Base, near Sacramento, in the early to mid-60s. We returned the favor by driving down to Ford Ord Army Base to visit with them. Both families had lime green 1957 Plymouth station wagons; and our times together were wild. We children, waited until we thought our parents were asleep and then sprung up at midnight and played the bongos, the organ, danced, howled and giggled when we were supposed to be in bed. We did everything but sleep!

When our family headed down the coast to Monterey, Uncle Jr., a fanatical football addict had three black and white televisions going to catch as many games as possible, which was long before the advent of ESPN. We saw the entire family one last time in the '70s when they had returned from Alaska, and were headed for their new base in Maryland. After that, we didn't see Uncle Jr. again for years until a fateful day in December.

Something happened to Grandma Mabel so we dropped everything and drove to her house to find a team of paramedics feverishly performing chest compressions.

In December 1984, I flew down to Georgia from Washington, DC to see my parents and grandmother. I recall that Sunday before Christmas I went to church with grandmother, holding her hand, and admiring how lovely she looked wearing a stunning suit that was black, white and hot pink with a matching hat and heels. I told her I would make Christmas dinner for her and my parents.

A few days later, the Cornish hens were on the counter being prepared for the oven and the cranberries were ready to chill when an urgent call came. Something happened to Grandma Mabel so we dropped everything and drove to her house to find a team of paramedics feverishly performing chest compressions. She was rushed to the hospital where life sustaining measures were continued but proved futile. We knew that the doctor who was assigned to her case didn't want to pronounce her dead, particularly on Christmas day, but did so late that evening after trying to resuscitate her for an extended period. Her death; however, was not in vain. Nor was her funeral a completely sorrowful affair. Death brought long lost family members to us, including Uncle Jesse who we hadn't seen in years, and another character would emerge that we would never forget.

A Most Unforgettable Character

A few months before Grandma Mable died, we met her older long lost brother, Joseph Johnson, better known as Uncle Buster. He was an amazing dynamo, who was bald, with a round belly and eyebrows that knitted together like the picture of my Great Grandmother Frances that hung on my mother's family room wall. His skin was a smooth tobacco hue and he smoked incessantly. His voice and demeanor was gruff, but the deepest interior of his heart was soft. He had had a hard scrabble life. Born in 1900, he left home at 14, hopping in box cars on trains, and traveling around the country, eventually joining the circus. He served time in jail, but I don't know all the details of that past life.

When my mother innocently tried to plan sleeping arrangements the evening after the funeral, it was hilarious. She incorrectly believed, that Uncle Jr. and Uncle Buster would be comfortable sharing the king size bed in her room. Both men shook their heads from side-to-side in unison. "I ain't sleeping with no other man!!!" Uncle Buster adamantly proclaimed.

Uncle Buster's presence, and personality made all the other pieces of our family history fit. My mom, a non-nonsense woman, who can be blunt, displayed some of the personality traits as Uncle Buster. So, we finally could say, "Oh, that's where that came from!" His arrival in Albany, made my Grandmother so happy because she had been waiting for his return for years and they had the sweetest reunion in August 1984. Big brother and little sister. My older sister was in from California with her little boy, Mackey and joined the family for a few days. We enjoyed hearing stories that Uncle Buster revealed about his mother, who was my great grandmother.

"She could throw any man clear off the porch!" Uncle Buster would seriously declare.

My sister and I thought Uncle Buster was genuinely interested in us when he asked about our birth dates. "What's your birthday, child? What's your sister's?" With intense concentration, he wrote down the numbers and repeated them, "Let's see. One, twenty-eight, fifty-nine. Eleven, twenty-six, fifty-two. I got it!" His bald head was beaded with perspiration as he looked at the numbers.

"I'm gonna hit it this time!" We soon realized that Uncle Buster had a penchant for playing the numbers and was banking on our birthdates to win.

Meeting Uncle Buster was a miracle because he wasn't too hot on the South for good reason. "When I left Georgia, they were calling me Nigger this and Nigger that," he said, reliving the bitter memory, "Now they call me Sir," he quietly stated, as if stunned by it all.

The world had changed since the time Uncle Buster had left to seek a better life in Philadelphia. Our time in Georgia was special, but four months later we would see him again for Grandmother's funeral. Uncle Jr. came too. He and Uncle Buster had never met and here they were connected through his sisters, my late Grand Aunt Adela, who was Uncle Jr.'s grandmother, and my Grandmother Mabel whose sudden death brought Uncle Jr. and Uncle Buster back to us. There are pictures of us all crying, arms wrapped around each other, eyes swollen from sorrow, but through our grief we found each other and a new incredible bond was formed. Uncle Jr. and Buster, though related, were like night and day.

When my mother tried to plan sleeping arrangements the evening after the funeral, it was hilarious. She incorrectly believed that Uncle Jr. and Uncle Buster would be comfortable sharing the king size bed in her room. Both men shook their heads from side-to-side in unison. "I ain't sleeping with no other man!!!" Uncle Buster adamantly proclaimed.

And Uncle Jr. readily agreed that it wouldn't work out for him either. So, Uncle Buster ended up sleeping in the downstairs recliner all night. Since they were non-church goers everyone encircled Uncle Jr., Uncle Buster and me to save us, but in our own way, we had personal relationships to God. After the time spent together, my uncles become permanent fixtures in our lives, attending my wedding and growing close to my sister's young sons.

My husband and I took a trek up to Philly to meet Uncle Buster's 77-year-old girlfriend the summer after our wedding. He had been previously married to a kind lady named Sarah who had passed away. When we arrived Uncle Buster's girlfriend, Vernetta, was a gracious host, but as for my uncle, not so much. When she said, "Buster get our guests something to drink," Uncle Buster replied, "Shoot, those Negroes ain't no guests!" However, he relented and brought us some orange soda and we had a wonderful visit. Before we hit the road, as was customary in the South and particularly for black folks, due to Jim Crow laws which kept us from cafes and restaurants, Ms. Vernetta sent us off with a bag of homemade chicken, bread and fruit, which reminded me of our road trips from California to Georgia in the segregated sixties.

Last Chapter, Last Verse

Uncle Buster's favorite phrase was, "I'm gonna hit you in the head with a brick, gator!" which I think was his way of telling me he loved me. He called every man, "Mack," which was what he also called his dog. And he always spoke his mind without a filter which I admired because he knew who he was in a very racially charged and oppressive society for black men who were brave, beautiful and yearned to be free. Being his own man was critical but dangerous in that era. Yet he had wisdom and common sense because he had lived so long under those conditions.

As my husband astutely noted, the other day when discussing my uncles' prowess, "Uncle Buster knew when to get out of town!" which was so true. In his youth, he was told by a sheriff to leave the county and never come back. "If any little thing happens around here, I'm gonna come looking for you." So, Uncle Buster complied to avoid being locked up or killed, at least in that town.

When I innocently asked Uncle Buster what toys, he received as a child, he schooled me on being poor. "Toys?!!! Toys?!!!" he repeated. "We didn't get no toys!!! We were lucky if we got an orange or some nuts at Christmas time!!!" There he was telling it like it was.

As an older man, Uncle Buster loved driving his Cadillac, fast! I thought I would lose my lunch the way he drove, and vowed never to get into a car he was driving. He crossed over lines while reaching for his cigarette lighter and literally rode inches behind cars ahead of him. One time he was pulled over by a trooper who asked for his license. Uncle Buster was so incensed that he grabbed his license back and drove off in a huff.

When I innocently asked Uncle Buster what toys, he received as a child, he schooled me on being poor. "Toys?!!! Toys?!!!" he repeated. "We didn't get no toys!!! We were lucky if we got an orange or some nuts at Christmas time!!!" There he was telling it like it was.

When my mother's white co-worker said, she was going to Philadelphia for a conference, my father, mentioned that, "Ruth has an uncle there," which was clearly information my mom didn't want revealed only because Uncle Buster might have closed the door on the woman and said, "I don't know no white people!"

To avoid that possible scenario, my mom explained that visiting him might not be a good idea because he was hard of hearing, which was an absolute fabrication, but was easier than to explain the truth.

Uncle Buster was able to ascertain and assess how to maneuver through life because he had witnessed and been through a lot. He knew the street-life, but had experienced a sweet gentle love with his first wife, Sarah. He adored his mother and a son who made him proud. When he met us, he held onto us. For what he had been through he was still savvy and knew how to survive and knew what to engage in and when to walk away, explaining, "When a brother tells me the sky is green, I agree, and say, yeah man, you're right," to avoid troubles or altercations.

It was a bonus that Uncle Buster lived only two hours away from us and Uncle Jr. lived in Maryland only a stone's throw from where we resided. Uncle Jr. lived long enough to hold my daughter in his arms when she was a toddler. He also gave us lovely gifts from the department store he managed. We had solidified a bond that was unbreakable.

I'm sure Uncle Buster and Uncle Jr. had some regrets, but they came to our lives and enriched them with their personalities, feats and most important to us – their love. My uncles made me laugh, and like my father were strong, black men who had lived through some difficult times, but were solid and true heroes to me.

At the end of Uncle Buster's life, he had to be admitted to the ICU unit, which he couldn't stand. Against hospital rules, he smoked in the room under the protective tent. He got so tired of being in the hospital that he grabbed his coat and hat and took the bus home even though he was supposed to stay there. He died at age 92 and lived his way on his terms. We miss him tremendously, and the eight years I was around him were full of laughter and family stories that were treasured pieces of history where those who had passed away, were reborn and vividly alive in our minds, through Uncle Buster's remembrances.

Uncle Jr. died a few days before his 65th birthday. Adjusting to life after the military wasn't easy. He worked too hard in Corporate America, and my mom worried about him. In 2001, he was buried at Arlington National Cemetery. Anytime my mom went to visit gravesites, she called everyone who left her a *party pooper,* but she was most upset about Uncle Jr.'s leaving. Although all my uncles' journeys on earth are complete they filled us with much to guide us, for they were long lost, but due to a brief shining moment we reunited, and they are supplanted in our lives forever.

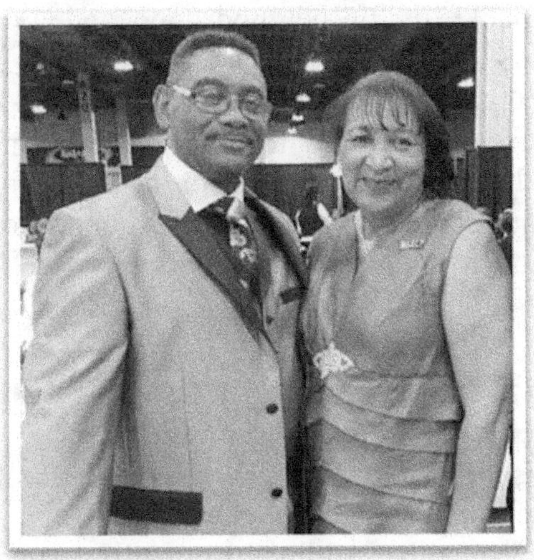

The Willie Fitzgerald Story

Portia Fitzgerald

Willie Thomas Fitzgerald, a strong handsome figure in stature and expression in his family and community, uses his God given talents to help others, despite any challenges that he may have encountered as he grew up in a rural, segregated, socioeconomically impoverished environment. Willie was born in rural Pittsylvania County, Virginia, to Willie Green and Rebecca Fitzgerald and he was the third child of four children.

Willie could tell then that he wanted his life to be more than just a limited perimeter, he wanted to learn, see, and explore more in life.

Willie often states that, "His family was poor, but they did not know it." He goes on to explain that he felt that way because most of the Blacks in his neighborhood and area in which he lived experienced what he did. They all worked hard, and were mostly tobacco farmers, sawmill, and factory workers. During his very early years, Willie and his family lived in a very small framed house that was a distance from the main highway, thus he and his older sisters had to walk in harsh conditions before they could get a ride to Central Elementary School, which was for Black students, grades first through seventh.

No Crystal Stairway to Leadership

Willie often would have to stay out of school and help with the tobacco, as his father supplemented the family income by working in the tobacco factory during seasonal times, leaving Willie, mother and other siblings to do the farm work. Willie's mother was a very strong, talented, Christian woman who instilled the same characteristics and ethics in her children. She used her limited 7th grade education and talents of cooking, sewing, and creativity to make sure that her family and their environment didn't look "poor." Willie's father, a US Army veteran, was not as fortunate to get as much formal education as his wife, but he was also gifted and talented in carpentry. He assisted or built many buildings and homes in their community, including the home that Willie lived in as he grew-up, located just outside of the town of Chatham, Virginia.

The influence that Willie's parents had on him along with his teachers and other influential leaders in his community had a great impact on his dreams and aspirations. Willie could tell then that he wanted his life to be more than just a limited perimeter, he wanted to learn, see, and explore more in life. After Willie graduated from segregated Northside High School, in 1965 in Gretna, Virginia, he was hired at Ennis Business Form, Inc. in Chatham, but not until he and his parents had been carefully investigated or inquiries made to influential whites regarding his character. Then after being given the o.k. by one of the whites,

Willie was hired as the first black for a skilled labor job at the company. His character and work ethics carried him far.

After leaving the job because of being drafted in the US Army and returning upon the completion of his two-year service duty, Willie went back to his job and utilized his leadership abilities to become the plant's Union president and soon thereafter, he was promoted to shift supervisor for the printing department, where he remained until he retired after 45 yrs. His journey as a leader on his job was not a "Crystal Stairway", for he encountered and witnessed many things along the way that showcased injustice, unfairness, and inequality; however, Willie was bold and brave and would always speak up for himself and often for others who often appeared too afraid to do so.

Through War and Love: A Father of his Own and Those Who Needed Him

During his term in the Army, Willie served in the Vietnam Conflict. There he received many leadership awards and commendations before being honorably discharged on March 31, 1968. He received the National Defense Service Medal, Vietnam Service Medal, Vietnam Campaign Medal, and the Sharpshooter (Rifle M-14) for his outstanding services. His last duty assignment was a 36K20 WIREMAN for HQ BTRY 1/27th ARTY APOSF 96268.

Two years after getting home from the Army and returning to work at Ennis, Willie married the love of his life, Portia Fitzgerald, on August 22, 1970. Even though they had been classmates in high school during their senior year, their admiration and love for each other did not grow until the earlier part of that year, then they planned a quaint, beautiful wedding at a very small church for which he was a member, Bell Grove Primitive Baptist Church in Chatham. Portia was a school teacher and they both lived and worked in the locality where she also retired after 36 years in the Pittsylvania Co. School System.

During that time, they had three children, Melanie, Stephanie, and Willie T. Fitzgerald, Jr.

Willie was an excellent father for his own three children as well as for many other children in the community. He would always have time to listen to them, support them in their initiatives, and even take them into his home and care for them as he did his own. On one occasion, an exchange student official called Willie and Portia to see if a student who had been brought to the US from Denmark could stay with them for a couple of days until a home could be established for him because at the last minute the family decided not to receive him. Willie, though apprehensive because the student was of Japanese descent, and had grown up in Denmark, still welcomed him with love and warmth.

Jan (pronounced Yen) Tanaka, humbly bowed and nervously greeted the family, while thinking, "How will I ever be able to stay over here, even for a weekend with this family in such a rural area?" The student was enrolled in the high school with Tommy, Jr. and grew to love the family and had high respect for his new guardian, "Papa Willie." Jan remained in the home for the entire school year and participated in all activities with the family, including church. He grew to love each member of the family and was sad when he went home. He even came back to the US on one occasion and went on vacation to NY with Willie and the family.

On another occasion, a classmate of one of Willie's girls came to spend a couple of nights with the family and ended up staying a few months because she could feel the warmth, love, and comfort of a strong caring family, as her own family was confronted with dysfunctional circumstances and graciously consented to their daughter being under the guidance of Willie and Portia.

Willie often said that what he witnessed while serving in Vietnam made him appreciate things more and have compassion for the children, thus he makes as his motto: "If I can help anyone else along life's journey, then my living will not be in vain." He tries to instill this attitude in his own children and others. Willie always wanted his children to be able to have more and do more than he was able to do when he was growing up. He is a firm advocate of the importance of getting a good education.

A Mission Still in Progress

Willie believes that whatever anyone does, he should do it well and be the best that he can be. Portia loves what her husband stands for and supports in him 100%. Their strong commitment to each other and compatibility is a great determinant for their successful marriage of 46 years. Others in the community speak admiringly of the relationship and do not hesitate to call on Willie for counsel and support.

"If I can help anyone else along life's journey, then my living will not be in vain."

Willie uses is boldness, leadership abilities, and concern for others as he performs his duties as president of the local branch NAACP. He has served in this capacity for over 15 yrs. He was inspired to do this because of dreams of Dr. Martin Luther King, Jr. and a local NAACP advocate, Mr. Clyde Banks, who was instrumental in helping him get his job at Ennis and making sure justice, equality, opportunity, and freedom were meant for ALL people. If it wasn't for the NAACP, we would not be able to enjoy many of the opportunities, rights, and benefits that we have today, however, Willie feels the mission is not accomplished and there is much work to be done.

Transformations

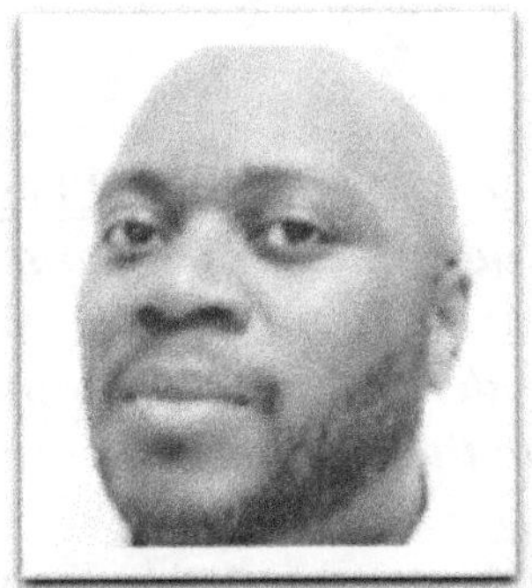

Author and transformed father, richard jones.

Daddy, Do Better

richard jones

Regrets...I've Had a Few
**The more I looked into my daughters' eyes, the more I longed
for them to see me as a father for which they could be proud.**

My three daughters reign supreme among the reasons I am blessed to be me. Many people have enriched my life, but none like those *little women* who simply call me *Daddy*. They inspire me more than anyone to be a positive presence in their, and others' lives. I love them more than words could ever convey, and I take incalculable delight in watching and helping them grow.

Regrettably, I have not always felt that way. There was a time when I believed that siring three daughters was a curse. I also was the kind of man I hope they will always avoid. I was manipulative and mean. I used and abused women in just about every way imaginable. However, the more I looked into my daughters' eyes, the more I longed for them to see me as a father for which they could be proud. Yet, the more I listened to them, the more I learned the abysmal degree to which I was a disappointment and disgrace to them.

Me-Against-Them
Consequently, I adopted a "me-against-them" mentality that only made me more antagonistic and jealous as a parent, and delayed my deliverance from the evils of domestic violence.

My daughters told me about the nightmares, headaches and tummy aches that accompanied my fits of rage. One even told me that she was no longer proud to call me *Daddy,* an admission that nearly ripped my soul to shreds.

My daughters did not care about getting material things, but how all in the family might get along. Although I was distant, even when I was close to them, they did not want me gone. They wanted me to get better; to do better; to be a better person and not just become a so-called better man.

My daughters' unrelenting love for me not only transformed my pitiful perspective on parenting, but also the way I think of, and treat women altogether. They were resplendent rays of sun under which my heart warmed to the idea of fatherhood.

Like many abusive men I thought I was a dynamite dad, even though I was a pathetic partner. So my initial reaction to the chastisement by my children was denial, defensiveness, and downright seething anger. I accused their mother of poisoning their minds because I refused to believe that they could feel and express such disapprobation without adult assistance. Consequently, I adopted a "me-against-them" mentality that only made me more antagonistic and jealous as a parent, and delayed my deliverance from the evils of domestic violence.

Still, my daughters persisted in challenging me to change. Their criticism was constructive too, because they vented wholesome expectations and not just their woeful frustrations.

One day our middle child even read me an excellent children's book about conflict resolution when she noticed that I was becoming angry with their mother. Yes, they wanted a different daddy – their father to become a *new man,* rather than a new man to become their father.

A Child Shall Lead Them
When I relinquished the role of the "know-it-all-have-it-all dad," I became receptive to my daughters' incomparably good influence as children with hearts made of Heaven's gold.

I wish I had changed sooner than later, but the day finally came when their speaking up, and speaking out, suddenly galvanized me into getting myself together. What I once perceived as insulting comments became inspiring critiques as I remembered the saints of ol' reinterpretation of the biblical expression, "a child shall lead them." Their loving me led to a radical revision of who I was.

My daughters loved me to wholeness. Their healing presence in my life was helping me overcome the malady and madness of being a misogynist and male chauvinist pig.

I made life hell on earth for many of the women who opened their hearts to me. However, *the devil* that *made me do-it,* was not some fire-breathing, pitch-fork-carrying, soul-chasing, havoc-wreaking, metaphysical overlord of postmortem retribution. It was a steady diet of formative and formidable social experiences that etched into my subconscious, a demeaning and demanding attitude toward women.

I had self-serving beliefs about what it means to be male in general, and *a man,* in particular. My initial role as a *hu-man* were scripted by negative social forces I could not resist until I recognized them.

<u>Love Lessons</u>
***It was not enough for my daughters to reach out with such
love. I had to reach back and reciprocate.***

My daughters' unrelenting love for me not only transformed my
pitiful perspective on parenting, but also the way I think of, and
treat women altogether. They were resplendent rays of sun under
which my heart warmed to the idea of fatherhood.

As I reached a profound awareness of my daughters' solidarity
with all *sistas,* I awakened to the powerful and practical realization
that I could not give them proper respect without also showing the
same respect to all women. Moreover, I was making indelible
impressions on them as the first man to love, and be loved by
them. I no longer wanted to bequeath my daughters negative
images and ideas of femininity, masculinity, love, friendship, and
human relationships in general.

It was not enough for my daughters to reach out with such love.
I had to reach back and reciprocate. In doing so, I learned to love
them and others for who they are, and sometimes, despite how they
are. I learned to look beyond others' faults and see their need for
someone, including me, to always help bring out the best in them. I
learned to respect those who did little or nothing to earn respect. I
learned that true love is the motivation and means by which I can
make the most of whatever moments I share with others. I learned
that to love is to choose hope instead of hate; forgiveness instead
of bitterness; selflessness instead of selfishness; kindness instead
of cruelty; and strength of character instead of weakness of mind;
and I learned that I cannot be much of anything unless love is
everything to me.

<u>Bone of My Bones, Flesh of My Flesh</u>
I just had to humble myself and parent.

It is not because they are cute and cuddly that my daughters are
Daddy's girls. It is because they are bone of my bones and flesh of
my flesh. Consequently, I would not love them any less, even if

they were the most obstinate children. However, they are as good to, and for me, as anyone in my life. I just had to humble myself, and parent.

When I relinquished the role of the *know-it-all-and-have-it-all* dad, I became receptive to my daughters' incomparably good influence as children with hearts made of Heaven's gold. I learned that it is truly a blessing to have children, because they are treasures in earthen vessels, and they too, can bless and enrich my life.

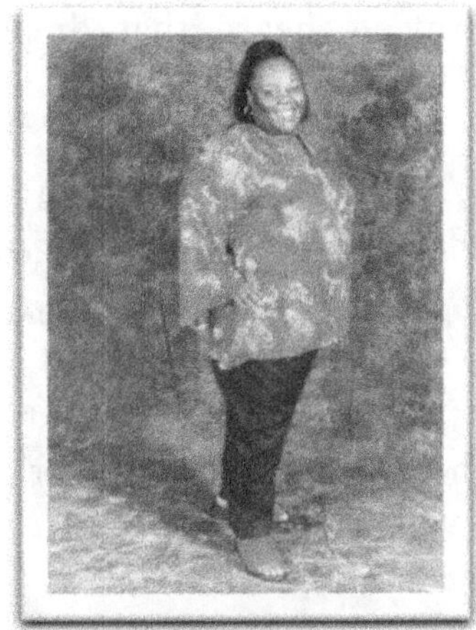

Author, Techina Jackson.

A Black Girl's Dreams Can Come True

TeChina Jackson

<u>Who Would Love This Black Child Back to Life?</u>
Although I've always heard that dreams can come true, I wasn't counting on that being my fate as my life hung in the balance.

I actually didn't get to know my father until I was in my late teens and on the verge of relinquishing my life. For many years I had been told that the man who was my flesh and blood, the first man that was supposed to care for, and protect me, didn't want, or love me.

My father's absence in my life preconditioned me to feel a sense of hate for him. So it should come as no surprise that from my perspective, it seemed like such a rare thing for a Black child to have a relationship with his or her father.

Although I've always heard that dreams can come true, I wasn't counting on that being my fate as my life hung in the balance.

At seventeen, as far as I was concerned, I had nothing to live for. I was ready to give up.

During one of the lowest and darkest points in my life, my father, who was then a virtual stranger to me, came to the adolescent psych ward where I was on suicide watch. At seventeen, as far as I was concerned, I had nothing to live for. I was ready to give up.

The Heart of a Father
"I don't want you to go. I need you."

The look in my father's eyes is ingrained in my memory. They held an expression I've never seen before, as tears flowed down his face.

"I don't want you to go. I need you," my father said, looking at me.

I was both shocked and confused. This came from a man that I rarely had seen, and yet, there he was telling me that he needed me.

Just when I finalized my resolve to leave this life, my father showed up and upset my whole program. That was the very first time that I had ever really seen the heart of my father. It was the day he stood up, and I saw the man that I had waited for all my life. That was the first time I knew I was his daughter, not only in name or by our similar features, but in spirit and love.

Through a brief encounter, my life had literally changed. A spark ignited, creating a close relationship with my father.

A Second Chance
I feel so fortunate to have a second chance with my father, who is now my best friend.

Since our initial meeting more than a decade ago, my dad and I have bonded so much. He has become my number one cheerleader and personal assistant. I am successful academically and in my personal endeavors because of him.

My father prays for me, encourages me, and checks me when I'm out of order. I'm so thankful for the man he is, and the relationship we have established. I wouldn't trade it for anything.

I feel so fortunate to have a second chance with my father, who is now my best friend. I'll always thank God for how He's blessed both father and daughter to be healed, and at last, lovingly reconciled.

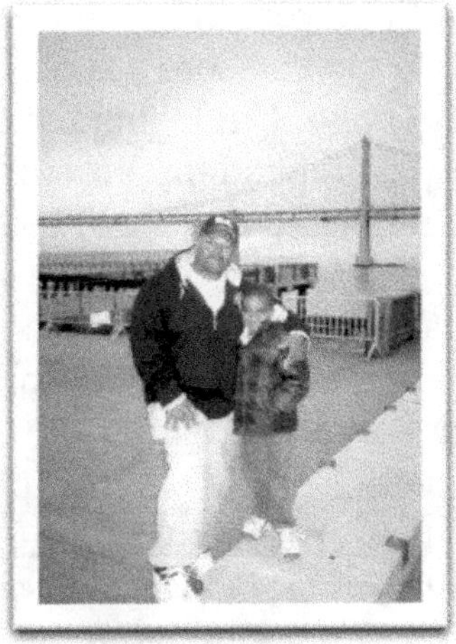

*The author and proud father
with son Jayson.*

I Wanna Go Everywhere You Go!

Leon Alexander Gray

<u>Who Wants Ice Cream?</u>
*If I want Egg Nog ice cream in my tummy tonight
I'd better go.*

It's Tuesday and the family has just finished eating dinner. My wife, Angela and I are having a friendly debate about whose going to buy ice cream. The freezer has a half gallon of Angela's favorite, Mocha Almond Fudge, which I bought on Sunday along with a half gallon of my favorite and seasonal appropriate, Egg Nog.

With Angela's favorite missing only two scoops, the Egg Nog ice cream was consumed barely an hour after dinner. It's also favored by daughters, Kristen and Tamera, our son, Jayson and the biggest consumer, our three year old granddaughter, Dymond, who had two helpings. I didn't even score a scoop.

Sitting with an empty bowl, I'm losing the debate. Angela wasn't budging. So I smiled and grabbed my keys. If I want Egg Nog ice cream in my tummy tonight I'd better go. Excuse me. I'll be right back.

I'm back, full and happy. The latest half gallon of Egg Nog ice cream is almost gone. I swear, it wasn't all me. The kids hit me up with spoons as soon as I returned.

<u>Proud to be a Father</u>
"Dad, I wanna go everywhere you go!"

When I was leaving for the store, Jayson hurriedly joined me. It was fine with me because he pretty much goes everywhere I go. It's been that way all seven years of his life. So it made me proud to be a father, more importantly, his father when he said, "Dad, I wanna go everywhere you go!"

It was one of those cherished moments, because although he's said it through actions, he'd never conveyed it in words before.

One of Jayson's favorite songs, *Brick House* was playing on the radio.

"Please turn it up, Dad."

It wasn't the Commodores classic, but a recording of the song by my band, LSB. Jayson is a big fan and our best roadie. As he bobbed to the music, I occasionally looked at him in the rear view mirror and reflected on life as the father of this precious child. I held my emotions in check until I began thinking about my own father. I wanted to go everywhere with him, but it was not to be.

I only remember playing catch with my father once when I was about six years old. It was a somber memory, but it never diminished my desire to have a son to play catch with him any time he desired.

My parents divorced when I was nine, yet it didn't separate my desire for my father to be a part of my life. I still wanted him at my events, but he was a "no-show," who broke promises. Sure we spent some time together and he offered words of wisdom and gave me a few dollars from time-to-time. And I still loved him, despite him rarely seeing his sons. However, without his leadership, I had to learn about manhood from mostly teachers, who invested in me beyond the classroom.

<u>**Forty Years of Unleashed Frustration**</u>
Although it wasn't a heated exchange, I lost control when he used a word that set me off…

Recently, I respectfully unleashed 40 years of frustration on my father for not being there for me. Although it wasn't a heated exchange, I lost control when he used a word that set me off, which I'll get to in a minute.

My nephew, Tristan came by one day seeking financial assistance. He's a great young man set to graduate from college.

"Hey Unc, I was wondering did you get a letter from Grandpa Leo? He was supposed to send me some money to help a young brotha out."

"Tristan, as much as I love my old man and he means well, he doesn't have the cash flow to come through. I hate to tell you how many times I've rushed to the mailbox only to be disappointed. I learned over the years to appreciate the surprises, like when he actually sent the money he promised. Overlook the broken promises with somber appreciation for his good intentions."

Fortunately, Tristan's father and grandmother came through for him. There was no need for me to call my father about it, because ironically he contacted me.

"I'll take care of things for Tristan," my father assured.

"Dad, don't make promises you can't keep." I was nearly fifty, talking to Dad man-to-man as a son with love.

"I don't want to say this, but...How come you weren't there for us growing up? How come you always promise to do something, like send money that rarely came in the mail, or never show up at an event? You'd send us a few dollars every now and then, but never when you said you would. I'm okay with that, but don't do that to your grandchildren.

"Son, let me first say this. When your mom remarried, I had to be tactical in my approach in coming to visit you."

When he said *tactical* I went into a frenzy. Keeping his distance was part of Dad's strategy over the years. My uncle and stepfather were a threat to him; but he lost me with his explanation of being *tactical*, because my stepfather died of a heart attack when I was 17 years old. Yet my father still never came forward to support me as I excelled.

"Son, I remember I came to one of your games and you hit that ball so far....I was like wow! Look at that boy. I remember when you were a little boy and I'd hit that ball to you and you'd run back and catch it. I just knew you were going to be good."

I fell silent trying to temper my comments with love. My voice trembled as I released a loud sigh.

"Hmmmm....I remember, because that was the only time you spent with me. You only came to one game, but I played in hundreds. We won the city championship, yet there I was, the only Black kid on the team without any parents or family in the stands. I don't blame Mom because she was working hard trying to raise three boys as a single mother. Where were you when I graduated college? Heck, I graduated twice, junior college and college...."

My voice was strong...bold.

"I'm not mad at you. So what if you didn't come see us. It didn't stop me from coming every weekend to listen to your sports and Korean War stories. You meant well. Even after you left us, I still love you very much and I'm glad you're my father! So let's just drop the 'tactical' theory and agree that it just didn't happen. You weren't there for us, and move on. You have another chance with your grandkids. Leave a different legacy with them. Don't make promises. Share your stories with them. It's ironic, but I learned to

sacrifice my life for my children because of your reluctance to do that for me. You've made me determined to be a good father!"

Stunned by my comments, my father called everyday for more than a week, deposited money in the bank for his grandchildren, and promised to come see them. Although old habits die hard, at least now, we share a common desire to be better men and better fathers.

A Somber Memory…A Better Legacy
Whether I succeeded, or stunk up the joint, I yearned for a father's shoulder to lean on, his attentiveness in listening to my rants, or simply his silent presence in the stands.

Both my fathers fell short of being great dads. When I was 16, my stepfather while in a drunken stupor one night, wielded his gun with intentions of shooting me, my mom, or himself. Frantically, my mother and I searched for the keys before he could unlock the gun.

A year after the gun incident, my stepfather had a massive heart attack and died. Even though we didn't bond, he wasn't that bad. At least he rescued us from poverty, positioning me to be successful. Despite his efforts, I chose not to be like my fathers. I excelled in baseball and the classroom while working a job. However, whether I succeeded or stuck up the joint, I stilled yearned for a father's shoulder to lean on, his attentiveness in listening to my rants, or simply his silent presence in the stands.

I only remember playing catch with my father once when I was about six years old. It was a somber memory, but it never diminished my desire to have a son to play catch with him any time he desired. In fact, I embraced the fantasy that has become a reality. God blessed us with three girls before Jayson. Do you think that stopped me from playing catch with them? Not a chance! Our daughters are gifted athletes and honor students.

So where does that leave Jayson?
Simply by my side…

Even though the boy can hit the ball far, he carries a football. Throwing 30 yard spirals to me harkens back to when I played catch with the girls. And then I think of the day I played catch with my dad.

I've looked past my father's shortcomings, deciding to love and respect him as my father. Instead of going through life without him coming to us, I made a choice to go to him. And I've continued to do so, traveling 70 miles round trip on weekends for the past 30 plus years.

I thank God for the strength and guidance to become a good father, a heart to forgive, and giving my father another chance to be a grandfather.

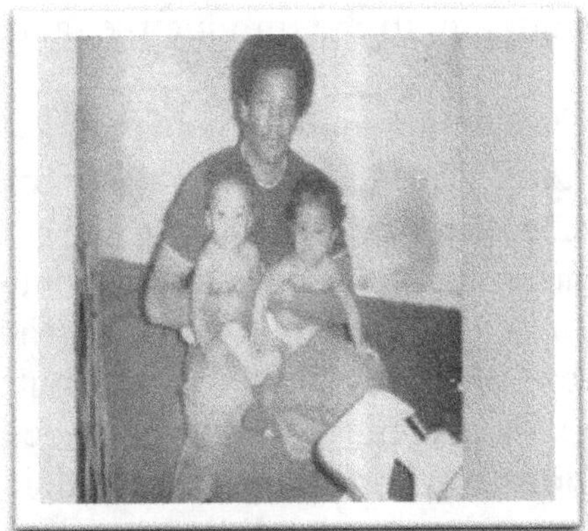

Author in first phase of fatherhood holding twin sons.

Phases of Fatherhood

Bernie Siler

<u>Not Ready to Be a Daddy: *Phase I*</u>
I had always heard that the stigma regarding Black men was they don't take care of their own children.

I was born and raised in Washington, D.C. and have achieved some level of success in life. A lawyer by trade, I have primarily practiced as a prosecutor in the District of Columbia. For the past five years, I have been on active duty in the United States Army as a JAG officer holding the rank of Lieutenant Colonel.

Throughout my education, training and career, I have experienced what I consider my three distinct phases of fatherhood. Before I became a dad for the first time, I had put my law school education on hold for a minute to be *irresponsible*. I wanted to experience all of the fun loving fantasies that I felt I had missed while studying to be productive and successful in the future.

To illustrate how unprepared I was in assuming the role of fatherhood, imagine a ridiculous agenda of running around with glamorous women, being targeted by the Los Angeles Police Department simply for looking like a young militant, having narrow escapes at sleazy nightclubs, getting into fights to protect my *honor,* and the like. Yes, that's what I put my life on hold to do. Well, while so engaged, it should have been obvious that this was a perfect formula to bringing an unanticipated *child* into the world. And sure enough, it did. My initial introduction to fatherhood came quite unexpectedly in 1975 when my twin sons, Max and Brandon were born in Los Angeles.

> ### *To what I considered to be my credit, I gave my sons' mother a few dollars every now and then, deluding myself into thinking that I definitely was not acting like the perceived stereotypical Black man...*

I had always heard that the stigma regarding Black men was they don't take care of their own children. So intellectually, I was well aware of my responsibility. But sometimes theory and actions part ways. I'll say that I didn't completely abandon my responsibility, but I came pretty close.

<u>I'm Not a Stereotypical Black Man</u>
Taking my hard earned money to give to a woman, never mind the fact that she was caring for my sons, was unpalatable.

I didn't see the boys for the first three months of their lives. When I did see them, there was a confrontation between me and their maternal grandparents, which gave me an excuse to continue being irresponsible. Without excusing my actions, their grandmother displayed empathy toward me after discovering my age. I was 23 at the time. Thereafter, there was a sort of coming together of the parties to try to do what was best for the boys.

Eventually, I began to spend more time with my sons and helped get their mother an apartment in Hollywood! Moreover, I acknowledged the boys to friends and family. However, my biggest issue in assuming my responsibilities was the payment of child support. Once again, the difficulty was not in understanding the principal, but carrying out the actions.

Taking my hard earned money to give to a woman, never mind the fact that she was caring for my sons, was unpalatable. Remember, I was spending my money on more important things, like taking hot ladies to Lake Tahoe, camping in the mountains with a hot babe, and buying a convertible Fiat to impress the ladies.

To what I considered to be my credit, I gave my sons' mother a few dollars every now and then, deluding myself into thinking that I definitely was not acting like the perceived stereotypical Black man. *I gave my baby mama ten dollars last Thursday. So don't be lumping me in that category of sorry Black men.*

Better Late than Never -- Stepping into Fatherhood
Shortly after the boys' fifth birthday, I was sworn into the Ohio State Bar. I took that opportunity to change a few things in my life, including being a more responsible dad.

Eventually I went back to law school in Ohio and the boys moved back to their mom's hometown of Chicago. There was some communication during that time and sporadic financial support from me. Shortly after the boys' fifth birthday, I was sworn into the Ohio State Bar. I took that opportunity to change a few things in my life, including being a more responsible dad.

My lifelong buddy, Lonnie drove with me to Columbus for the swearing in. Afterwards, we went on to Chicago to take the boys back with me to spend part of the summer in Washington, D.C. where I was living. This would be the first time they would meet their paternal grandparents, which turned out great! The child support issue became reasonably satisfactory for all concerned, but most importantly I became their dad.

Visits continued on birthdays, Father's Day and other occasions. At age 11, they briefly lived with me in Washington and again during their high school years. I felt that the latter time was particularly pertinent, because they were coming into manhood.

Having grown up in Washington, D.C., I was relatively street savvy but also a gentleman and a professional. The ability to balance the two is often what makes or breaks young Black men. I felt that I set an example of having the right combination of gentlemanliness and toughness for them to see. I now enjoy a good relationship with my 32 year old twin sons.

I Really Want to be a Dad: *Phase II*
Now I was really confused. Not only was I willing to be the father I should be, I had extraordinary credentials to do the job.

I married in July 1985, and in August 1986, Joshua was born. In contrast to my first phase of fatherhood, Josh was a welcome infusion into my life because I was ready by then. I saw him come out of the womb and the whole bit.

The experience with Max and Brandon prepared me for Josh. While it started out differently because he was born in wedlock, my previously honed skills would soon be put to the test.

Around Christmas 1986, my son's mom and I separated. Soon a new and unexpected situation blind-sided me. In contrast to the constant demands by the twins' mother to step up to the plate and be a man, I found myself being stymied by Josh's mother in every effort to do the things that a loving dad would do.

I've never been 100 percent sure as to what was driving the train to keep me out of Josh's life. I just knew that I wasn't allowed to see my son unless his mom was around. Yet, I had so much to offer, and desired a bond with him. Now I was really confused. Not only was I willing to be the father I should be, I had extraordinary credentials to do the job. My professional success alone, served as a good basic example. As a matter of fact, I was commissioned as a 1st Lieutenant in the Army right about the time he was born.

I had an exciting life to introduce Josh to. I was an avid sports fan and athlete who was invited to training camp with the Patriots, Cowboys and Washington Federals of the USFL. I had been a winner on several television game shows and was able to travel to exotic places relatively cheaply with military benefits. Additionally, I had all types of unique interests and successes outside of my career, such as being a Civil War historian, lecturer and re-enactor, which I knew I could enjoy with Josh.

I felt that I had a wealth of good experiences to share with my son and thought how lucky he was to have a dad like me; an opinion that obviously was not shared by everyone. Although I was not abusive to his mom, I may not have been the best husband. But marital dissension or not, that had nothing to do with the love I had for my son.

A Battle to be a Part of My Son's Life
The irony is that the first time around I waged a battle to be irresponsible.

As time passed, court battles were the order of the day. They weren't about getting me to pay child support because I always paid, but to let me be a part of my son's life. You would have thought I was some drug dealer, with an extensive criminal record, the way my son's mom resisted my efforts to be one-on-one with Josh. Curiously, the purported reasons as to why she resisted in allowing me to play an active role in my son's life were never proffered in court.

This saga continued until Josh was in his mid-teens when it became obvious to him that he had a good and caring dad and our interaction no longer required his mom's intervention. Our relationship was like it should have been all along, a little late, but much better than never.

I was given every opportunity, if I had been so inclined, to throw in the towel and use the lack of cooperation from his mom as an excuse not to be a responsible dad. Today Josh, who makes me very proud, is a fine young man of 21 attending college. The irony is that the first time around I waged a battle to be irresponsible. And the second time around I engaged in just the opposite type of battle to demonstrate that I wanted the responsibility of being a father; and was well-equipped to master the role.

Perfect Formula for Fatherhood: *Phase III*
All of the experiences of raising the boys, whether good or bad, have all been blended together into what comes close to a perfect formula for fatherhood.

Entering my third phase of fatherhood is happily a much shorter saga, if in fact, it is a saga at all. This time I became a dad completely by choice. I did foster care a few years ago with Connie, who is my daughter's mother. Not long afterward in April 2006, we officially adopted Kirsten as our bubbly little girl.

All of the experiences of raising the boys, whether good or bad, have all been blended together into what comes close to a perfect formula for fatherhood. Kirsten is a joy. We have mutual adoration for each other. I'm as one-on-one as I need to be with her. For me it's like living my childhood over again; going to the same zoo, the same baseball stadium, playing in the same parks where I played in the very city where I was raised. The only thing missing is her paternal grandparents whom I'm sure are watching us from above.

So goes my experience as a Black father. And now, as the kids say, "It's all good."

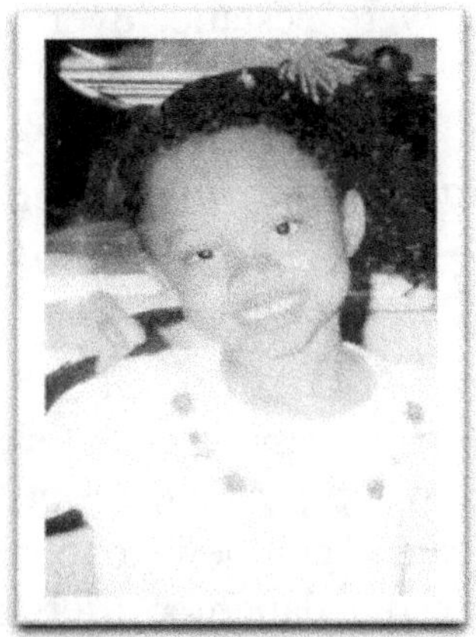

Author's daughter an inspiration named Sydney.

Finally a Child to Love

Peter S. Vanderpool

<u>Over the Moon</u>
When you are without a child, and so desire to be a daddy, father, protector -- you are grateful for whatever package God delivers to you. No complaints, no regrets, no returns.

Two years after my wife and I lost our first child in April 1996, beautiful Sydney entered our lives to bring joy to our empty house, comfort to our empty hearts, and a tiny soul to lie in our empty arms. Although we'll never forget our first, whose life on earth was just one scant hour. She no doubt, will live on forever within us.

When you are without a child, and so desire to be a daddy, father, protector -- you are grateful for whatever package God delivers to you. No complaints, no regrets, no returns. All I wanted to know was she breathing. Wrap her up, we'll take her. So when

Sydney was born we were ecstatic, over the moon, and quickly overwhelmed.

Some might have been devastated by the diagnosis, but we kept going like it would be okay. Remember we were thrilled to have a child.

My wife still teases me about how I swaddled our poor baby in blankets in of all places, Albuquerque, New Mexico in the middle of August. "We were new to parenthood and probably more overprotective of our daughter after the tragedy of our first born. Unaware of the various stages of development, I didn't know that babies can't initially turn their heads from side-to-side, so there I was testing our baby, dropping items to see if her eyes would correctly follow or if she could see me standing on the side of her. I made noises to see if she reacted. I was going to ensure my baby was okay. Yes she had ten fingers and ten toes, but I wanted to keep her safe if it was the last thing I did.

I Heard Your Baby Crying All Night Long
One night Sydney cried so much that it prompted a little five year old neighbor to tell my wife, in his sassy sing song voice, "I heard your baby crying aaall, niiight, looong!"

The first night we brought Sydney home was in a word: chaotic. We had the best laid plans, but Sydney wasn't having it. She cried and woke up maybe 30 times or more. My wife and I slept at the end of the bed with no covers, because we knew we would be getting up anyway. Instead of "good night," my wife turned to me and murmured, "good minute," for there would be no rest when Sydney was in the house.

I remember we tried everything to soothe our baby. "Get the baby's bottle!" my wife yelled, in a half crazed and half-dazed kind of way. I brought a roll of masking tape, because I was without my glasses and obviously didn't understand the request because it was 1:00 am in the morning!

"No! Her bottle!" my wife implored. So I grabbed a huge bottle of Evian water. "Please put on your glasses, honey!"

Without the cobwebs cleared and my vision fuzzy, I reached for my glasses, but discovered they were my wife's specs. After several more minutes of fumbling, and Sydney squealing, I finally gave her the right bottle. It was absolute hilarity and we were enjoying every minute of it, though severely sleep deprived.

We couldn't understand Sydney's fussiness and tried everything to calm her down. One night Sydney cried so much that it prompted a little five year old neighbor to tell my wife, in his sassy sing song voice, "I heard your baby crying all… night… long!" And my wife, who was nearly 40, and clearly lacking sleep quickly replied, "Well I heard your daddy playing his music aaall, niiight, looong! So there."

<u>How Can Anything be Wrong with Her?</u>
She looked just like a healthy, beautiful baby girl, but the problem would persist.

Nothing seemed out of the ordinary to our pediatrician when we reported the restless nights Sydney was having. She was easily agitated and we just couldn't figure it out. Any outings or parties were cut short. There was no time for idle chit-chat or mingling because Sydney would cry or act out. Seconds at lunch buffets weren't going to happen. So food was quickly consumed. Finally after several visits to physicians over the years, we were told that Sydney had Pervasive Development Delay and speech and language problems on the Autistic Disorder Spectrum. Although she was late to speak, she was observant, and to us and her African American teachers in pre-school she was *off the chart smart.*

Some might have been devastated by the diagnosis, but we kept going like it would be okay. Remember we were thrilled to have a child. So something like Autism wasn't going to destroy our dreams. Yes it is difficult at times, but we are riding on *God's wings* for courage, grace and guidance in raising and nourishing

Sydney. She is absolutely beautiful. We are grateful because I am a father, and my wife gets to mother a child.

<u>Just Right</u>
Unwilling to throw our child away, we have vowed to give her all the opportunities we can to help her thrive.

To us, Sydney is just right. It was other people who began asking why isn't she doing such and such? Some interrogations were brutal. Well "she does but she takes longer to do it," we responded, before abandoning the need to explain. Just like anyone else we are a family.

We really couldn't even comprehend Autism and how others would react to those who struggle with it, but we weren't going to give in to it. Our child was bright. She knew things that some of the experts didn't know she knew.

By entering elementary school, both Sydney and our lives have been upended in some ways. Of course we've seen growth, but we've also seen our child try mightily to adapt.

Year-after-year produced an uneven education and dire comments, like, as one teacher put it, "The other children think she's kind of weird," or "She can get a high school certificate (in lieu of a diploma)." The latter comment was voiced when she was only eight years old. There were at least ten more years left to educate our daughter in school, and she was already being counted out.

Why couldn't anyone see what we saw?

Unwilling to throw our child away, we have vowed to give her all the opportunities we can to help her thrive. She loves airplanes, going to plays, all types of music from Opera to Jazz, staying at fancy hotels, splashing in the pool and dancing. She also likes to read (sometimes) and learn about different, states and continents. When we talk about history and current events she wants to know more. Recently she turned to us and said, "I'm tired of doing the same homework."

We know she can learn in her on way, in her own time. She may not know how to easily interact socially, but at home, in the environment where she is safest, she is sharp and continues to make gains.

When Sydney is asked to do chores, she coyly looks at her mother and replies, "Daddy will do it." I admit that I am a little soft and my daughter does have my number. Sydney challenges, is challenging, and still needs to be challenged by those who don't understand how bright she is.

Inquisitive, wonderful, and lively, that's my girl! I'm constantly awed at how she handles what the others say she can't do. She is aware of how others treat her, but she copes fairly well with a very stressful life due to a neurological system that is always in a state of alert. Sometimes Sydney fears the unknown, and intense anxiety makes it difficult for her to relax, focus and interact properly at all times, but in her calm moments she has such clarity, sweetness and peace.

There have been many occasions when our little girl apologizes for what she cannot always control. "I don't mean to be upset or scared. I will try. I promise," she's been known to say. Sydney is a child who wants so desperately to have a normal life. However, her mother and I have taught her that it's okay not to be like everybody else, because we love her for who she is. She has strived valiantly to use whatever skills she can when the world seems too big and frightening. At nine she is bravely taking a step at a time.

Don't You Guys Know Anything?!!!
Sometimes Sydney asks so many questions that at times we simply can't answer them all.

Our Sydney does have a little attitude from-time-to-time. It goes with the territory. When she asks, "Daddy, have I been a bad girl?" Naturally I shrug my shoulders and respond, "What do you think?" She smiles and swings from side-to-side, then softly murmurs, "Noooo."

Sometimes Sydney asks so many questions that at times we simply can't answer them all. So when the question comes up we say, "We don't know, Sydney."

Not one to be easily pacified, she huffily responds, "Don't you guys know anything?"

"Yes there is one thing we know, how much we love and adore you."

So our fight continues. Yes, we are tired of the throw away mentality of the school system. There are some who really care, but too many don't take the time to know and observe the potential of a beautiful gift from God named, Sydney. We are inspired by her. And only hope that others' could see what is right there before them – an inquisitive little human being, who can excel if nurtured!

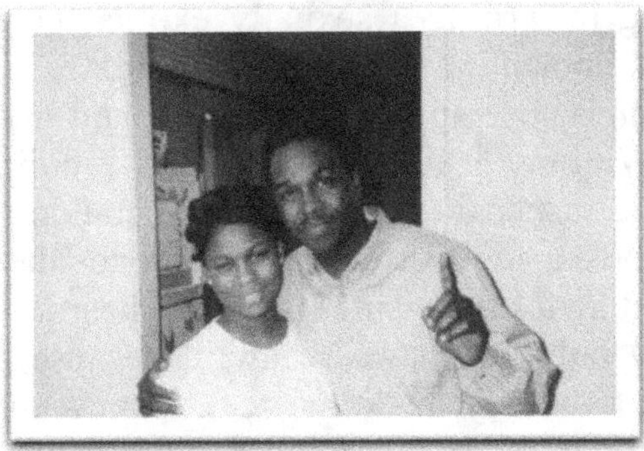

Author with her father, Mr. Ray Gailes.

The Man Who Never Gave Up

Tracy Gailes

<u>My Most Treasured Male Figure</u>
Reflecting back to that day when I was 12, I find it amazing that my father had such a presence in my life …

"You gon' have to tell Ray," was one of the most dreaded phrases to ever leave my mother's lips. Ray Gailes is my father, and while I didn't know him well at the time, I still remember the trembles that shot through my body when I was told that I had to report to him about my inappropriate behavior in school.

Reflecting back to that day when I was 12, I find it amazing that my father had such a presence in my life even though I only saw him every other weekend as the court had ordered.

Through all of my delinquent behavior, my dad didn't give up and send me back to where I came from.

Admitting to writing a sexually explicit note at school was definitely not something I looked forward to revealing to my father; the man whose approval I sought, and my most treasured male figure. With my head hung down and avoiding eye contact, I handed him the suspension notice which I couldn't bring myself to explain. He took a few seconds to look over the paperwork and began the most awful chastising I had ever heard.

What my father said wasn't awful because of his choice of words, it was how they made me feel. I know that if my mother would have spoken the very same words, I would have just rolled my eyes and been thinking about what I was going to do the next day.

Somehow, with my father, I was left with a feeling of nearly indescribable shame, dishonor and guilt. At that moment, I resolved NEVER to do something so terrible as to cause that level of disappointment and disapproval to be cast upon my soul again. However, as children soon forget, I continued my rebellious phase which eventually led to my packing my bags and starting a new life with my father the following school year.

<u>Mister Bojangles and Me</u>
As we rode in the car, my dad would sing "Mi-ster Bo-jayn-gales…!"

Before I was officially in my father's custody, I valued him and have very vivid memories of my early childhood with him. As we rode in the car, my dad would sing "Mi-ster Bo-jayn-gales…!" in a voice that reminded me of those old time preachers who would sweat and spit all over the pulpit in Jesus' name. He would play gospel and secular music and sing away. To this day, I believe that I'm the only person in my generation that knows almost every verse of every Sam Cooke song that there ever was.

Story time was fun with my dad. My favorite book was *Little Brown Bear*. When he read me that story, he imitated the characters' voices filling me with much amusement. I loved that story so much that I memorized it in its entirety. My dad actually thought that at age three, I could read! That's when I was the sweet apple of my dad's eye, long before my rebellious stage.

<u>A Little Terror Called Tracy!</u>
I put my father through emotional ups and downs, yet he fought on.

When I moved in with my father at 13, I was a *little terror*. My father tried everything to get me back on track. He sent me to various schools because I was always getting suspended or expelled. Through all of my delinquent behavior, my dad didn't give up and send me back to where I came from.

I committed some of the most deplorable acts including blatantly disrespecting my dad's household and wife. I put my father through emotional ups and downs, yet he fought on. He instilled values that many people have long forgotten.

Regarding curfew, my favorite quote from my father is, "You don't need to be bumpin' around at night." On honesty, he'd say to me, "I was born at night, but I wasn't born last night."

Although he was reluctant to give me the *sex talk*, my father hinted in other ways the *dos* and *don'ts* of womanhood. He frequently schooled me in other lessons of life as well, including survival, respect, family, and consequences. My father even counseled me about what proper attire to wear according to season.

<u>Why Didn't I Grab My Coat?</u>
All I kept thinking after all the trouble I found myself in was, "Why didn't I grab my coat?"

One cold December evening, my dad came home to find that I had left my coat on the couch. I told him I was going to a football game, so his concern prompted him to try to reach me. Sure enough, I was somewhere that I wasn't supposed to be. All I kept thinking after all the trouble I found myself in was, "Why didn't I grab my coat?"

There were many trying times, but the perseverance of this strong Black man was not in vain. Three years later, a conscientious young lady was emerging. I was starting to enjoy life in the right way. Even now, I love to listen to the wisdom and knowledge of my father, who is a historian, Bible scholar, and active in the community.

I Don't Know Who or What I Would've Become
I don't know where I'd be or who I would have become without him.

My father and I sit on the veranda and have intellectually stimulating and rewarding conversations now. I strive to be like him in many ways, though he insists that I must strive to be better, which is no simple feat. I admire him and seek his counsel at nearly every turn. Although I'm not a little girl anymore, I will eagerly plop down beside him embracing all that he has to offer me as a loving father.

By the time I entered college, I started realizing how important my father was to me and what a difference he had made in my life. I believe that had I remained in my mother's household, I would be living a life devoid of structure (unless I consider the possibility of the cell block structure) and spiraling out of control.

On myspace.com I named my father as my hero. I deeply hold this to be true. I don't know where I'd be or who I would have become without my father.

Back in the Days Code of Conduct
While the values of society are declining, in my house, the "back in my days" code of conduct were upheld.

It wasn't until a few months ago when I received a call from a close friend that I understood how blessed and privileged I am.

"You know, you're lucky," she said.

"Huh?" I replied.

"I was just thinking. You're the only girl I know that has both of your parents. I don't even know that many women with their fathers in their lives. You're fortunate. Well anyway, I just wanted to tell you that."

In the Black community today, fathers are hard to find, and good fathers are even more difficult to locate. Too many men have fallen by the wayside. This goes to show why I feel my father is worthy of praise.

While the values of society are declining, in my house the "back in my days," codes of conduct were upheld. Today I can truly appreciate that. I intend to pass on my dad's compassion and dedication to my children, whose father I want to be just like my daddy.

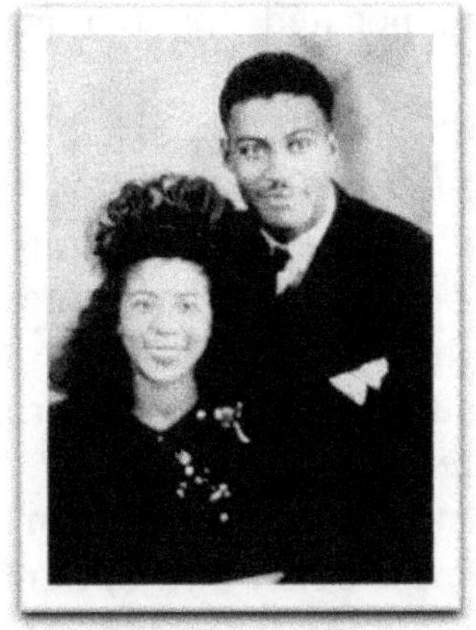

The author's parents.

I Didn't Know

Virginia "Honey" Carter

<u>Difficult to Know</u>
I always felt that when I was a young girl, my dad was just mean. Unlike my other siblings, I shut him out until one weekend in the summer of 1995.

I know Daddy loved us, but as a father of six, and an only child, challenging times were ahead. Private and particular, my father wanted things done his way. He was difficult to get close to. Albeit financially astute in caring for us, and charming and delightful to cousins and friends, there was another side of him that perplexed his family.

Daddy wanted my mother to stay home so she'd be there when he returned from work. His insistence that we eat dinner together at 6:00 p.m. negated any opportunity for after school activities.

My dad was a strong-handed disciplinarian. In spite of that fact, we enjoyed our family time on his terms. At the crack of dawn my father had my sister and I up ironing or preparing breakfast (never the boys). When he wanted quiet time, he got it. When he'd go bowling, we were glad he did. Unfortunately his bowling escapades caused friction with our mother. After 33 years of marriage, she wanted out.

I always felt that as a young girl, my Dad was just mean. Unlike my other siblings, I shut him out until one weekend in the summer of 1995.

An Unexpected Journey to Discovery
The blood drained from Daddy's face. After an unbearable silence I managed to ask the doctor, "What can be done?"

My car broke down on a road trip to see my son play in a basketball tournament in Southern California. Repairs would take a week, so I called my father who lived in San Diego to ask if I could stay with him. I was reluctant to do so because I'd recently sent him a letter about our difficult past.

After sending everyone home on the plane, I rented a car and headed south. When I arrived at my father's home, I was surprised by the number of similarities that we shared. From being excellent money managers to keeping our garages organized, we were identical in habit.

The following Monday, Daddy asked me to accompany him to his doctor's appointment. When his name was called, I remained seated, reading my book.

"Will you go in with me?" he asked.

I had a sinking feeling because Daddy looked worried. With x-rays in hand, the doctor placed them on the lit reader. His words were sparse, "You have pancreatic cancer."

The blood drained from Daddy's face. After an unbearable silence, I managed to ask the doctor, "What can be done?"

When the doctor suggested surgery to locate the cancer, Daddy agreed to the procedure.

<u>Why Daddy?</u>
My eyes met his, and questions started gushing from my mouth like water from a faucet.

After leaving the appointment with his doctor, my father and I stopped by a restaurant. I wanted to have a heart-to-heart talk with him about the letter I had written.

When I queried my father about it, he said, "I never read it. I burned it."

My body began to quiver. "Why would you do that?"

"I just didn't want to hear it," he replied, stirring his coffee.

Daddy's face tightened. I started to shake my foot beneath the table, and my stomach became uneasy, not knowing what to expect.

I thought I'd finally get answers. I was the only child who was estranged from him when he left home. One day my mother told me that Daddy asked about everyone, and he specifically wanted to know about me.

"Never tell him anything about me, my children or my business!" I snapped.

Even though I was mindful of Daddy's condition, I couldn't squelch my desire to have my concerns addressed.

"Daddy, I have some questions I need to ask you."

"How many?"

"I won't lie. I have several. Are you up to it?"

"Just tell me all your questions and I will see if I can answer them."

My eyes met his, and questions started gushing from my mouth like water from a faucet.

"How could you walk out on a marriage without regard as to how our mother would financially survive? Why did you think your

physical discipline needed to be so harsh? Did you really love us? Did you have regrets about having so many children? Why didn't you attend any of our high school graduations? Did you think that being an only child made it difficult for you to be our father?"

Daddy's face tightened. I started to shake my foot beneath the table, and my stomach became uneasy, not knowing what to expect.

"I'm not going to answer your questions individually, but I worked hard to provide for the family. I wasn't given a blueprint as to how to raise you children; it was learn as you go. I was raised by my grandparents because my mother had me at 14 years old and went about her way. I tried to do my best and there might have been times I had selfish moments, but I was the father."

We both sat silently. He kept his eyes toward the ceiling as I tried to comprehend it all. Then I began to recall that Daddy was not only an excellent provider, but an outstanding electrician, often working daily eight to ten hour shifts. Companies vied for his services, and he made damn good money.

I didn't want to push any further because I didn't know what was going on in Daddy's mind. For the first time; however, I saw a side of my father that I connected with. His comments gave me much to think about. He even alluded to spending more time with us.

I wanted to ask, *Why now?* But I didn't.

As we walked from the restaurant he muttered, "I'm sorry."

<u>A Time to Gather</u>
Nearly eleven months after his surgery, the words "I'm not dead, but I'm dying," came in a whisper through the phone.

Back at my father's house, I picked up his photo album and my heart dropped when I saw photocopied pictures. He had been absent from our family for some time and must have made them when he was invited up by my nephew to see a HBO fight and stayed with me.

When Daddy's surgery was performed, all of his children, including our mother, Lu La, were gathered to learn that his condition was terminal. The only one missing was our brother, Jeff, who died as a result of street violence in 1975.

At my father's request, we all reunited during Thanksgiving, and for his upcoming 73rd birthday in April 1996. This time our circle included grandchildren and great grandchildren. Both events were grand celebrations.

A few months later I was on my father's deck during a warm summer day. Unsure of how to broach the subject of his funeral arrangements, I said, "You know, I told my children when I die, I wanted to be cremated and placed in Jeff's grave."

Daddy didn't say anything. Thinking that I had overstepped my boundaries, I got up to go inside. Before I got to the door, he reached out towards me.

"Can I be buried with Jeff too?"

"I don't think that would be a problem at all," I replied.

"You know, I always thought you to be very responsible. I saw you as my hero."

My father's comments caught me by surprise. He went on to discuss his bank account information and what he'd set aside for his funeral. Then he offered me his 1978 *Dodge Tradesman* van.

Nearly eleven months after my father's surgery, the words, "I'm not dead, but I'm dying," came in a whisper through the phone. The family rallied to care for Daddy, deciding to take shifts. Shortly after my sister and I arrived, he stopped breathing.

After calling 911, we tailed the ambulance, running red lights. Daddy was a "no-code." It appeared that our first shift would be the only one needed. Our father spent his last Saturday listening to his favorite jazz and blues music through a headset.

I stayed the night at the hospital, sleeping on a cot. At 5:00 am in the morning, I bolted up and said, "It's time."

I have no idea why I said what I did, but an hour later my father was dead at the age of 73. As was his request, Daddy was cremated and laid to rest in the grave of his son.

A Legacy Revealed

Like my father, I had apparently shielded my love from my children, as I worked long, hard hours to focus on survival as a single parent.

The revelation of my father's legacy didn't' hit home until I was driving my daughter to Xavier University in New Orleans.

"Mom, you don't love me and Austin."

I immediately pulled over. Like my father, I had apparently shielded my love from my children, as I worked long, hard hours to focus on survival as a single parent. Although the discipline I wielded was modified, I was not a warm and fuzzy mother. I too, was hard to get close to. I recognized that I had other traits and physical attributes that were similar to my father's.

Reflecting back to the time I spent with my dad opened my eyes. There were things I never told anyone. The most surprising was how my father felt about me. Despite a struggle to find a connection in our troubled relationship, I honestly didn't know that I was his hero until the very end.

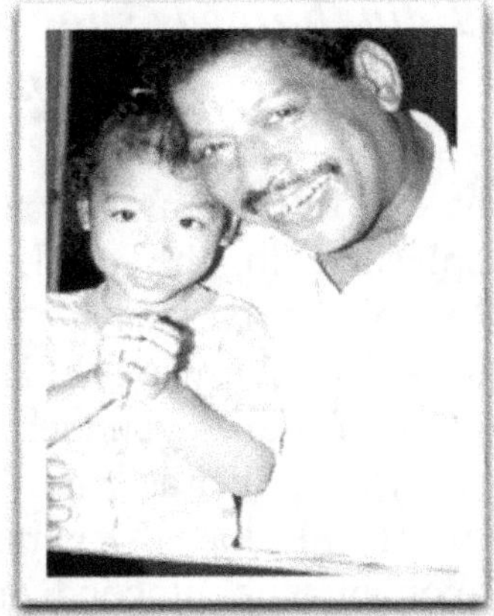

Author with Dad, Mr. William Loveless.

To Be Pale In Comparison

Apple Loveless

A Night to Remember
The strong smell of chlorine, the persistent mosquitoes, and the occasional old woman who pinched our cheeks became too overwhelming.

After retiring from the United States Army, my father, William M. Loveless, started a business in the Philippines and married my mother, Floredy, who is a Filipina. I was born in Manila and lived there until age 12. Although many years have passed, I vividly remember an event that occurred when I was nine that forever changed my sense of self-worth and my perception of who I am.

A couple of years ago my dad recalled the incident that brought me to tears when I was nine, and asked if I

remembered it. I did, but was shocked that I had said those words to him.

The balmy night was full of laughter as people milled around the grounds and splashed in the pool. It was the birthday celebration of Mr. Reynolds, who was my father's best friend, and my best friend, Hanni's dad. We were the only children in the sea of tipsy adults, except for Hanni's younger sister, whose existence we ignored because we viewed her as a spoiled child.

The strong smell of chlorine, the persistent mosquitoes, and the occasional old woman who pinched our cheeks became too overwhelming. Hanni and I desperately wanted to escape.

Fortunately our moment came when the house maid told us to go change out of our wet clothes. So we raced each other to the house, and as usual, I won, being the oldest and the fastest.

<u>Imitation Beauty</u>
The whiteness of the powder clearly contrasted against my skin as different shades of brown emerged.

Hanni and I grew up with the same excitement of many girls whose mothers were proud of their own looks – mothers that possessed an array of cosmetics that we longed to delve into; colorful concoctions that our mothers applied carefully – religiously.

We watched in awe as our mother's made themselves up. Sometimes they even made us up to resemble life-sized dolls, or we *borrowed* their make-up when they were preoccupied with gossiping with one another.

After getting dressed Hanni and I began imitating our mother's rituals until we saw a pretty guest named, *Miriam who was freshening up. Intrigued by her looks we attempted to copy her beauty routine. Fortunately, she put up with us, and even smiled as we both slathered on layers of lotion like she did. We put on her perfume, dabbing a little on our wrists and necks; then placed a small amount of baby powder into our hands before applying it evenly to our faces.

Miriam had a creamy white complexion and Hanni, a slight tan that lightly intermingled with her naturally pale features. On the other hand, my skin was as brown as dry dirt. When I looked in the mirror I was horrified by what I saw. The powder had created an obvious half-formed mask. The whiteness clearly contrasted against my skin as different shades of brown emerged. I turned to Miriam for help and she let out a quick laugh before she could stop herself. Hanni laughed too, which didn't help matters. The powder on her skin was barely visible.

Miriam was surprised and amused by the way I looked, but I was shocked and appalled by the ugly outcome. I scrutinized her lovely face for any traces of the powder. However, she blended in only a fine amount to her milky skin, and I couldn't help but notice that her face was beautiful, unlike mine.

Bitter, salty tears rolled down my face leaving pasty trails against my cheeks. I ran to the bathroom and tried to wash the powder off, but scrub as I might, it only got worse, turning the consistency of glue. In a rush to clean my face, I may have contributed to a more hideous outcome. And then again, maybe the results were hideous because I had rubbed a nice large handful of powder on my face in a desperate attempt to be as beautiful as Miriam.

My Disgrace

My dad quietly glanced at my face. After a few moments of silence he asked, "Do you want to go home?"

I was so upset by the turn of events that I lay sprawled on the bathroom floor sobbing uncontrollably as Hanni watched helplessly. "Go away, Hanni," I murmured through my heartache. Although she was only seven, she knew something was seriously wrong, and ran to retrieve her mother.

Though kind, Hanni's mom was very commanding. Within seconds she managed to drag me out of the bathroom in all my teary shame. When I explained what happened she disappeared to tell my father because my mother was too busy enjoying herself to be bothered by such nonsense.

My dad quietly glanced at my face. After a few moments of silence he asked, "Do you want to go home?" I managed a nod. So he gently lifted me into his arms and I buried my face into his chest determined not to let any of the guests see my disgrace.

I Think I Broke My Dad's Heart
I didn't know it then, but I think that I had broken my dad's heart.

Oh what strong feelings of pride I had back then! I thought that moment in my life to be my worst ever. I cried hard in my dad's arms as he wove his way through the merry crowd. I only paused to wipe my nose against his shirt or cringe quietly when strangers asked, "What's the matter?"

Finally when we were away from the crowd my dad asked, "Why did you put the powder on your face?"

"So I can be white like Miriam. I just wanted to be pretty," I replied in a muffled voice.

My dad carried me all the way home without saying a word, while I cried myself to exhaustion. I didn't know it then, but I think that I had broken my dad's heart.

Just As I Am
Dad said he had to leave the Philippines because he worried that I wouldn't know I was beautiful just the way I am.

When I was 12, my family moved to the United States so that I could further my education and become something other than a nurse, store clerk or housewife, which were some of the aspirations of many women in the Philippines.

A couple of years ago my dad recalled the incident that brought me to tears when I was nine, and asked if I remembered it. I did, but was shocked that I had said those words to him. He smiled at me, which seemed both pleasant and painful. Then he revealed that due to the events that occurred during the night of the party, he definitively decided to move our family to America after my elementary school years were over.

Dad said he had to leave the Philippines because he worried that I would struggle with low self-esteem and would never realize what I was capable of. It also concerned him that I wouldn't know I was beautiful just the way I am.

To this day I don't consider myself an amazing beauty. I know I'm not perfect. Although it would be nice, physical perfection is not one of my top priorities. With the racial diversity that spans the United States, I've learned to like both my body and face the way they are. I like my skin color.

My last boyfriend once told me that one of the things he liked most about my physical appearance was my smooth, brown skin. I smiled and thought, 'Thank you Dad.'

Miriam is not the actual name of the character in the story, but the person was real.

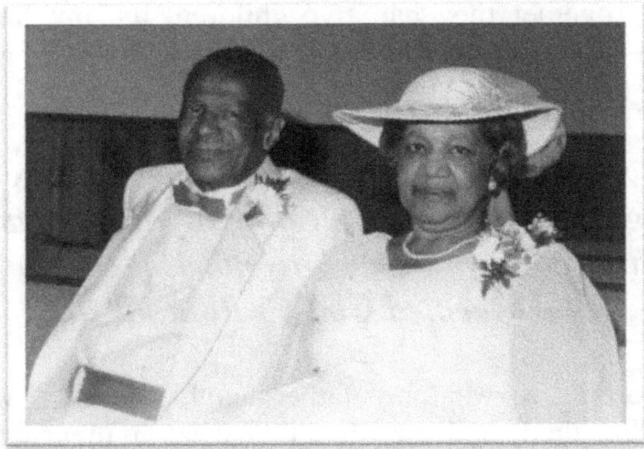

"Daddy" St. Cyr and Grandmother.

Dad, Daddy and Me

Derrell Roberts

Not the Daddy Type
According to what my father had taught me, men worked and provided for their families.

Okay… the title is confusing but hang in there. Herman Roberts Jr. is my dad. My daddy was Mr. Edmond St. Cyr Jr., who also happened to be my grandfather. Confused? Don't be, I never was. During my childhood these two men were very different in who they were and how they viewed fatherhood. Yet when I became an adult, they were very much alike in their philosophies and how they impacted my life.

A native of New Orleans, Herman Roberts Jr. was the only child of Louise Roberts, a devout Christian woman who fiercely loved her son. Grandmother didn't think any woman was good enough for him, and that included my mother Elizabeth, who he married. Together they had five children, but my father wasn't really the daddy/husband type. This isn't a knock on my dad, but you have to follow the story to understand.

My dad, who was an immature womanizer, even though he had five children with my mom and had three children from a previous marriage, changed when he accepted God's will in his life.

According to what my father taught me, men worked and provided for their families. Modeling what he preached, he was a taxi driver, bus driver and a longshoreman who never seemed to miss work, but in his dedication he wasn't able to attend my school recitals, band concerts, football games or basketball games.

Wait. Back up a minute. My dad did go to one of my basketball games. Had my best game for the Willie Hall Panthers too, but Dad was sitting in the wrong gym because he didn't know the color of my uniform. By the time I saw him and invited him to the next game in the right gym I was too tired and spent. So I played like crap. Imagine, minutes before I had played my most inspired game thinking he was watching, because I wanted him to see that his son could play. I think I still try to do well and impress my Dad, even to this day.

<u>Enter Daddy, Mr. St. Cyr If You Will</u>
More and more Daddy started to be the voice I listened to in my teen years.

In regard to being an involved father, my dad really didn't have a good role model to guide him, considering the era he grew up in and all. So I learned to forgive him. Even when he and my mom broke up when I was 12, I still forgave him. That's when Mr. St. Cyr, my grandfather and the man I called "Daddy," stepped in.

He and my grandmother visited New Orleans often enough that I always knew their home in Los Angeles was a refuge if I needed it.

My mother, who passed away in March 2008, was the greatest mom God ever created. Although she tried to be both a mother and father to me, she could only be my mom. Like most teenage boys I wanted to explore life, express myself and be independent.

Growing up in the St. Bernard projects in New Orleans wasn't always the safest place to explore but I never went to jail, or got someone's daughter *knocked up*. However, that in no means absolves me of any wrongdoing. I was just fortunate those things didn't happen. *Thank you God!*

More and more Daddy started to be a voice I listened to in my teen years. When my oldest brother Earl, who some figured would end up incarcerated, thrived while living in our grandfather's home, I left for Los Angeles in June 1976 with my mom's blessing.

Big Man, Big Heart
I wanted to be like him in every way. I still strive to be that type of man.

Daddy was physically big. In fact everything about him was big – his persona, his heart, and his love. He had the respect of everyone. As the plant manager of an elementary school, he was also the president of the school's Parent Teacher Association which seemed a bit odd since he had no kids at the school. But he was Mr. St. Cyr and that seemed to matter most.

With our regular heart-to-heart sessions, Daddy helped me make some of my best and toughest life choices regarding college, politics, and love. We talked sports, community activism and even whether O.J. Simpson did it. Daddy went to his grave thinking that the Juice was innocent. I, on the other hand, had a different take on that one.

Daddy encouraged me to vote because of those who died and sacrificed their lives for me to have that right. So it was a duty I took seriously, which grew into a love for politics. He seemed most proud when I was mentored by the late Assemblymen Julian Dixon, who later became a Congressman. Truthfully, even then, my main mentor was Mr. St. Cyr.

The Emergence of a Transformed Dad
Herman Roberts is the living example of how God can work in a man's life.

Unfortunately, Daddy died too soon from emphysema but he lived to see me graduate from college. I wanted to be like him in every way; and even now, I still strive to be the type of man he was. As life moved on I was able to reestablish my relationship with my dad, Herman.

After graduating from college while on my way to Washington DC, I had the chance to sit with my Dad over a drink at a Jazz club in New Orleans. Funny how an oyster shooter, a Schlitz beer, and age can get you to ask the tough questions, like "Why did you leave my mom?"

My dad's response was not one of blame but was reflective of his life. "Your mom and I were at different points in life," which was the part of the explanation I held onto. Herman Roberts is the living example of how God can work in a man's life. My dad who was an immature womanizer, even though he had five children with my mom and had three children from a previous marriage, changed when he accepted God's will in his life.

The Third Time is the Charm
Each of us secretly thinks that we are my dad's favorite child.

My dad's third marriage is to a wonderful woman who gave him three more children. With the inclusion of my brother Earl and Connie's daughter, Stephanie and as the primary daddy of her four kids, my dad has 13 children in all.

So the guy who was an only child has certainly learned how to be a great role model as a father and grandfather. He's been described as "A deacon at church, a pretty good husband, a good friend and a heck of a dad." Just ask the 13 kids he raised. Each of us secretly thinks we are my dad's favorite child.

My dad is the reason I established a relationship with my daughter some 19 years ago. Even after her mom and I ended our relationship, Kjar (key-air) and I stayed together. Today I am her dad in every conceivable way. While she was growing up I tried to attend all of her school events and walked her down the aisle when she got married.

The Ultimate Example of What a Man Should Be
A man takes care of his family first and helps others after that.

If I live to be the type of man my grandfather was, and type of man my father grew to be, I would be extremely contented. Two very different men gave me the ultimate example of what and who a man is, and should be: *Responsible to those in your life. Respectful to all you come in contact with. A man takes care of his family first, and helps others after that. He does not run away from his weaknesses, rather confronts and overcomes them. And a man is willing to give without expecting a reward in return.*

The truth is that by striving to live up to each man's expectations, which I will continue to do with full intention, I know I will be a combination of the best attributes of what it means to be a an ultimate man and good father.

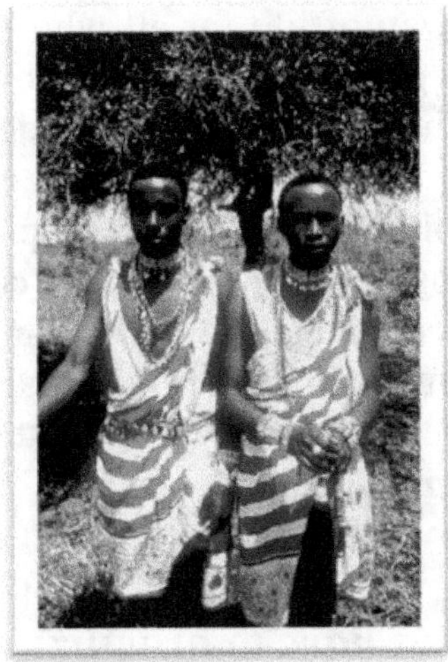

Maasai groom and best man.

Maasai Fathers

One Man's Mission to Merge Two Traditions

Stephen Ole Kesire

In Reverence to the Father

They are taught to revere the elders (ancestors, grandfathers and fathers) who are honored as leaders for their wisdom and knowledge.

I am a Maasai, a descendent of the nomadic tribe of Kenya, East Africa, the most remote group of people in the region. I come from the Oloshoibor in the Ngong, Kajiado district and was brought up in the strongest traditions of my ancestors. My parents, Meiponyi Kesire and Sarah Meiponyi ensured that we observed every detail of the rituals that they received from their fathers, which dictated the way of life for all who practiced them. Passed from generation to generation, the way of the Maasai must be strictly adhered to in accordance to the elders, who are the *father figures* of the tribe. They command the greatest respect in the community. Any violation calls for severe punishment.

It is the responsibility of the whole community, every man and woman, to correct and shape the children. As the leaders, the elders keep a watchful eye on the youth, and are keenly invested in the upbringing of the boys, who are expected to transition through four essential stages before reaching manhood: Boyhood, Moranism, Youth, and Eldership.

As a group, boys have to organize themselves and kill a lion using spears and swords. By holding the tail of their prey they show that they are ripe and ready for circumcision, and hence, prepared to become Morans, a stage all desire to reach.

Leading Boys Into Manhood
Boys are not allowed to sit down when men are standing.

In my village we live in a manyatta, which is a traditional home (dung-hut), which several families share. All the boys stay together and mostly sleep in one hut. Olayioni or boyhood is a stage where one is under the supervision of the elders to keep the traditions of tending to cattle, sheep, goats and taking care of their flocks. Caring for one's flock is essential to the Maasai. Boys are taken out in the bush where they are trained to survive in the wilderness against hyenas, wolves and other predatory animals.

Boys do not go to war because they are considered children until they are 22. However, they are taught to revere the elders (ancestors, grandfathers and fathers) because they are elevated to a position of authority for their wisdom and knowledge. Those coming into manhood must greet the elders by bowing and touching the elder's head as a sign of respect and submission. Boys are not allowed to sit down when men are standing.

As a group, boys have to organize themselves and kill a lion using spears and swords. By holding the tail of their prey, they show that they are ripe and ready for circumcision, and hence, prepared to become Morans, a stage all desire to reach. After killing a number of lions, the elders come together to consider taking the group to the next level and determining who should go and who should not.

In becoming Morans -- warriors of the community, young men must be circumcised all at the same time. Each has to have a number of birds on his head as decoration after the procedure. The significance of this ritual is to increase a youth's skill of throwing sticks and spears in times of war. After a year for recovery, they are primed to ascend to the next stage toward manhood.

Strong, courageous and experienced, the Morans (Ilmurran) are ready to stand on behalf of the community. With the duty of defending their people from warring communities and wild animals, they have the utmost respect for the elders. A word from an elder can cause a thousand Morans to bow down in respect. They believe that elders hold the blessing for their future.

Occasionally in ceremonies the elders bless the Morans. When one Moran goes astray and does something that is not acceptable in the community, he has to make some wine and call the elders to come and bless him in repentance and speak a word.

Morans continue in their role until a new, energetic age group rises to take over and the older Morans can retire to achieve the role of eldership. The newly anointed Morans then perform a big ceremony in a manyatta, bringing the whole community together. They are then allowed to marry and have children. After the blessing of the elders, one is then allowed to graduate to a leadership role as an elder, the most honored position. He can now make decisions with the others on matters regarding the future of the community and is the last word for the people. As a model for generations that will follow him, he must be disciplined in his every word which carries the weight of life or death. An elder must run his own family well, organize ceremonies and graduations, and is the guardian of the whole community.

Parting with Tradition to Embrace Fatherhood
Maasai fathers didn't really care for their children. There was no love.

Although women and children have tremendous value, they are not highly regarded by Maasai men. This is where I part ways with tradition. I am a different father to my children, Deborah Nashipae 7, Keziah Nosim 4, and Benjamin Lempiris 2, (a fourth child is expected soon), and husband to my wife, Leah. I love them.

As I was growing up, I recall that there were many restrictions for the wife, and the practice of ritualistic circumcision for young women was common. Although some traditionalists still want to maintain it, the practice is slowly being abandoned, and now girls are attending school.

In the Maasai culture, men were kings and women were to tremble before them and just be there for the men. Failure to do so brought harsh punishment. The community believed the only way to rule a wife was to forcibly beat her. Wives were to be beaten twice or thrice a week to make sure she stayed humble to her husband. She was not allowed to laugh and rejoice with him. The man had to put on a stone face to scare the wife. Sadly, they weren't allowed to eat together or walk together. A woman had to walk at least a hundred meters away from her husband.

Maasai fathers didn't really care for their children. There was no love. When a man came home the children became aware and knew how to behave themselves. No noise. No entering a house where the father was present. That's part of the reason why the men married many wives, or at least two, so that when the man is in one house, the children can occupy the other.

Since I've seen and gone through so much rejection, not having anybody to care for me, it has been my greatest concern to be very close to my children. I went to school in the '80s and early '90s because my father was forced to send me by the chief. He never knew nor cared about what goes around in school. Even though he paid for my secondary school, I remember being sent home when it wasn't enough. I had to stay home a whole month until I collected fees in the amount of about $5.00 US dollars. This repeated interruption affected my education. Now I vow to take my children to the best school.

Deborah Nashipae, our first born attends a private school for which I pay a lot of money, but I want her to get the education I did not receive. Next year I have to move to a bigger town in order for the rest of my children to go to a better school. I take time with them to love and care for them and if I am not around then their mother is there with them.

Due to the love I have for my wife, I have broken all the harsh Maasai traditions. We walk holding our hands together, eat together and share family matters together. She is the assistant pastor in the church I lead. When I am not there she takes the whole responsibility of running not only the local church, but of the other churches that are under my care.

Many times we have gone into the hotel and ate together. In the beginning, the Maasai ran out of the hotel amazed that a man like me can go so low as to eat with his wife. With our actions; however, we have managed to influence the community and change a lot of things. Now all of our church members do the same.

The Transformation of the Maasai
It might be difficult to keep the traditions that the Maasai are known to have followed for years, but I have a vision.....

I started a church with women. It is a place where men and women clap their hands together unto the Lord. This to the men was unacceptable. Yes, I taught the wives to respect and honor their husbands despite what they go through. Some of the women watched helplessly as their bibles were burned. One of my leaders had her bible burned too. Only one page survived and it was from the book of Job.

The Maasai bible has a drawing of Job and the suffering he went through. Today all the women that we started with at our ministry have husbands in church now. They have seen God through their wives. This has changed the community towards us and the CHRIST we serve.

Having gone through all the traditions of the Maasai, I realize it was a good, simple life except for the way women and children were treated and a few other traditions that were disagreeable. What I embrace is the leadership, personal responsibility and acceptance of all communities despite weaknesses. Even though my time for Moranism was cut short because I was attending school, I want to see much of what I learned preserved such as the way of dressing and the respect for the elders. It might be difficult to keep the traditions that the Maasai are known to have followed for years, but I have a vision to start a Maasai cultural center where our children can see and learn about their rich cultural heritage and prosper from each community.

Today I am a Christian leader who trains pastors and raises my children with my wife, to walk in the way of God. I believe in teaching and giving them my time because I want to raise leaders full of vision, love and sensitivity toward others; and share powerful traditions of my upcoming as well as those principles I've adopted that will extend a new respect and love to our wives and children.

He Taught Me

Frank Withrow

My father is the key to my success
He told me, "You are my child
And you will do you best!"

He can give you the look and you'll understand
You better do right or you'll feel his hand

My father is my hero, role model and king
And to please my father, I'll do anything

He taught me how to share and how to love
He taught me to believe there is a God above

He taught me to treat folks fair and equal
And lend a hand to elderly people

He taught me how to enjoy my day
And to think problems through when they come my way

He taught me education would help me achieve
But common sense is what I really need

Father, you are the best of the best
And you are truly the key to my success

Daddies' Girls

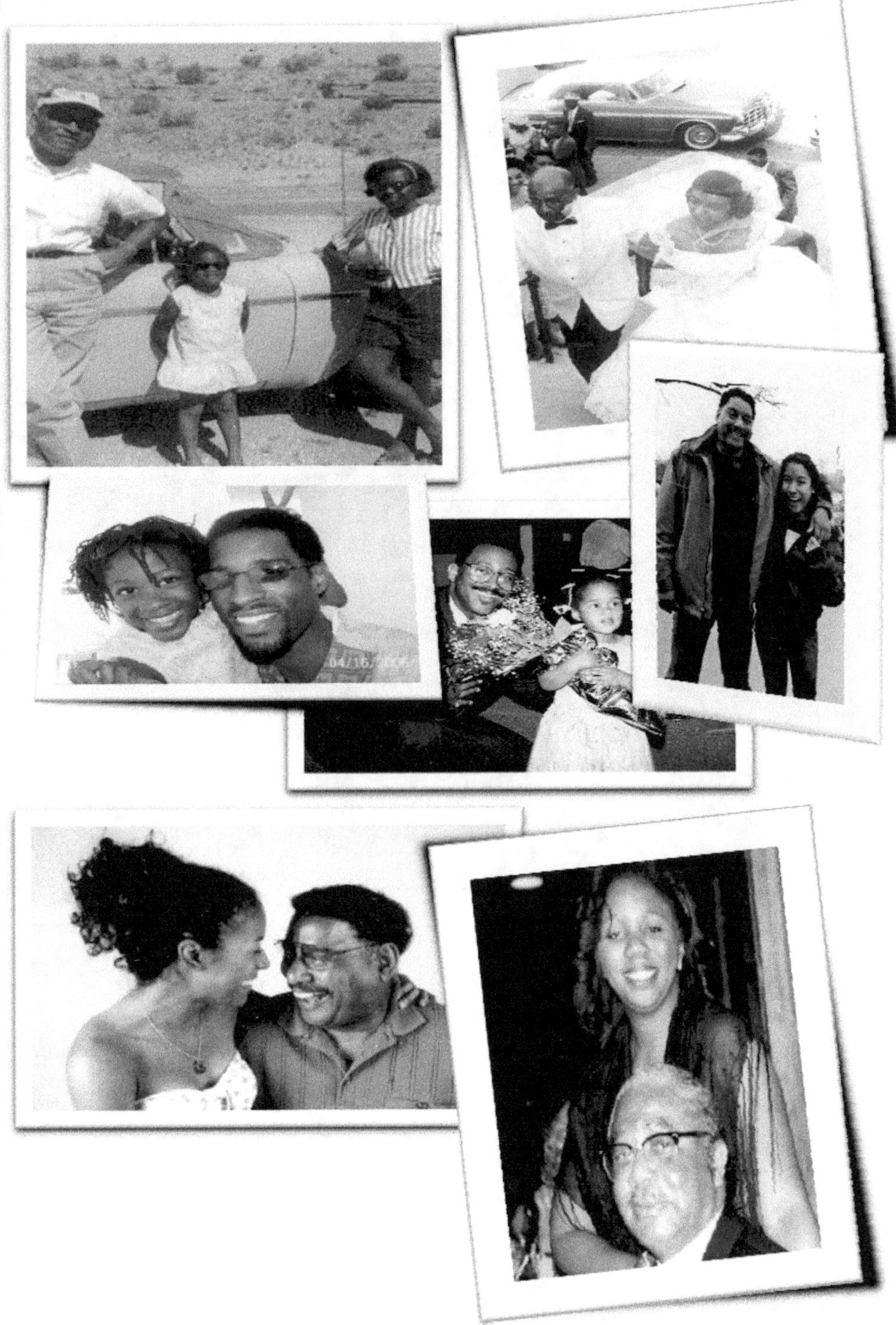

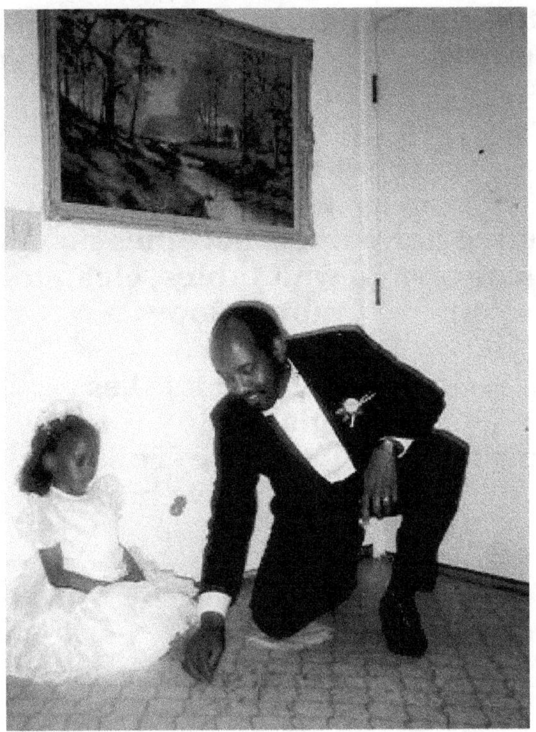

Frederick Holmes playing jacks.

The Beauty of Black Fatherhood

Jeri Marshall & Joslyn Gaines Vanderpool

Being a father to a black girl is
the best role in the world,

Our daughters, black angels, darling girls
bring us to manhood and help us mature,

**A black daughter
helps her father discover his potential too,
and forces him to do things he vowed
he'd never do –**

**but to look into her
eyes, as she watches you
define her path, it becomes no matter of
concern to wait tables, clean toilets,
mop a floor ...**

**whatever it takes
we'll gladly do for her,
even raise our level of consciousness,
and aspire to give her more.**

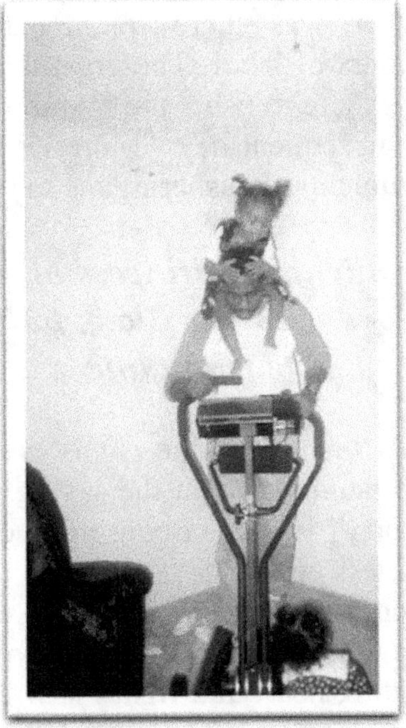

Author helping her Black father, Mr. Eduardo Barrow, exercise.

The Guardian That Walks with God

In gratitude to my Black Father

Genesis E. Barrow

Once upon a time in a land called Panama, a little boy was born. His skin was deep brown -- his future was bright. Given the name, Eduardo Emmanuel which means a guardian that walks with God, this boy would grow up to be strong and become my father.

My Black father was there for my mother during her pregnancy and 36 hours of labor. The great thing is that he, along with my mother, was there to usher me into this world and my first day of school, and subsequent days. More importantly, my Black father has been instrumental in ushering me to Christ.

And I'll have a Nubian princess of my own one day who will be in love with her Black father like I am in love with mine.

My Black father taught me the *rights and wrongs* of loving and being loved. He taught me that the saying, "love means never having to say I'm sorry" is a lie. Being in love means saying you are sorry when you mess up.

My Black father is still teaching me that when a man loves a woman, a woman he will sometimes hurt, he will move heaven and earth to heal her hurting heart and right his wrong if the man who loves the woman is really a man.

I love my Black father, who will be surprised because sooner than he thinks I'll finish middle school, high school, then college, and start my career; and marry a man with deep brown skin who will love me just like Christ loves the Church. And I'll have a Nubian princess of my own one day who will be in love with her Black father like I am in love with mine.

I thank my heavenly Father for blessing me with my Black father and my two Black grandfathers. I thank you Father for *Abuelo whom I can see whenever I want. And I thank you for my Granddaddy who watches me constantly through the crystal waters.

*Abuelo – Spanish for grandfather

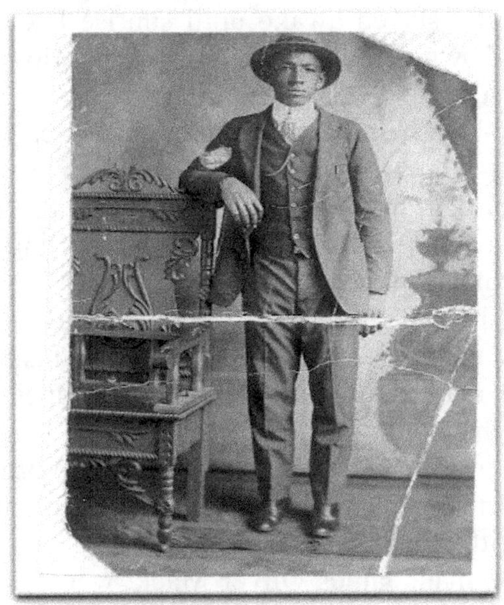

Author's father Mr. James Daddy-boy Mack.

Daddy-boy

Ethel Mack-Ballard

I called him Daddy-boy, my little Daddy-boy, not because he was small, he was average height, five foot eight or nine, but compact, and well-muscled, with skin the color of rosewood. His arms felt smooth and hard like the wood.

Daddy worked hard as a master molder in an iron factory on the west side of Cleveland. Before leaving home at dawn he always came into our rooms, first to kiss my brother, and then me good-bye. I'd wake just enough to recognize his scent. He smelled of cigars and shaving lotion.

When Daddy put his arms around me for a hug, he was cautious and gentle because he was so strong. Every morning he would tell me if I stayed awake until sunrise I would see fairies dancing in the dew among the ribbon grass and flowers, and then I could "touch magic."

My Daddy-boy believed in touching magic. Magic for him was something tangible like the peach trees in our backyard, his vegetable garden, my mother's flowers, and the Kentucky blue grass he mowed each Saturday morning. Everything that grew was a little miracle of touchable magic.

My father helped teach me to read the way he taught me to pay attention to nature. I would sit on his lap in his big overstuffed chair while he read aloud the evening newspaper -- front page, editorials and the comic section, pressing my hands against the pages, guiding my fingers over the sentences. Words were magic. Words told stories, expanded the imagination, recovered the past and gifted us with knowledge.

This gentle man, James Oliver Mack, who seldom raised his voice, and never raised a hand to his family, was a combat veteran. My father's *Negro* unit fought with honor in France during World War I. Upon returning to America, they received little recognition from their native country.

In 1919, my father and mother married. Eleven years later my brother was born, and I came four years after him in the midst of the Great Depression. Despite the hardships and deprivation of the '30s, my parents, through perseverance and hard work, managed to purchase their first home.

The thought of our house brings back my first fully conscious memory of my father holding me on a wooden rocking horse in my parent's empty bedroom. As we viewed the swaying leaves of a huge Lady Cigar tree through the window, I hear my father's laughter; feel his hands keeping me safe and secure. My childish giggles mingle with his voice as I cry, "Home! Home!"

Memories of my father are a constant companion. I think of him in scenes. Me insisting that my Daddy-boy blow behind the bedroom door and into my closet to make sure the Boogey Man can't come into my room, then singing a Scottish ballad with his clear tenor voice, *"You take the high road and I'll take the low road, and I'll be in Scotland afore ye,"* lulling me into sleep and safety. Memories of me sitting on the basement stairs watching Daddy shovel coal into the huge black furnace spewing tiny explosions of sparks; or Daddy changing the burnt out tubes in our big console radio so I could listen to *Let's Pretend Fairytale Theatre*.

With my hand tucked into the pocket of Daddy's overcoat, we walked to the Imperial Theatre to see *The Wizard of Oz* -- a memory that stays with me, because Daddy loved Technicolor Hollywood movie musicals. This was magic you could see and hear…magic you touched with your imagination.

Remembrances of me collecting the rings of smoke from Daddy's cigars to adorn my fingers and using the empty boxes to store my paper dolls are ever present; as well as me following my Daddy-boy into the back yard for what he called "a little adventure." Our small adventure was him showing me a bird's nest in our neighbor's Maple tree or bees gathering honey from hollyhocks growing along the side of the house. It's all the little things -- the accumulation of small moments.

Growing up meant growing away -- too old now to sit on his lap or call him my little Daddy-boy. Too old and self-absorbed to go on "little adventures" but also there was the comfort of knowing, without acknowledging that he would always be my *safe haven*.

In this uncertain world, in these uncertain times, my childhood memories of my father's relationship with me are my strength when trouble, worry, or fear prevails. I will always feel protected as long as I can call on those memories. Now in the closing years of my life, I like to think that when my time is nigh, it is my little Daddy-boy who will come to guide me safely home.

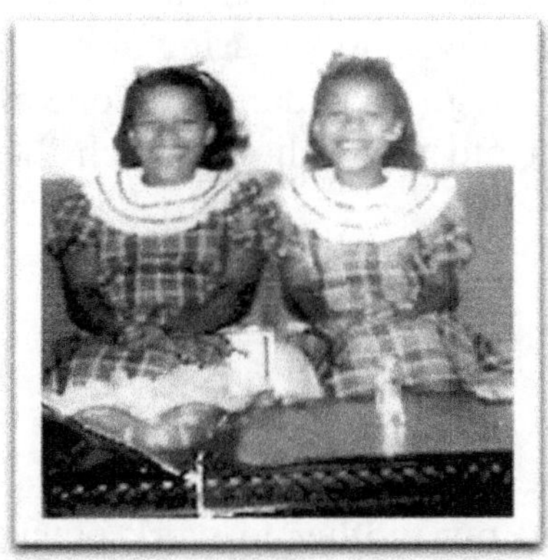

"Daddy's Little Princesses," author and sister Gwen.

Larger than Life

Patricia E. Canterbury

Dapper Daddy
My father was a fine dresser; one of the few who wore a topcoat (a holdover from his days in New York City) to Mass.

My father, Robert Johnson, was born in Schenectady, New York at the beginning of the 20th Century. He displayed the manners of a man of the 19th Century. I never heard him swear, although I'm sure he did, but *never* in front of women and girls. When he got angry he'd take a walk down the road (an actual *dirt* road) to cool off, then come back home and be Daddy.

My father was a fine dresser; one of the few who wore topcoats (a holdover from his days in New York City) to Mass. Daddy also wore fedoras and believed in tipping them to all the women as he passed them on the street, in the grocery store, in church, or in his pool room. Yep, in the late '50s and early '60s Daddy owned a pool room where boys and men stood when girls and women entered, where there was no swearing or smoking.

Smokers had to go outside! Everyone did, stating that "Mr. Johnson's a strict old man who'd snatch the *black off you* if you broke his rules."

An Olds Man
Every other year my father and mother purchased a new Olds until the late '70s.

Daddy allowed my mother to work outside the house but only two days a week. She was a bookkeeper who somehow made it home in time to have dinner ready every day. By trade, Daddy was an airplane mechanic, an occupation he learned as a member of the United States Army Air Corps; however, his true love was automobiles, especially the Oldsmobile '98.

Every other year my father and mother purchased a new Olds until the late '70s. Daddy taught my sister and me to drive when we were 14. He said, "If you're ever in a situation where you need to get out of a place and come home, I want you to know how to drive." Of course, learning to drive those steel boats was a huge thrill.

Beware of Little Princesses Carrying Big Guns
Even though both of Daddy's little head strong, steel-willed princesses hated hunting, we were given 30.06's which were way too large.

Daddy wanted to ensure his daughters could defend and protect ourselves. So besides knowing how to drive, we were also taught to shoot.

Even though both of Daddy's little head strong, steel-willed princesses hated hunting, we were given 30.06's which were *way* too large. However, a 30.06 is a big deterrent, even if it has spent most of its natural life stored in the hall closet. Although it was the only gun in the house, there were special occasions that it was put to very good use.

As was customary in our household, every one was required to meet Daddy and Mother. If rowdy boys came over to the house, Daddy would take out the old 30.06 and give it a nice cleaning *in front of the boys*. To say that all of my high school friends were terrified of my gentle, sweet Daddy is an understatement.

Even though Daddy told us to do exactly what our southern cousins did whenever we left the house we were visiting, he was terrified that his little princesses would say something to invoke the wrath of some of the older southern Whites...

<u>The Nuns Didn't Have Anything on Daddy</u>
I was taught by nuns who were less strict than Daddy.

Daddy and mother used the dinner table to discuss current events in which my sister and I were expected to be up on all the latest news. We were encouraged to discuss why we felt a certain way and be able to defend our point of view.

Growing up on a 20 acre farm 15 miles south of downtown Sacramento, Daddy felt that we might be spoiled farm kids. As 4H members we raised lambs, but Daddy insisted that we needed to learn to live with city folks; it was a good thing because we moved to midtown when I was in the sixth grade. No more hour long drives from the farm to the Catholic school where I was taught by nuns who wore habits and were much less strict than Daddy.

<u>"Colored" Water Fountains Don't Contain Purple Water</u>
My sister and I learned that the "Colored" water fountains we saw down South did not contain purple water as I once believed. They were for US!

Daddy would say that we needed to learn to deal with all types of folks, and to that end, we traveled every summer to visit cousins in Tennessee, Missouri, Mississippi, Louisiana, New York and Montana.

Even though Daddy told us to do exactly what our southern cousins did whenever we left the house we were visiting, he was terrified that his little princesses would say something to invoke the wrath of some of the older southern Whites whom he said, were "still trying to get the enslaved folks back."

My sister and I learned that the *Colored* water fountains we saw down South did not contain purple water as I once believed. They were for *US!* We were shocked! Daddy explained to *keep US in our place we had to drink from the Colored fountain.* I was too young to understand why, because the water tasted the same as back home. It was a particularly long summer with lots of discussions.

For the Love of Fireflies, Thunder, and Country Life
Daddy taught us to ask questions about everything; to love family, even the crazy ones, because they told the best stories; and to love fireflies, thunder, and country life.

My sister and I learned to hide in basements during thunderstorms while visiting the Midwest, but immediately forgot when we returned home and threw open the windows and ran out into the rain, "because lightening only *got ya* in Kansas."

Daddy taught us to ask questions about everything; to love family, even the crazy ones, because they told the best stories; and to love fireflies, thunder, and country life.

Since Daddy hailed from New York State, he delighted in telling us stories of race tracks, (he loved horses and was disappointed that we couldn't afford to raise them on our farm). Daddy also enjoyed the night clubs and theater-life; thus he and mother drove to Oakland or San Franscisco every other month. It's no wonder Daddy always wanted to write plays. He kept a note pad by the side of his bed to jot down thoughts of plots or song titles. However, he never completed any, nor shared them with anyone other than mother.

Daddy was larger than life, and believed that his children could be anything they wanted to be. He only lived to be 76 years old. In 1984 he died, and I miss him every day.

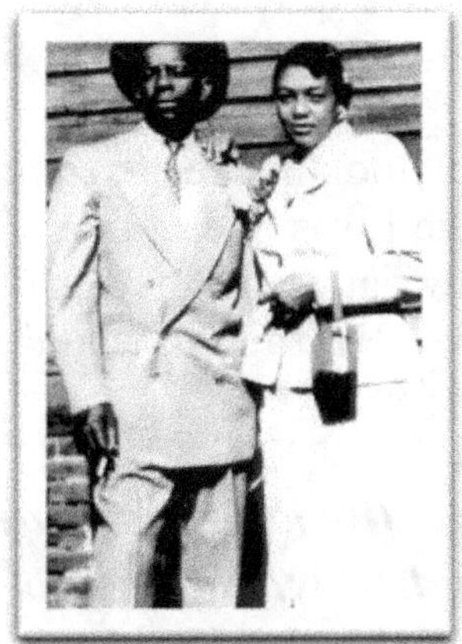

Author's parents. On the left, "The smartest man in the world," Mr. Daniel Paul Dorn.

Kindergarten

Staajabu

<u>I Didn't Know that I was a Girl</u>
I found out that I was a girl when my mom told me I had to start wearing dresses because I was going to start kindergarten soon.

I was born in 1943 in a row house around 10th and South Street in Philadelphia, Pennsylvania. Delivered by a mid-wife, I was registered five days later at Thomas Jefferson Hospital. I'm not sure why, but for some reason I didn't really understand that I was a girl until it was time for me to go to kindergarten.

When I was little I went everywhere with my dad or my brother, Hubert. I loved them both. I wore a tee shirt, bib overalls and a baseball cap most days. Before I was five years old, Daddy taught me how to push a wheelbarrow, use a knife, ride a horse, pick okra and feed the chickens. I also helped my daddy build houses.

Sometimes Daddy took me deep-sea fishing where the men on the boat treated me like I was one of them. Daddy put a small plug of tobacco in my jaw, gave me a can of beer, and turned my baseball cap sideways. He said it would keep me from getting seasick. And it did.

> ### *Well, my dad was the smartest man in the world and I always thought I was going to grow up to be just like him.*

When my daddy carried moonshine to his customers, I rode next to him on the front seat of his truck. Since we were inseparable, I even recall Daddy setting me up on the bar to conduct business with the bartender at night clubs and bars. My legs would be swinging down from my perch.

I never saw my father drunk or out-of-control at any time. Like a boulder, Daddy was tall, strong, muscular and Black. He was always so neat in his dress, even when in coveralls. And he always smelled clean. They called him "D.P." for Daniel Paul Dorn, and I was "Little D."

Victoria is a Very Long Name
Unlike Lil' D., Victoria is a very long name, but I wanted to write it so that my dad would be proud of me.

I found out that I was a girl when my mom told me I had to start wearing dresses because I was going to start kindergarten soon. She also said I wouldn't be going with my dad anymore because school was very important and he wanted me to be smart. Well, my dad was the smartest man in the world and I always thought I was going to grow up to be just like him.

"Your name is Victoria and you have to learn to spell and write it before you start kindergarten," my mom told me.

Unlike Lil' D., Victoria is a very long name, but I wanted to write it so that my dad would be proud of me. So Hubert taught me to read and write.

__I'm not Talking...__
We lived in New Jersey and the rest of the kids didn't talk anything like me.

I refused to talk at all in kindergarten; therefore, the school had meetings about me. My mom and dad had to discuss with my teacher why I wouldn't talk.

"When I talk, the kids laugh and make fun of me," I told Daddy when were alone together.

We lived in New Jersey and the rest of the kids didn't talk anything like me. I talked just like my mom and dad who were both from down South, and had thick, southern accents.

My dad was a quiet, thoughtful man of few words. After I told him about the first time I spoke in class, and the other children laughing at my accent, he told me it was all right if I didn't want to talk. "But if I was you," he said, "I would pay real close attention to how they talked and if you want to be real smart, learn to talk like them and show them a thing or two."

And I did.

By second grade, Daddy would only pick me up on some weekends. He and Mom were not getting along very well and they explained to me that they were going to break up. When Daddy arrived I would have been up for at least two hours sitting on the steps of our row home with my beat up baseball cap on. He never disappointed me either.

After things really got bad between my parents, I was old enough to catch a bus and meet Daddy at the diner in the town of Glassboro where he lived. We would eat and talk. Sometimes he would give me money for whatever I needed. He knew I would give it to Mom. And I did.

<u>Oh the Wonderful Things He Said</u>
"You're going to grow up to be a very beautiful, very smart young woman," Daddy would say.

Daddy would always tell me how beautiful I was when other kids, even my older sister called me names like *"you fat pig"* or *"you black dog."*

"You're going to grow up to be a very beautiful, very smart young woman," Daddy would say. And I did.

My dad was highly respected. Some folks were even afraid of him. They said things like, "He worked for the Mafia," and "He would kill you quick as look at you." I never found out where all those rumors came from. All I know is my daddy never lied to me about anything. He never hit or hollered at me, and he taught me more about life than anyone else. He was the smartest man I've ever known and he never had a chance to go to school – not even Kindergarten.

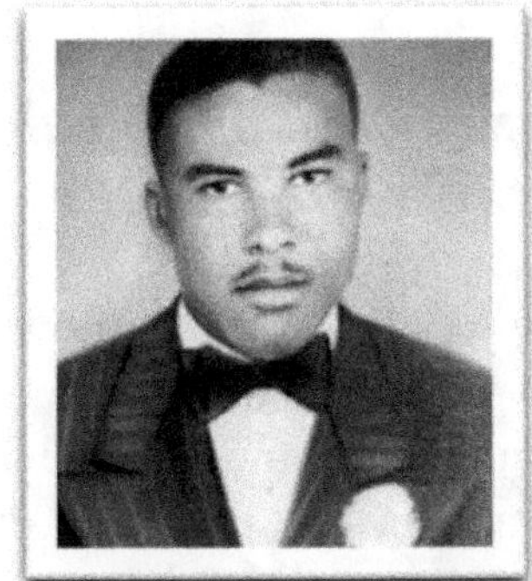 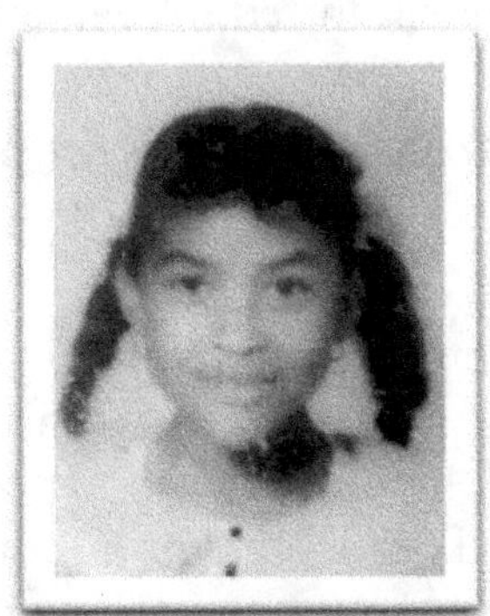

Author and "Daddy's Girl" next to her father, Rev. Jimmie Thrower.

A True Man After God's Heart

Cloteal Thrower Herron

Daddy's Girl
***Daddy would boast with pride when people commented,
"What a beautiful name for such a beautiful baby."***

I am so blessed to have had a father like Jimmie Thrower. I believe it is every girl's desire to be *Daddy's little girl*. And without a doubt that's exactly what I was.

I loved my daddy so much. When I was born Daddy proudly proclaimed that his firstborn was "the most beautiful baby girl the Thrower family had ever, ever, ever--EVER seen." He named me *Cloteal* after his girlfriend in Bible College. Daddy would boast with pride when people commented, "What a beautiful name for such a beautiful baby."

"I named her after my girlfriend in college," he would reply proudly.

Momma always gave him *the look*, but with grace and confidence retorted, "Yeah, but I got the man."

Daddy refused to let Momma work outside the house as a "maid for them White folks."

I often wondered *why on earth* would Momma allow Daddy to name me after another woman? Over the years I've come to realize that she loved him more than *any name*, and that he loved and respected her all the more, for permitting him to do so—*and* she let him *brag about it* too. This was true, unconditional love.

<u>Anointed Name of Honor</u>
It was my grandparents desire to name their new baby boy after this great country preacher man …..

Daddy and I were both born in the country: Strong, Arkansas. He was the youngest boy of 11 children -- eight boys and three girls. Although the family said that Daddy was born "sometime in October," his birth date is listed as November 26, 1925, which was the day he was formally named. Until then he was known as *Man*, which was written on his birth certificate.

It was my grandparents desire to name their new baby boy after this great country preacher man named Reverend Jimmie Hornbeck. So upon the reverend's return to Strong, my father was anointed, "Jimmie."

<u>An Unnecessary Ending to An Exceptional Life</u>
The small Black community protested when the hospital would not treat the preacher, but their pleas were in vain….

Daddy grew up in a very poor family on a farm. However, they were "rich in spirit," and were very proud, decent, and humble folks. The community of Strong respected the Thrower Family. My father came from a long line of men of faith, who were called to teach God's *Word*. His daddy, Grandpa Minor, in addition to

Granddaddy Wallace, Great Granddaddy Richmond and Great Great Granddaddy Aaron were preachers.

Nearly seventy years ago while out *preaching the Word of God* on horseback, my Grandfather Minor became ill, and was refused medical attention at a *Whites Only* hospital. The small Black community protested when the hospital would not treat the preacher, but their pleas were in vain. After all, Jim Crow tradition was Jim Crow tradition, even when a life hung in the balance.

My daddy was 16 years old when his father died that night in 1941. My grandmother, Mary Charlotte Thrower became a young widow who would never remarry. She honored Grandpa's memory until the end. Grandmother passed away in 1987 at the age of 98. Daddy was devastated; now both his parents were gone.

<u>A Father of Firsts</u>
Because he had a college degree, and his White co-workers didn't, Daddy was later promoted to shipping and receiving supervisor.

Daddy excelled in school becoming the first in his family to graduate from Bible College in Little Rock, Arkansas. Later he would continue his education graduating with a B.A. in Black studies and a M.A. in counseling from California State University, Hayward, which has since been renamed California State University, East Bay.

After I was born in 1951, Momma and Daddy moved to Milwaukee. Shortly after arriving they got a call from my daddy's brother, John Henry, who was beginning a church ministry in Oakland, California. So Daddy and Momma packed up and headed to California to *labor in ministry* with my Uncle John Henry and my Auntie Grace.

Glorious Kingdom Primitive Baptist Church first service was held on December 29, 1951, which symbolically, forty years later in 1991, would be Daddy's *"Going Home Celebration."*

After Momma and Daddy settled outside of the Bay Area in the small community of Vallejo, Daddy was hired as the first Black janitor at the Shell Oil Refinery in Martinez, California. As a hard worker who was personable, Daddy quickly gained the respect of his co-workers. Because he had a college degree and his White co-workers didn't, Daddy was later promoted to shipping and receiving supervisor.

Eventually, Daddy and his best friend, Jerry Higgs would use his prior janitorial background to start their own business, *Jim and Jerry's Janitorial Service*. They were a huge success, landing jobs that many Blacks never had the chance to bid for throughout the Bay Area.

Brilliantly Being What His Father Was Denied
Since his father passed away when he was a young teen, my daddy wanted to be the father to us that his daddy didn't have a chance to be for him.

Daddy enjoyed fatherhood. From 1952-1964 more babies were born to Mae Omie and Jimmie Thrower. I have four siblings: Romona (deceased 2000), Jimmy Jr., Arnold Keith, and Shawana. Since his father passed away when he was a young teen, my daddy wanted to be the father to us that his daddy didn't have a chance to be for him.

Determined to make a good life for us, it was important to Daddy that he be a good provider and faithful servant. I recalled him holding down three jobs, all at once to support his family.

Daddy refused to let Momma work outside the house as a "maid for them White folks." He knew how broken his own mother's spirit had become when she had no choice but to labor as a maid for many White families following Grandpa's death.

Daddy served in many capacities, and was engaged in his church, the community, and his children's lives. My father was a minor and major little league coach for both of my brothers, one whom played professionally for the Oakland A's and the St. Louis Cardinals. As president of the Wilson Park Little League, Daddy motivated the boys to excel in school and sports. He also encouraged the coaches and parents to support the boys in all aspects of their lives.

<u>Getting His Brag On</u>
Daddy's pride in us was a gift. It gave us self-assurance, confidence, good esteem, personal insight and inspiration.

My father's love for his family was very evident. He let everyone know how proud he was to be a father, and how proud he was of his children. We were *good kids*. Relatives would joke that they were *sick of him* always bragging about his kids. Daddy did brag a lot about us, almost to our embarrassment.

Daddy's pride in us was a gift. It gave us self-assurance, confidence, good esteem, personal insight and inspiration. We knew we could do and become anything that we desired in life. The only thing that *could or would* hold us back would be ourselves.

All of my siblings and I have a healthy sense of esteem, purpose and service that we have passed along to our children. If he were alive today, I know Daddy would be *getting-his-brag-on* about his children, grandchildren and great-grandchildren.

<u>Oh How He Loved and was Loved in Return</u>
Daddy was a real public servant and hero who loved helping people.

Many loved Jimmie Thrower. Small in stature, but big hearted and spirited, he was a wonderful father, husband, pastor, community activist and friend to many youth. Daddy was a real public servant and hero who loved helping people.

On many Sunday mornings he would go to the Greyhound bus station and bring the homeless to our house. Momma prepared a big breakfast for them. Then they would bathe or shower, and Daddy would give them twenty dollars before taking them back to the bus station. His only request was that they help someone else along the way.

During the early '70s there were race riots in our community. So Daddy, who was generous and well-respected, organized clergy from different denominations, to walk the hallways at the two local high schools. Their presence served to ease the racial biases and tensions. As a result of this effort, he was encouraged to run for public office; but Daddy knew his calling was in *ministry* and not *politics.*

I Am My Father's Child
Momma tells me, "You're just like your daddy, trying to help somebody when they don't want to help themselves."

Daddy was publicly acknowledged in a community celebration called, *This is Your Life,* a chronicle of all his community deeds. I will never forget the humility or the look on my daddy's face when his family, friends, school personnel, and local public figures surprised him with this distinguished honor.

I take pride in being a servant and champion for *at-risk* children and families. Momma tells me, "You're just like your daddy, trying to help somebody when they don't want to help themselves."

It's in my blood.

I'm proud of my rich spiritual heritage and legacy. Like the previous generation of men in my family, my brothers, nephews, husband and son-in law labor in ministry. I praise God for blessing my life.

I know I have *favor* because of the seed Jimmie Thrower, a powerful and mighty man of God, planted during his short life.

Daddy was called to *Glory* on December 29, 1991 at the age of 66 from prostate cancer. He had two *Home Going Celebrations.* One was in Vallejo and the other in his birth and final resting place, Strong, Arkansas. More than 1,000 people came to pay their respects, sharing stories and testimonies of how my daddy had changed their lives.

Elder Jimmie Thrower was a true man after God's heart. Oh good and faithful servant, your work was not in vain. I am my father's child.

I love you Daddy!

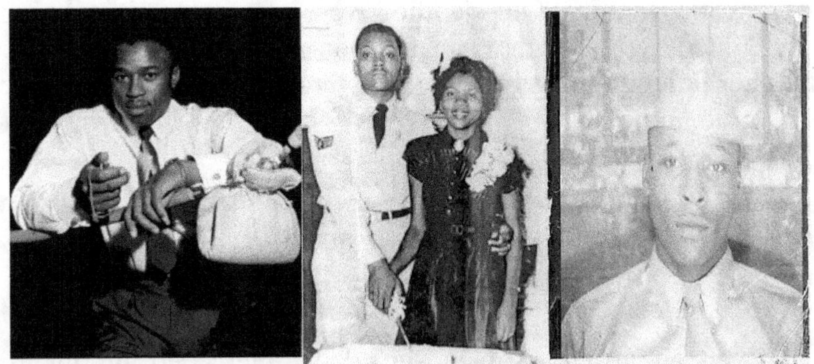

Honorary father, Mr. Wilbert Gerald on the left. Author's mother and father, Mr. Morris and Mrs. Ruth Gaines on their Wedding day, June 11, 1950. Honorary father, Mr. Edgar Willies on the right.

Our Black Fathers: Brave, Bold and Beautiful!

Joslyn Gaines Vanderpool

<u>I'm Making it My Business!</u>
"If anything involves you, I'm going to make it my business!"

Our fathers had respectable names -- Edgar, Morris and Wilbert to name a few. Throughout our childhood they echoed this, and other self-assured phrases, "If anything involves you, I'm going to make it my business!"

My girlfriends and I adored our daddies who didn't exactly believe in *giving us our space*. Sometimes they'd pick up the other phone during a serious gossip session and interrupt. "It's a school night girls; time to hang up the phone and go to bed."

We had daddies who watered the lawn a gazillion times or mowed the same blade of grass over and over again to monitor any boys in the vicinity. Our daddies were always nearby. At times, they'd step right on the dance floor and tap our dates on the shoulder to let them know that they were getting too close or it was time to go home.

Our daddies had to create a life where their children were embraced, if not by society, then, at least they were determined to be there for us.

Even as grown women our dads interceded in our lives. Sometimes they'd arrive at our doorsteps unannounced and refused to leave if a male companion was present. They were still holding on and claiming their role as the first men in our lives.

<u>What'd You Say?!!!!</u>
Yes! I do believe I was sent into orbit, but at least Daddy let me live!

Black daddies are something! It doesn't matter how old they are, or whether they are on a walker, wear a pacemaker or are arthritic, those brothers could, can and will move, if their children are foolish enough to challenge them. If they're really mad, they can run on fumes alone!

One of our daddies chased his teenaged son all the way down the street when the young man momentarily *lost his mind* and used profane language in reference to his father. His daddy was too mad to ask, "What'd you say?!!!" Although he was nearly 60, you'd think that he was the second coming of Jessie Owens, rounding the corner and leaping over bushes to catch his child. At 13, I nearly drove my father to that end.

On a lazy summer afternoon my father told me to do some chore that I thought was simply beneath me. So I blithely suggested, "Why don't you do it yourself?"

He obviously was a loving man because I'm still here to talk about it. Yes! I do believe I was sent into orbit, but at least Daddy let me live!

Besides asking, "What'd you say?" our daddies were perplexed by what we were wearing, doing, and more specifically, thinking!!! Our Afros, platform shoes, psychedelic clothes, funky music and outrageous dances were off the hook, but not to our daddies.

When one friend's father heard his children singing, *Tear the Roof off the Sucker,* he threw down his hands in resignation and lamented "I'm working to keep the roof over your head, and you children want to tear it off. That's just crazy!"

<u>Why Does Everybody Hate Us Daddy?</u>
Daddy held me in his arms as I broke down in tears from the vicious insults that wreaked havoc with my esteem.

Our daddies told us things like, "Don't worry, baby. It'll be alright" when we'd ask, "Why aren't we allowed to go to the pool or library?" or "Why can't we drink from the clean water fountain?" or "Why did that man call you a boy, Daddy? You're not a boy." Although they tried to placate us, we knew that our hurt haunted them.

While our family was stationed in Japan in the early '60s with the U.S. Air Force, my sister, the only Black child in her elementary class suffered from her teacher's demeaning treatment towards her. When my father appeared at the school, "dressed in full military regalia," as my sister proudly recounts, Daddy told her, "You don't have to stay in that class, sweetheart" and transferred her to another teacher.

Back stateside, my father rescued me from my daily second grade hell of being called a wide range of derogatory names, the "*N-* word" being the most prominent racial slur directed toward me by some of the other children.

Daddy held me in his arms as I broke down in tears from the vicious insults that wreaked havoc with my esteem. At that moment, like many of our Black daddies, he assured me that I indeed was *somebody*. Then he gave me courage in a few powerful sentences. "You're special. Anyone who calls you names is speaking from ignorance because they don't know you and how beautiful our people are."

Daddy even got the dictionary and looked up the "*N*-word," which at the time, was defined as a coward. "You're not a coward, Joshie. God loves you, and so do I, and your mother. So the next time anyone says that to you, set them straight. Let them know that we're all special in God's eyes."

My dad's words have been life sustaining. Due to the encouragement I received, I could survive and would never need the approval of others to exist.

Our Black Warriors
Super bad! That was the essence of our daddies --Black men of steel. Superman didn't have a clue about what Black daddies could do!

The pain our fathers carried was brilliantly hidden in the quiet recesses of night where they must have grieved alone. If they were treated badly we didn't always know it. Our daddies had to create a life where their children were embraced, if not by society, then, at least they were determined to be there for us.

Our Black fathers were bold, brave and beneficial to our lives. With their omnipotence, we knew that they would protect us. To ensure the survival of their families, they sometimes endured intolerable treatment in the workplace and in the world. Their intelligence, abilities and service to their country, were insignificant to many, except the ones who recognized their worth: their families.

All of our daddies served in the military in places that freed them temporarily from America's bigotry. As heroes, they fought in World War II, Korea, and Viet Nam.

Super bad! That was the essence of our daddies --Black men of steel. Superman didn't have a clue about what Black daddies could do!

The Wonder Years
We were happy Black girls secure in who we were because of what we'd been given....

Our daddies made us laugh. Mr. Wilbert let us ride inside the open trunk of his fabulous 1964 Bonneville. We giggled hysterically each time we hit a bump in the road.

Mr. Edgar took us to the lake, barbecued burgers while we splashed in the water, and drove us to the Dairy Queen in his new lemon hued Cadillac. When he asked if we wanted to eat in his car? We nodded affirmatively. Sure enough, he shook his head from side-to-side and said solemnly, in his deep throated baritone, "Not in my car."

There were so many activities our fathers chauffeured or accompanied us to. Anytime our parents released us to the public, they'd warn, "Don't be so loud." Immediately ignoring them, we laughed until we dropped. We were happy Black girls, secure in who we were because of what we'd been given: pride, faith and belief in self.

On trips to baseball games it was *all good*. Doting daddies plied us with hot dogs, popcorn, helmets and mitts just to have their children next to them. Remembrances of Jackie Robinson joining the *Bigs* were recounted as well as stories about other larger than life heroes of the Negro leagues. Even though my dad was a life long Dodgers fan because they were the first to break the color line, he cheered for Willie Mays fading back in the outfield, *going back, waaaaay back,* stretching his lithe, lean body to catch the ball at the wall in a moment of Black excellence.

In those wonder years, our daddies took us to church, assured us that we were bright and gave us a strong sense of racial pride.

During the holidays, gifts were abundant because our fathers knew that their Black babies deserved the best Christmases too.

To connect to our roots, road trips were taken. The journeys were important, and at times, dangerous due to the volatile racial climate. Bringing home good grades was expected. Sometimes our daddies acted like we did *just okay* in an effort to keep our egos in check, but we overheard them boasting to anyone who would listen about how smart their daughters were. And when it was time to drive, all of my friends and I looked to our daddies to help us secure our licenses.

I can still picture my father's thick eyebrows furrowing together when I asked if I could begin driving at 15.

"Noooo sireee!" he said adamantly, shaking his head. "I'm not about to turn you loose in a car!"

Somehow, Dad's reaction made me feel like an unbridled stallion that needed a team of handlers to steer the car! Despite earlier objections, our daddies took us to deserted parking lots where they taught us how to do two- point-three turns, and parallel park. Weekend-after-weekend, they patiently instructed us until we proved to the state of California, and more importantly to our daddies, that we were fit to drive.

It's a Shame
Back in the day, each daddy was free to lecture, advise, admonish, teach and embarrass us.

One day in 1974, my sister's friends came by in their "fly looking" attire and began dancing. At that moment, my father came in the living room, placed a Bible on the coffee table and tapped it twice for emphasis. Daddy was never subtle.

Not my sister's ally in those days, I even empathized with her and was so mortified, that I could have slipped under the coffee table where I'm sure she already was. Suffice to say, the party was over. When the coast was clear, the group discreetly left. It was a shame because our daddies didn't care who was there when they scolded and schooled us.

The lessons our fathers imparted were for everyone as was demonstrated when my friend came by. I'd been assigned the mundane task of raking leaves. As I started to walk off the job, I heard my father call out, "Where are you going?"

"With Barbara."

"Oh no you're not. Give her a rake too!"

'How embarrassing!' I thought.

Barbara's father returned the favor years later by interrogating me about why I carelessly left my wallet on the front seat of my car. So we were never free. Where one daddy left off, another was in the anchor lane, ready to take the baton of teaching, advising, and of course, embarrassing us.

Just Beat Me Already!!!!

The one thing we hated was a *Daddy lecture.* To make sure that they made their point, they'd ask, "Did you hear me?" We dared not respond in the way that we really wanted to. '*Yes we heard you. You only said it a hundred times. Dang! Why don't you just beat me already!!!'*

Today, we'd give anything to hear them again as they shared their words of wisdom.

<u>Daddies' Girls</u>
Each father was a part of our lives and cheered our victories.

We were literally daddies' girls, not just our own daddy's daughter. Each father was a part of our lives and cheered our victories. When I was accepted to UC Berkeley, all of my girlfriends and their daddies and mamas were proud, and parties where thrown in my honor. One of my surrogate fathers even came to my graduation with his wife, grandson and his daughter, my friend. My family was there too. With degree in hand, my daddy hugged me tightly, and whispered in my ear, "I'm so proud of you."

That night, both my parents knelt beside me and tucked me in so tight that I couldn't move beneath the covers. The day's events symbolized an accomplishment for all of us, including my girlfriends, and their parents, because each girl was excelling in a world that told us we couldn't.

<u>No Doesn't Always Mean No</u>
Our daddies stretched as far as their powerful arms could reach and gave us the moon.

For us a Black daddy's "no" didn't mean, maybe. It meant NO! At least sometimes it did. We knew our dads had big hearts by the outings they took us on, the gifts they brought us, the lessons they shared and the generous hugs they provided. Our daddies stretched as far as their powerful arms could reach and gave us the moon.

Principled, confident, God-fearing men -- our daddies were a dream. I'll never forget my father and all of the honorary fathers that touched my life. All have died in our circle, except one or two daddies, but they were, and still are: Our Black Fathers: Brave, Bold and Beautiful!

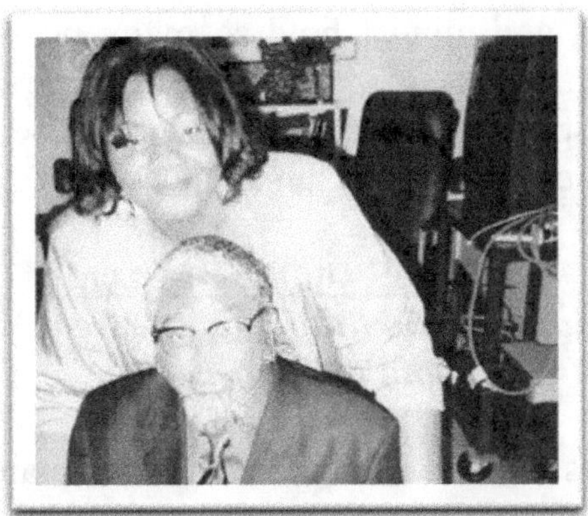

Author with her father, Dr. Josephus McGee, Sr.

To Know Him Is to Love Him

Jacqueline Webb

The way that my father loved my mother set a standard for me; and I will not, and cannot accept anything less.

The Man Who Could Deliver Smiles
When I think of this big, tall, gentle man, I can't stop the smile that spreads across my face….

Handsome, strong, loving, kind, funny and stern – that was my father. If I were to paint his portrait, it would be a wonderfully vibrant and striking picture of a very strong Black man, who loved his wife, children, parents, brothers, and all of his extended family.

To sum it all up, my father gave tremendous love, and was dearly loved.

In my heart and mind I hold so many positive memories of my father. When I think of this big, tall, gentle man, I can't stop the smile that spreads across my face because that is what he delivered to all he encountered: an abundance of smiles.

What's in the Bag Dad?
A champion bargain hunter, my dad could find clothes and food for us all...

My parents had to find deals to adequately care for ten children. A champion bargain hunter, my dad could find clothes and food for all of us.

One time, my dad came home with a particularly interesting bargain that will never be forgotten. It was a bag filled with wieners -- chicken wieners to be exact! (Did I mention that I used to think that we were a test family?) Well, we boiled those wieners and the water turned green. We even tried baking them and the green discoloration still wouldn't go away.

Even though it's been many years since we were exposed to that interesting delicacy, some of my siblings to this day, cannot stomach chicken wieners; but there was one adventurous kid who thought those wieners tasted pretty good -- *me!*

The Way My Father Loved My Mother
The way that my father loved my mother set a standard for me; and I will not, and cannot accept anything less.

Through his life example, my father taught me how I must be treated by the man who says he loves me. Anything short of this would show a lack of respect for the memory of such a great man; a man that I will love forever -- my father, Josephus McGee, Sr.

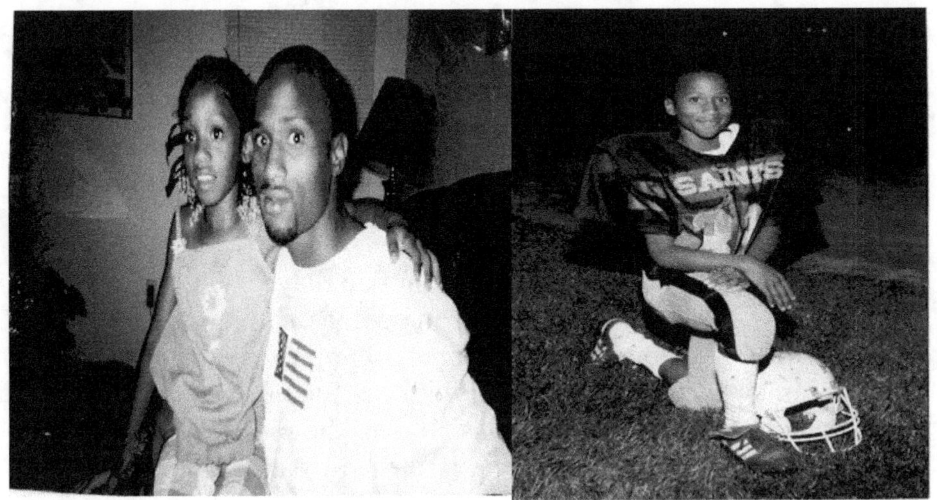

Author with father, Mr. Ben Griffin. Father as a young star in his lucky red shoes.

Lucky Girl, Lucky Shoes

Breanna Griffin

<u>In Step with My Father</u>
I knew I could soar with a part of my dad grounding me in the form of those magical shoes.

My dad has a lucky pair of shoes: red Adidas with white strips on the side. According to my Grandmother Anita, I was destined to wear them one day. When I was younger, I tried them on every few years with the hope of inheriting some of my father's greatness. I knew I could soar with a part of him grounding me in the form of those magical shoes. Today, they fit perfectly and I fly around the track in step with my father, striving to emulate his essence and achieve some of his many accomplishments.

For being in his thirties, my dad is in great shape. Born in 1977, Daddy excels in all types of things like baseball, basketball, football, and fatherhood. I want to be just like him because he most definitely is the talk of the town. When people ask me his name, I say "Ben," and they know the rest.

"Griffin," they say.

And I say, "Yes."

"Man, you should have seen your dad play."

Well I have, and he's taught me a lot of things that I know right now. On average, Daddy scores 30 points every game. I saw all of his tapes, and newspapers with his picture when he was in high school and college. Dad was all over the place! I wonder why he isn't in the *NBA because he is the best basketball player I've ever seen.

Daddy says nice things to me and "wants the best for me."

<u>He Makes Me Laugh</u>
Every time I talk to my dad, we laugh.

Besides being an athlete, my dad is a coach, personal trainer and a great man who would give up anything for his family and kids: Deion, 10, Isaiah, 4, and me, Breanna, 12. Deion lives in Texas and sees Dad during the summer. I visit my dad on weekends and when I'm off track during the school year; and Isaiah lives with him.

Dad is a great storyteller, and loves talking about his grandfather and one particular cousin. Every time I talk to my dad, we laugh. Like the time during his childhood when his cousin wet the bed while Dad was in the bunk below. My dad told on him and his cousin said he was just sweating because it was so hot.

My dad's birthday is July Fourth, which is the same date as his great uncle's. Grandma Anita used to take him to the park on Independence Day and bring a cake and other party favors for Daddy's special day. Since the park was full of people who were barbecuing and celebrating with their friends and families, Daddy mistakenly thought they were there for his party too. To him it was a blast!

<u>Too Old to Be a Flower Girl</u>
Sometimes I wonder when he's going to get married.

Ben Griffin is well-liked and fun to be around. Tales about my father's exploits as a boy are well known, and everyone enjoys telling stories about him, just as he loves sharing and keeping us laughing with the stories he recounts. Everyone on the block knows him because he is very caring.

Daddy says nice things to me and "wants the best for me." I think about him too. Sometimes I wonder when he's going to get married. When he does, I only wish the best for him, even though I'm a little too old to be a flower girl.

Being a morning person Dad wakes up at 4:00am and goes to work cleaning out houses so someone else can move in. Because of all he does and all he means to me, I am a lucky girl. I LOVE YOU DADDY!

*NBA: National Basketball Association

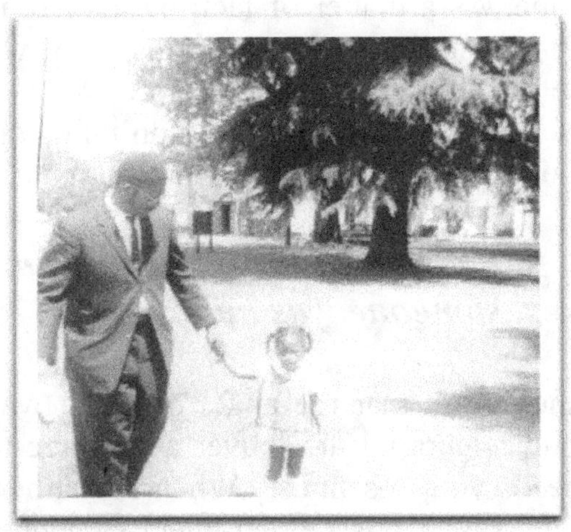

Author and her father walking in the park on a Sunday afternoon.

When Heaven Calls

Alberta Barrow

<u>Not Before I See My Son</u>
In his quiet strength he surveyed the room.

I saw him leave. The moment he really left was before the long nights in the hospital stretched into days. His moment of departure was at a birthday party that I nearly missed. We were sitting around the table laughing and talking. In his quiet strength he surveyed the room. Then his eyes began to moisten, but his tears were held in suspension.

"Are you alright?" I asked.

Without a single utterance, my father just looked at me like it was the last time. As a matter of fact, he looked at all of us that same way. My oldest sister told us to sing, as it was the day that my great niece was turning two; but before we could comply, my father lost his balance. Although he didn't fall or faint; he just simply leaned over and rested on his beautiful mate, my mother.

When my father looked for all of his family to say his last good-byes, someone was missing.

I sometimes think that the angel of death walked up to the table during our celebration to deliver a message to our beloved, "The Father needs you, Josephus." When my father looked for all of his family to say his last good-byes, someone was missing. Since he didn't see all of us there, he began to cry, but ceased because the Father spoke to the angel and revealed that my father wouldn't take his last breath until his son came home from war.

My brother Israel was in the eye of the storm in Iraq when our father was transitioning. So the Army granted him an early release, but knowing and faithfully believing that Daddy would be there for him, like he always was, Israel stayed on not wanting to place his troops in a difficult situation. As if scripted, Israel made it home in time to see our father, who could now truly rest in peace.

<u>Holding On For Dear Life</u>
"Now daughter, you need to stay and help your mother."

When I was little, I'd cling to my father's leg because I wanted to go with him, but he knew the day would come that I would try to hold on to him for dear life, and would need to remember him saying, "Now daughter, you need to stay and help your mother."

There were many days I would sit and wait in front of the screen door and watch him drive away and wait right there with great anticipation for his return, as he pulled up in front of the house. I thought my father must have known I would return to my old habits where I'd watch the sky waiting for him to appear with Jesus, because the dead in Christ shall rise and meet Him in the air. Since Daddy knew that that wouldn't be good for me, he taught me that Jesus said to *occupy **until** I come (Luke 19:13)*. So I'm heeding my father's powerful instructions until we meet again.

<u>Finally, Assuredly Leaving</u>
His leaving could best be described as supernatural.

My daddy, who was the biggest, strongest, most honorable man I ever had the pleasure of knowing, lived his life with integrity and left this life the same way. His leaving could best be described as supernatural.

I suspected my father knew that a few days after my 39th birthday he would leave this earth for a place not made by hand. Because of the way his ending transpired, I believe he knew that his Heavenly Father needed another angel. Since he had already done tremendous works on earth and he saw his son once more, my father could finally and assuredly say good-bye to all of those who were significant to his incredible life on earth, and ascend to join the rest of the angels who were awaiting his arrival.

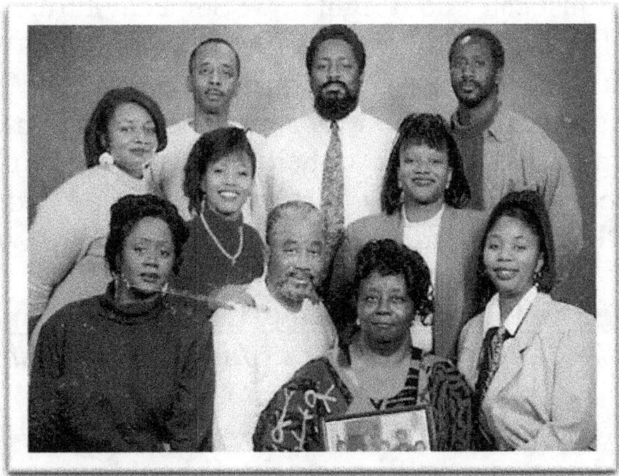

Author center row, far right, with her parents (center) and siblings.

Tomorrow I'll Be Stronger

An excerpt from my daily journal

Vanessa Rushing

Everyone is Looking for Me to be Strong...
Good morning Lord, please tell my Dad I love and miss him a lot!

Alana came for a visit last night, a very nice visit. She lost her dad five years ago. She like Moma and the sisters, think that I should keep a journal. They say it will help so here it goes...

My conscious prayer is, "please let me be strong tomorrow." Today I find it hard to let go. I can't explain it nor do I want to gather up the strength to try. My dad's passing has been so unbelievably hard and I find myself in such an unfamiliar place. Everyone (Derek especially) is looking for me to be strong, smile and sing. I just can't do it right now. Someday I truly believe I will and it will be heartfelt -- just-not-today.

Donise wants to get together once a week to play Chess. Dionne wants me to sing on the new gospel praise team at her church. It's all to keep me busy and from being depressed. Carol even invited me to Wednesday morning Bible studies. I nod and just think to myself, OK, but tomorrow, when I'm stronger.

<u>Maybe I Should Just Cry, Cry and Cry Some More</u>
It's like the words to Stevie's song, "I wish those days would come back to me."

I don't know, maybe Lisa is right. I should just scream and let it all out. Jackie and Ann, even Berta told me how they cry for what seems to be hours. As for me, it's been a few minutes here and a few minutes there. Who knows, maybe if I do what everyone is doing and saying and just cry, cry and cry some more I will feel better. <u>But</u>, then I think what if it works for them but not for me and I slip away into a deep sadness that I can't come out of.

It's so strange for now. I want to just be in my bed by MYSELF! Yet no one at my house will let me. Everyone here thinks I need to be with someone. I wonder if that's how Moma felt when we were younger. I remember her wanting to go somewhere and I would say, "I'll go with you." How funny! It's like the words to Stevie's song, "I wish those days would/could come back to me.'

I'm glad Alana came by last night. She didn't say lets talk about what you're feeling. She said, "write down your emotions so that you can express yourself in a journal." She's right. Why do people say, "talk about it?" I can't find the words to express how sad I am. Sure others have lost loved ones, many girls, also "daddies' girls" have lost their fathers. But I LOST MY DAD! Is he in a better place? Yes. Is he rejoicing there? Yes. Is he out of pain? Yes. But, I miss him. Not only do I miss my daddy, I miss me, I miss my mom, my sisters and even my brothers.

It's been good writing and expressing myself. I'm going to pray, read my Bible and go to work. I know that I, along with my sisters will be OK. The prayer for me is also my prayer for them so I know tomorrow we'll be stronger.

A Lasting Legacy: Goodnight Sweet Prince

Sha-Toyia Anderson

From a Near Tragic Birth to a Beautiful Beginning

It was 1988, Ronald Reagan was president of the United States, the champion of ice figure skating was Debi Thomas, the first African American woman to advance that far in the sport; and I was born, which was the most important event of the year.

The woman who brought me into the world was very strong minded, but her mind was cooked like bacon when it's overdone. Smells great, but, wasted, in her case from the amount of alcohol and drugs she consumed. Born premature, I couldn't breathe on my own. Tubes were placed down my little throat and my tiny heart pumped against my chest begging for life, begging for a chance to become a winner.

Troy was 6'1, with dark brown skin, and a face like an Egyptian Pharaoh. His smile was so perfect that your heart just melted like ice cream, and his afro, well -- it was so big that it was its own country and he loved to pick that afro into impeccable perfection every day.

My mother, who was not my mother, died two weeks after my birth, but my whole life was set up for greatness and God made sure that I, the miracle child was made of strength. He chose Katherine Jones, a woman with a pure heart, beautiful golden skin and full curly hair to be the mother out of a million mothers in the world to fully embrace me as her own. She would give me life, after a nearly tragic beginning, and offer unconditional love and lovingly take care of me and my father.

Everything was set in motion for me because Katherine Jones, and Troy Anderson were the greatest parents a child could wish for. My father was born June 6, 1967 and raised in the Del Paso Heights area of the north side of Sacramento, California, which is better known as the *DPH*. Troy was 6'1, with dark brown skin, and a face like an Egyptian Pharaoh. His smile was so perfect that your heart just melted like ice cream, and his afro, well — it was so big that it was its own country and he loved to pick that afro into impeccable perfection every day.

Enter the Candy Man—Exit the Sweetest Father

My father was loved by everyone and supported his family with dignity. He was a hardworking African American man who was a martial arts performer, security guard, lover, teacher and compassionate to any individual he met. More importantly, he was a believer in God.

All the children in my neighborhood in the Del Paso Heights area knew of my father and he always came out of nowhere walking up with a brown paper bag full of candy and made sure all the kids got candy that was equally distributed. Even if there wasn't enough, this angel made it enough for every child. He taught us to love one another and respect our parents and he put the "L" in love because everyone loved him and his legacy of peace. He would provide protection and love for his entire family and friends and most of all his wife Katherine and daughter, "baby shay".

On a hot summer night in Del Paso Heights, my mother and I were relaxing in the comfort of our home. The smell of honey, strawberries and kiwi scented the air as she showered and washed her hair, and I watched and listened as she hummed, "Can't nobody do me like Jesus."

"Get up!" I commanded, looking at my father, but he didn't and my heart beat grew smaller and smaller. I thought maybe my heart would stop beating if he didn't get up. I wanted to cry, but the tears never came out, being six years old and watching him not getting up didn't make sense but he looked peaceful and I didn't want him to get up if he was tired.

The peaceful moment was short-lived, replaced with the eruption of gunshots popping off like fireworks. Suddenly the night turned as cold as blue ice and we began to shiver. My mother ran outside butt-naked to find a horrific bloody crime scene. Like her shadow, I bolted too, steadying myself behind her wearing my Little Mermaid pajama dress with my long thick pig tales anointed with Black Magic hair grease and my chocolate skin slathered in pink baby lotion. I watched my mother cry, scream, curse. She couldn't take the sight of this martial arts performer lying in the street shot dead with bullets riddling his body.

Shattered glass was everywhere. My father's brown Ford Pinto with my name on the side of the driver side and mother's name on the top of the hood moved away slowly and my father's Egyptian face was frozen in a blank stare. The 27-year-old lay there dead.

"Get up!" I commanded, looking at my father, but he didn't and my heart beat grew smaller and smaller. I thought maybe my heart would stop beating if he didn't get up. I wanted to cry, but the tears never came out, being six years old and watching him not getting up didn't make sense but he looked peaceful and I didn't want him to get up if he was tired. So, I let him sleep with his eyes open and I didn't cry cause I knew he was just sleeping. My family members grabbed me and covered me to shield me from the bloody scene, but the man who shot my father, made sure to say aloud that he was the murderer of my father.

Though I couldn't see the scene anymore, my hearing became perfect like I had always been blind all six years of my life, but my hearing senses led me to hear all of the crying and commotion of my father's death.

A True Representation of Love and Success Like Father Like Daughter

My beloved father was killed because he was black and the security guard who killed him let it be known in court that it was because he was black. It was simply a hate crime and this man didn't agree with the color of my father's skin so killing him while he was on his way home from work to be with his wife and daughter made perfect sense to him.

Good fathers are overlooked and mine was so valuable in my life. Sometimes I cry but my tears now are tears of joy because I'm happy to continue what he represented with love, grace, strength, integrity and positivity.

The man I knew as my father left me when I was six years old. I loved when we rode on his motorcycle. With him I laughed so hard I nearly choked. Life was beautiful because he was in it. I could call on him and he would come and make sure I had everything I needed. My mother always reminds me of the dream he had for me, which was simple (to be successful at everything I do no matter what it is. Be great at it and love it).

Good fathers are overlooked and mine was so valuable in my life. Sometimes I cry but my tears now are tears of joy because I'm happy to continue what he represented with love, grace, strength, integrity and positivity. After my father's death, my mother made sure to raise me right. She remained strong, prayed every day for me to have a successful life and future; and made certain that through my father's legacy that I would live without allowing negativity to intervene in my life.

My father's dream was to teach martial arts fighting, take care of me and my mother and watch me blossom as I grew older. My mother reminded me of all the good my father did because that was the only way he knew how to be. He represented love and peace. So here I am in love and peace, a representation of him. I am an image of Troy Anderson and I walk the earth feeling like a proud daughter by being in college and pursing my dreams. My father is the catalyst to my success because I strive every day in every way to take care of my mother and myself as he would do if he were still alive.

After my father's death, my family on my father's side won a million-dollar wrongful death lawsuit. Although, I was unaware of it, I'm not worried. I am happy that justice was found for my father and the man who killed him was sentenced to prison. My father's death has left my body feeling empty at times now that I'm grown, but a father so loving as mine is what I want to be an example of. People will know what and who he was. So, I will carry on like Troy Anderson. His love never perishes, his legacy is what I live by and my admiration for him will always remain deep in my heart.

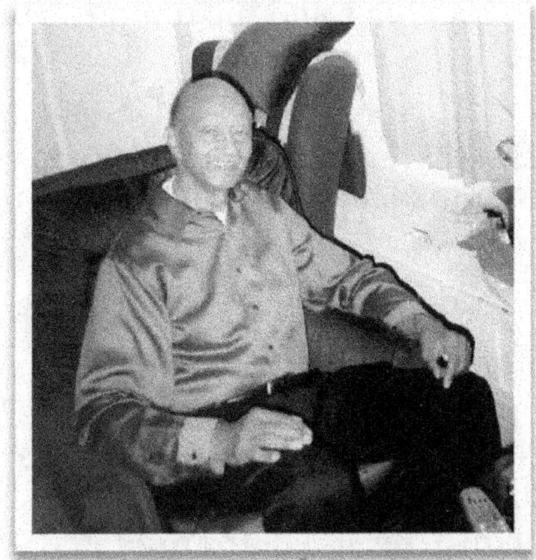

My Dad, My Friend, My Hero

Roshaun Fowler

The Principles of Farming in Forming a Love for Life

Even though he grew up during the Great Depression on a 300-acre farm, my father, Wilbert Lee Fowler never lacked for, or expressed wanting anything. Born on August 26, 1933, in Little Rock, Arkansas, he was the only child born to Doris Marie and Willie Lee and raised in a multi-generational home with his parents, four aunts, two uncles and his Grandmother Carrie.

My father loved life on the farm, loved walking through the corn field barefoot with his shoes tied around Sunny's neck, loved the soil between his toes and the fresh ears of corn, which he fondly recalled.

My father's grandmother and his mom traveled to town, over fifteen miles away from their farm to do "day work" (cleaning homes, babysitting, etc. for white families) all week long, except on Sundays which was considered a day of rest. They would leave the house before daylight and return after sundown. The men also worked from sunup to sundown tending the farm, milking the cows, feeding the hogs, taking care of the mules and the horses, as well as, plowing the fields and gathering in whatever was in season. So, my aunties who made clothes by hand and were excellent quilters became my father's primary caretakers while his mother and father worked.

Work was not just reserved for my father's elders. He was responsible for feeding his dog Sunny, as well as the chickens and geese, which can be attributed to an excellent work ethic that he maintained throughout his life. He also remembers the hogs, which hung inside of the smokehouse, primarily because of the thick sliced pan bacon that he enjoyed with his Sunday morning breakfast. The array of vegetables and fruit trees, including the Granny Smith apple tree was a source of income for the family, allowing them to maintain the farm; but it also was a source of joy for my father because his grandmother made scrumptious apple turnovers for him.

The farm sustained the family, providing just about everything they needed, except items that they had to purchase in town. Although my father's grandfather died prior to his birth, it was my Grandmother Carrie who conducted the business transactions in town. She was the matriarch and her family respected and trusted her decisions.

From Life on the Farm to Finding the Love of His Lifetime

At the age of five, my father, a curious and inquisitive student, began attending school with his Uncle Ted in a one room schoolhouse. His Uncle Ted was twelve years old and this would be his final year of instruction, as the highest grade taught by the schoolteacher was the sixth grade. Since they wanted a better life for him, his parents decided to leave Arkansas when he was just nine years old and relocate to Oakland, California in 1942. His Aunt Mary and Uncle Walter were happy with this major decision, mainly because they already resided there. Despite my father not wanting to leave his Grandmother Carrie nor the farm, he was excited to ride on the Southern Pacific Train to California. His Grandmother Carrie prepared his favorite apple turnovers and provided enough provisions for their three-day trip.

Upon their arrival at the West Oakland Train Station, my father fondly remembers receiving his first silver dollar from his Uncle Walter. He and his family resided in a boarding house where they shared the bathroom and kitchen with two other families. Opportunity was the reason for my father's parents move to Oakland. They wanted to provide their son a better life, which included going to high school and possibly even college.

Being conscientious with a strong work ethic that was rooted during his time on the farm, my father was a hard-working young man who believed in helping his family out in any way he could. So, he had a paper route, shined shoes and ran errands on his bicycle. He also took his education seriously and did not disappoint his parents, because he graduated from McClymonds High school in the Spring of 1951; and while attending City College in San Francisco, he was inducted into the United States Navy during the Korean War. However, prior to his enlistment he met the girl of his dreams, my mother, Rose Marie!

When my father's cousin Donald introduced him to my mother, sparks flew. My mother possessed all the qualities he was looking for in a wife. She was beautiful, intelligent and very strong-willed. Plus, she was an excellent cook, which also made my father fall madly in love with her! Thus, before enlisting in the Navy, he proposed to the love of his life and she accepted. My parents were married on February 9, 1954. When I look at their wedding pictures, it is easy to understand why they fell in love. Daddy was a handsome man and Momma was a gorgeous young woman. From their union, five beautiful daughters were born and lovingly cherished.

My Father – My Foundation

After my mother passed away, my father being a strong gentle soul, made sure he was always there for us as our rock and our foundation.

My sisters and I were raised in Oakland, California, residing with our parents, and our Collie, named Laddie in a wonderful two story Victorian home. My grandparents lived on the lower level and we lived on the upper level. We had a huge backyard which consisted of two single storied duplexes and a garden with fruit trees. Our home was surrounded with a chain linked fence which gave us an even more secure feeling.

One of my fondest memories as a child was waiting for my father to come home from work. He held two full-time jobs (it was his work ethic again). His day time job was as an electrician at Western Electric and he worked at a meat packing plant during the grave yard shift. Therefore, when he came home from his first job, I was ready to greet him with my jacket on to go with him.

I was a Daddy's girl from a very young age and everyone in my family knew it. My father always took the time to listen to me with intent. He was never too busy or exhausted to listen to what was on my heart. He even agreed to call me by another name, which was not my birth name. The name I chose was Pixie Ann, because she could fly and make herself disappear. I was only five years old and this cartoon character appeared larger than life to me.

My mother forbade my new name and I reluctantly had to obey her. Therefore, as fate would have it, twenty-six years later, I was affectionately introduced to my youngest niece as Aunt Pixie. Apparently, my mother had never forgotten how important this name meant to me. However, hearing my mother teaching my niece to call me by this name was short-lived. She died less than three years later. After, my mother passed away, my father being a strong gentle soul, made sure he was always there for us as our rock and our foundation.

My Dad is the epitome of the quiet giant. It is through his silence and gentleness where I have I learned to be at peace with myself and others.

Once while going through a difficult period with my father, I remarked, "You never end our phone conversations by saying, I love you."

My father grew silent and then he explained, "I thought you knew by my actions how I felt and that was sufficient."

"Mother, always said she loved me, and it's very important for me to hear it from you."

I am elated to say that my father once again, listened intently and heeded my heartfelt request. It has been almost twenty years, since we had that conversation but he continued to end our conversations with "I love you." And I responded as only a daughter could by saying, "I love you more than you will ever know."

Our relationship has not been a perfect one. It has had its share of ups and downs. But, through it all, I have learned so very much and it resonates with me wherever I go. My father's pearls of wisdom, or more accurately the lessons that my father has taught me are priceless! The ones near and dear to my heart are: *"Let your Yes Mean Yes, and your No Mean No, and always be a woman of your word; Always put family first; Believe in yourself and always follow your dreams; and lastly, always look forward to a better and brighter day!"* My Dad is the epitome of the quiet giant. It is through his silence and gentleness where I have 1 learned to be at peace with myself and others.

My father has always been there for me, even when I was no longer living in his household. He reminds me in a quiet way I am his daughter and he will always be there for me, even though he has recently passed on and assumed wings as my guardian angel. His unconditional love for me and my family has been phenomenal, and therefore I am grateful to call him, Daddy!

Herb Blackman Jr.—The Man Who Engineered Love

Rene McGaugh Blackman

When I met Rene, in January 2017, I sensed something was weighing down her spirits, I guessed right when she said she was missing her father who had died six years earlier. She shared how incredible and loving her father was, and I thought he sounded gentle and strong like my father, a military man who was intelligent, educated, and giving. She kept notes detailing the first day she learned of her father's diagnosis of cancer and she wrote of the days, weeks, hours and months she and her family spent seeking out doctors and getting medical tests, and the grief and stress attached to those efforts to find a successful treatment for her father. She was a daughter who was on a mission to save her strong, "best daddy in the world". What she shares is a story of love that lives on. --J.G. Vanderpool

The Best Dad in the World

Dad called me daughter number 2. As a little girl, I had this blanket that I took everywhere. I even stood by the washer and dryer waiting for it to come out. As soon as the dryer stopped I grabbed it and rubbed it against my face, despite my parents' efforts to wean me from it. At the time, I was six years old and the blanket became very raggedy. Then something began to happen to my blanket. I noticed that it was getting smaller and had shrunk to the size of a hand towel.

"Why is it getting smaller?" I asked my, dad. "Because you are getting bigger," he responded. Many years later he confessed that he secretly had been cutting off the blanket. And we both laughed about it.

Dad and I engaged in many activities together and his love was always predominant. Being very athletic and in excellent physical shape, Dad played tennis, ping pong, and went jogging with me. He liked to bowl and was on the Church league when we lived in Detroit. On Fridays I went with him, and he gave me money to bowl with my friends. We even talked about taking flying lessons.

Dad enjoyed answering all my questions, which inspired me to become an engineer. He also strongly encouraged me and supported my career choice when being a woman, and a black woman at that, was unheard of in the field of engineering; but he was familiar with roadblocks and obstacles and knew that he had to engineer his own dream if it was to come to fruition.

Generosity, kindness and concern for others were major characteristics of my dad, and I learned much about giving from him. He was selfless and contributed to many causes, charities and individuals. He tutored and helped youth with their pursuits, served his country with the United States Air Force, and was a member of the Tuskegee Airmen Club in San Diego.

I'll never forget what my dad did on his way home from work one day. When he saw an elderly homeless woman in the alley pushing a grocery cart, he turned his car around met her in the alley and gave her $20. He told me if grandma, his mom, were in that situation he would want someone to do the same for her. Giving back was effortless for him and he often talked about making his favorite green beans for a homeless shelter for many years. He also donated blood for many years until he was in his seventies. Mom would often say that dad's arm had a pump that went to the blood bank. It inspired me to donate. I give on the average 3 times a year

Engineering a Dream

Dad was not only a Civil Engineer, he was a PE, a Professional Engineer. Even as a little girl, I was always interested in his work. I would ask him questions like "How does the gasoline in the car make the car run?" Dad enjoyed answering all my questions, which inspired me to become an engineer. He also strongly encouraged me and supported my career choice when being a woman, and a black woman at that, was unheard of in the field of engineering; but he was familiar with roadblocks and obstacles and knew that he had to engineer his own dream if it was to come to fruition.

It was in the era of segregation, and colleges in the South where he resided were not opening their doors to black students. So, he found a program that would help pay his tuition if he attended a school in the North, and he chose Howard University and excelled. However, despite is strong abilities and talents, he would face racial discrimination and later in life, ageism, as no one would readily hire him, but he persisted until he found engineering work, breaking barriers and finding success on many occasions.

When I was ready to learn more about the field of engineering, it was my father who nurtured my dream. On Saturdays when I was in high school, he took me to DCEP (Detroit Pre-College Engineering Program), which prepared students for college, who wanted to major in that field. Years later when I became an engineer and married, Ronnie, who also is a Civil Engineer PE, my dad was proud. Our oldest son Ryan, is following in my father's footsteps as well. He is pursuing computer science/ computer engineering degree. Like his granddad he is a community oriented person. His goal is to open room and board housing in the community for the disabled so they can receive basic care. Ryan has also served in the military in the Navy for five years. Our youngest son, Aaron graduated from an ivy-league school, Cornell University with a bachelor of science degree in Applied Economics and Management. Like his granddad he is very smart. Aaron took his studies very seriously. He was able to graduate in 3 ½ years without having to go to summer school.

When Angels Waited

My dad never felt sorry for himself even after being diagnosed with small cell cancer. He remained upbeat and continued to attend church. I even went with him to a Tuskegee Airmen meeting where I had the pleasure of being introduced to a group of very nice people. Niki, my sister, and I went to a college fair with dad in October. He was the oldest person representing Howard University, and the only person wearing a suit. Despite his illness Dad was energized talking to the students about the university encouraging them to apply and passing out brochures. He strongly believed that all young people should have the opportunity to a college education and successful life.

It was the end of his life, but my dad planned a major milestone surprise birthday for mom in October which was a great success. A special smile came across his face when he saw how happy and surprised Mom was. He played tennis as long he could. And he also took Niki, and I to and from the airport as long as he could; and there were also several occasions when dad would drop me off at the airport after having a chemo treatment earlier that day.

On Saturday morning, the day before my dad died, Mom and I got a call from the hospital to get there as soon as possible. When we got to the hospital his blood pressure was very low. A few minutes later his blood pressure sunk more and he didn't have a pulse. The doctor and nurse expected Dad to die shortly. With the aid of another pint of blood, his strong faith in God, strong will, and deep love for his family, Dad rallied back. He held on so that Niki, who was coming from Detroit could see him.

The ER nurse who treated him the night before came to visit dad in the comfort care room Saturday evening. The nurse was truly amazed and shocked that he was still alive. He said something to the effect about Dad having turned a big corner, it could have gone the other way. He also said he had never seen anything like that before.

Niki got to the hospital a few minutes after ten on Saturday evening. We were truly amazed Dad held on for 3 ½ hours longer so that we, as a whole family, could be with him for the last time.

Dad, you, were the best father a daughter could have had. You are with the angels at peace. Love you Dad, always.

One Man Show

MECCA

Joslyn Gaines Vanderpool

On his road to nowhere,
a brother unloved in America,
hemorrhaging red rivers of neglect,
searched far beyond forever
and found Mecca....
His hearth seemingly emptied,
His dignity ravaged by racism...
His manhood largely ignored...
A brother embraced his mantle
carried on the wings
of midnight by the spirit of the
Igbo Warrior coming to
infuse him with the quiet reserve
and steel of his ancestors.
A brother in America,
fierce, unwavering,
displaying that he is shrouded
in nobility...Brave, self-contained
like the Savanna, he comes verily
to cultivate his dreams, that were
denied for centuries
at the apex of his soul.

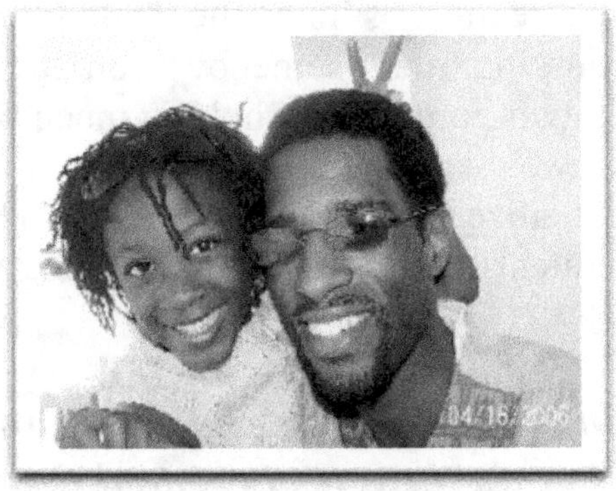

Author with daughter Tiyanane.

Fathering and Falling Out of Love

With Your Child's Mother

Clarence Emmanuel Griffin

<u>A Father's Letter of Advice on Divorce</u>

There are many of us who strive to witness a time when every child that resembles us can say, "My father was a good man, and I know he loves me because he made sure he was there.

Two years ago my letters would have been vastly different. I was a happily married man in love with the mother of my only child. Now I find myself on the brink of severing all ties with her.

Our daughter is a vibrant, articulate, curious and outgoing bundle of God's brown sugar. She is my motivation, my therapist and my inspiration. I could not imagine what life without her daily hugs and kisses would be like. Yet, here I am on the verge of staring that reality right in the face.

Having grown up in a family run by a single mother of four, I know what 'that reality' is like; the feelings of insecurity that something is missing, that somehow you are incomplete, and everyone with a two-parent household is much better off, happier, etc. Though it was emotionally damaging to see my parents separate, I also realized it was for the better. Their marriage was riddled with frequent fights and life-threatening violence to which I bore witness.

It is essential to let your children know through your actions, that the love that created them with their mother is still there, just manifesting in a different form.

On the other hand, my child has never heard her parents raise their voices at each other. I, for one, have always feared that my experience as a child would have an impact on my problem-solving methods, or that I would solve disputes in a fashion similar to that of my parents. As a result, when I found myself in such altercations I'd always walk away. A drive would usually calm me down. Upon returning, I was ready to talk through the problem with my estranged wife.

<u>When a Child Asks</u>
"No matter what happens between your mother and I, you should know we love you and always will."

So what can I say to a six year old girl whose parents may be headed for divorce? First of all, I've realized that when children are ready to ask the question, they are ready for the conversation.

Yesterday my daughter asked if her mom and I were getting divorced. It turns out she had asked her mom the same question the day before. I told her, "No matter what happens between your mother and I, you should know we love you and always will."

My response was enough to calm my daughter's nerves for the moment. However, I dread the impact it will have. The gravitational force of her sadness will pull at my heart so fiercely that I may consider changing my decision, but know that when it is time to move, one must do so.

By staying, the feelings of bitterness and resentment will grow, and the child will eventually see those emotional punches that parents, out of love and frustration, can throw at each other. Those punches may in turn, hit the child in ways that will last well into adulthood. I know. I have my scars. So I will do whatever I can to spare my child from an affliction such as mine.

Fortunately, my daughter and I share a strong bond. We are inseparable. Nevertheless, I know I will have to make an effort to spend more quality time with her. Life is complex and relationships tend to enhance that complexity. Due to our age, we're 33, it is probable that both her mother and I will start new families. In that case, we will have to figure our way through those uncomfortable feelings of priority, time, and who gets what, and when.

To any father or mother who finds themselves on the verge of making such a decision to sever the relationship, remember that when you are ready to answer the child's questions truthfully, you are ready to move on to the next stage in your adult life; however, your child has to know that as you move to another house or home, that wherever you go, they will be with you and that your love for them will be unchanged. Letting go of the marriage does not mean letting go of your love for them.

Learning to Fly All Over Again
Now I find myself flying solo all over again.

After seven years of marriage one becomes quite attached and accustomed to a certain routine. Our beginning occurred at the University of Zimbabwe where I was working my first job out of college as a program assistant.

My soon to be ex-wife was a third-year student at the university as well as a friend to a co-worker. About six months after being introduced, we began dating. For three months we went through the traditional Shona process of courtship and marriage.

The first part of the process was the mile plus walk in the midst of summer, through the hills with 40-50 pounds of food to *meet the aunts*. Next there was the five-hour session of meeting the parents, neighbors, cousins, and the rest of the community. What followed was the negotiation of the actual Lobola (or what is commonly referred to as bride price), though in this case it was more of an appreciation for the parents hard work in raising their daughter.

I was emotionally stretched to say the least, and made a promise never to have to repeat what I had gone through again. Letting go means letting go of this story, which in many ways has been part of who I am – a story that inspired me to think I could do anything, like *Dumbo's feather*. However I find myself, as many of you may find yourselves, having to let go of that thing that has so far helped define me. Now I have to learn to fly all over again.

As I go through my learning process, my advice to you is as follows: Take your time. Listen to that voice within that says you will be fine and whole again; and that no matter what, you will be a father to your children regardless of the situation. There are some contracts that cannot be voided, and fatherhood is one of them. Its abdication is not an option.

Many of us strive to witness a time when every child that resembles us can say, "My father was a good man, and I know he loves me because he made sure he was there." Being present, loving, and making memories means putting your pride aside, and not judging your ex for leaving. It also means remembering that one of the best gifts you can give to your child is love, and a template of success demonstrated in your everyday life.

<u>A Final Word of Advice ...Show Up</u>
Like any good public relations person will tell you,
showing up is 80 percent of the job.

If there is anything that should be taken away from my advice, it would be to remember to show up. Like any good public relations person will tell you, "Showing up is 80 percent of the job." Only those who are there can take part in the work. And raising children is indeed work, and an investment that can bring satisfaction.

Your children are going to have their heads filled with information regarding thoughts of the world, and of family and relationships. Therefore, it is essential to let your children know through your actions, that the love that created them with their mother is still there, just manifesting in a different form. So make sure from an early age, that your childrens' thoughts resemble your sound teachings.

Good luck,
Clarence Griffin

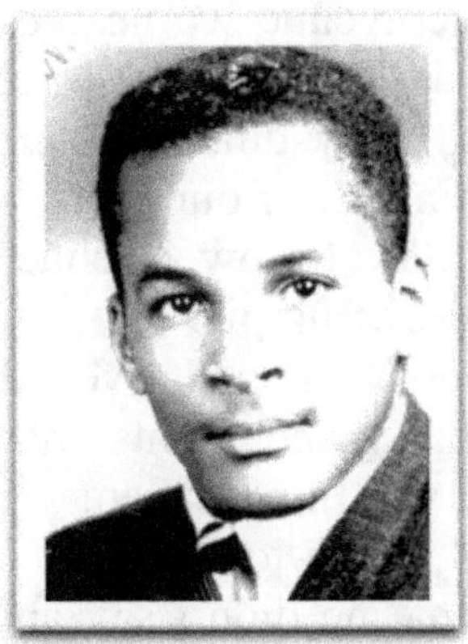

Cool Cat, *the author's courageous father.*

Destiny Driven

A Legacy of Belief and Courage

Denise Turney

<u>How Much Money Do You Have Cat?</u>
The way my father saw it was that if he just believed that he could do a thing then the thing could be done.

It was 1970. The white station wagon wound down Dow Avenue, the only street I had known as home for as long as I could remember. Sure, I was young, only seven years old, but I was inquisitive. I took in everything. What I had seen and heard over the years left me concerned. I desperately wanted everyone in my family to be okay.

Thank God my father, who my siblings and I nicknamed 'Cat' – short for 'Cool Cat,' knew that his children had the innate ability to triumph, to reach our highest goals.

At the end of the avenue we neared the cobblestone bridge. On the other side was the grocery store where my sister, three brothers and I ran to after dinner. Armed with the quarter our father gave us for eating all of our food, including our vegetables, we'd race to the bottom of Dow Avenue and cross the bridge to buy our favorite: *Hostess* fruit pie.

The station wagon bumped over the cobblestones as we headed to our paternal grandparents' house. It was a place my siblings and I thought was like Heaven.

I leaned forward, close to the back of my father's neck. He hated that, but this time he didn't say anything. It was a time of healing for us – our circle had been broken.

"How much money do you have, Cat?"

There. I asked it; although I tried not to. I needed to ensure that everyone was okay. I had this nagging feeling that my father didn't have enough money to take care of us.

My father turned to me with a soft smile and said, "I have fourteen hundred dollars in the bank."

"Is that a lot of money?"

My father stifled a chuckle. "No."

I stared at my father with a blank expression. He saw in my face what I dared not say. What he said next gave me courage. It gave me the same inner-strength and confidence my father gifted me each time he took us to the park on Saturday mornings where he ran up and down steep rolling hills and laughed and played with us. I felt so loved then.

"It's not a lot of money, but it's enough." A second later his smile widened. "We'll make it, Denise."

My father wasn't a "touchy feely" kind of man. He didn't hug us a lot when we were young. He hardly ever said, "I love you." However, he was a doer who expressed his love by enjoying life with us. As I searched his face there wasn't a hint of doubt or a trace of fear. At that very second I believed him.

The station wagon reached the end of the street. My father flipped on the blinkers and turned right. In a few more blocks we would be at our grandparents' house.

<u>Standing in the Gap</u>
My mother had recently passed unexpectedly, breaking our circle.

I wondered about the obstacles my father faced? Why was I concerned about how much money he had? There were five of us: two brothers, my sister, me and our father. A few years later our family expanded to include our beloved baby brother. With five mouths to feed, five people to clothe and keep a roof over their heads, my father had a great deal of responsibility.

Besides confronting the KKK or victories on the race track, we watched our father care for the five of us as a single parent. We watched him cook, do laundry, and find joy in being with us.

My mother had recently passed unexpectedly, breaking our circle. She had been a stay-at-home mom who endured lengthy and painful bouts of mental illness. So my father was flying solo. However, through it all, he stood in the gap.

<u>A First for South Knoxville</u>
For thirty plus years my father's dealership was a successful enterprise, making him the first Black man to own and operate a business in the area.

Our father took us with him nearly everywhere he went. On weekdays he worked long hours at the National Cash Register Company. Years later he opened his own trophy shop which floundered.

Undeterred by the setback, my father moved us from Dayton, Ohio to Tennessee where he opened up a car lot in South Knoxville. For thirty plus years my father's dealership was a successful enterprise, making him the first Black man to own and operate a business in the area.

But I'm getting ahead of myself.

As a seven year old, I thought it would take a million dollars to keep our family going. I worried that we would starve! My father, whose real name is Richard, didn't see it that way. The way my father saw it was that if he just believed that he could do a thing then the thing could be done.

Go Speed Racer!
We overhead the experts say, "He's a good driver, but that car's engine is too small. He's not gonna win."

Money didn't factor into the equation where my father was concerned. It was courage, confidence, and passion that mattered most to him. That belief came through nearly everything he did. It was the reason that he won trophy after trophy with the smallest race car in the city.

We'd go with my father when he went to local official drag racing sites. On racing days the bleachers were packed with spectators. The pit area was stocked with race cars and crew members, but my father didn't have a crew. He worked on his car alone – a small white Austin Healy.

We overhead the experts say, "He's a good driver, but that car's engine is too small. He's not gonna win."

Well he did win. My father never lost a race and he'd race anyone. His success despite the odds helped build my confidence and strengthened my courage.

No One Can Tell You What You Can or Cannot Do
"Whenever someone tells you that you cannot do something, what they are telling you is what they think they cannot do."

My father listened to his heart and mind. He didn't live his life based on what others told him that he could or couldn't do.

After I became an adult, and had achieved successes of my own, my father told me, *"Whenever someone tells you that you can't do something, they are not talking about you. Nobody knows what another person can or cannot do. Whenever someone tells you that you cannot do something, what they are telling you is what they think they cannot do. They may not have the courage to face their own fear, so they project it onto you. They speak right to themselves while they think they are only talking to, or about you."*

<u>Not Even the KKK</u>
Like most hate organizations, the KKK relies on creating fear in the people they target.

Not even the Ku Klux Klan intimidated my father. He refused to allow them to run Mr. T's Auto Sales out of South Knoxville. When the Klan decided to hold meetings behind my father's business, he didn't flinch; but he told them in regard to their gatherings, "Fine, but you best not come on my property."

My father let the KKK know that he didn't fear them. His philosophy was if they didn't bother him, he wouldn't bother them. Although he was not forcing anything on them, he did have the expectation that they WOULD respect him. Therefore, the Klan had to change their fear tactics or simply leave him be, because my father was not going to move his business.

Like most hate organizations, the KKK relies on creating fear in the people they target. They want their victims to be *very afraid*. Consequently, after confronting many that are afraid, they are at a loss when they encounter those that are not, like Harriet Tubman, Fannie Lou Hamer, and my father, who had a certain way of carrying himself.

Even though the Klan continued to hold meetings behind my dad's business for awhile, he stood his ground. Eventually, some of them went on to be loyal customers of his. This was due in part to my father's ability to develop relationships with people of various racial and ethnic backgrounds.

<u>We're Almost There</u>
Our father gave us the fuel to pursue our own lifelong destinies.

Besides confronting the KKK or victories on the race track, we watched our father care for the five of us as a single parent. We watched him cook, do laundry, and find joy in being with us. Our father gave us the fuel to pursue our own lifelong destinies. He led with grace knowing that it would pay off. He didn't complain. He saw to it.

Even now I can picture it. The station wagon speeds up. Another block and we'll be at our grandparents' house. My father smiles, reaches out and places his hand on my shoulder.

"We're gonna make it," he says.

He's right.

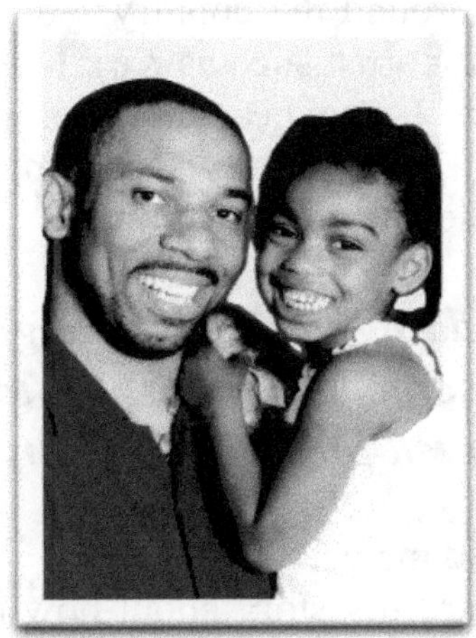

Father of the Year, *with most prized gift…daughter Tyra.*

Father of the Year

Terry Freeman Moore

Don't Applaud Yet
I was a father like many others I know, who were being denied the opportunity to fulfill our roles as dads. Yet, we desperately wanted to be in the lives of our children, nurturing and raising them.

In 2005 I was named, *"Father of the Year"* by the Center for Fathers and Families in Sacramento, California. Due to this distinguished award, I am well known around town for being a great and consistent father. People ask to take photos of my daughter and me together because of our strong bond of love. I've written poems about her and our relationship as well as the struggle it took to be with her.

Our saga has garnered several awards and I've been booked for engagements all around the country. Fortunately, I've had the opportunity to open for artist such as Kirk Franklin, Maya Angelou and Yolanda Adams. I also head a father support group called *Daddy's Here* which helps fathers spend more quality time with their children, regardless of the situation.

Instead of adding to the disparaging statistics of Black father absenteeism, I wanted to be present and accounted for regarding my child.

But don't applaud me yet.

You haven't heard my story about how my relationship with my beautiful daughter, Tyra almost didn't happen.

<u>Like the Days of Slavery</u>
I was almost left out in the cotton field looking through the window, watching my daughter's life pass by without my physical presence to love and support her.

After separating from my ex-wife, I felt like a victim of what slave masters forced Black fathers to do – relinquish their children. Whatever love to be exchanged, hope to be engendered, dreams to be realized between enslaved Black father and child could never come to fruition under oppressive circumstances.

In my case there was no slave master severing the bond between father and child. Rather it was those that I respected and loved. I was almost left out in the cotton field looking through a window watching my daughter's life pass by without my physical presence to love and support her.

Instead of adding to the disparaging statistics of Black father absenteeism, I wanted to be present and accounted for regarding my child. I was a father like many others I know, who were being denied the opportunity to fulfill our roles as dads. Yet, we desperately wanted to be in the lives of our children, nurturing and raising them. So I took action to avoid this monumental crisis that separates fathers from our own children and breaks our hearts in two.

Bittersweet Victory
My father finally got to spend time with his beloved granddaughter.

Albert Moore Jr. was a precious man, and my beloved father. Sadly, he passed away six months after my daughter was born. Despite his failing health and our desperate pleas to let him see his granddaughter, he was only allowed to see her twice before his death.

Before it was too late, the court system ordered my ex-wife, the woman I had made sweet love to in order to get our angel here, to release and share our child. My father finally got to spend time with his beloved granddaughter. But that second time was less than 24 hours before he took his last breath.

On the day when I was handed my daughter to be alone with for the very first time, it was beautiful. The first thing she did was smile at me. The moment was slightly more beautiful than my father's final night of life with her. As she sat on the bed looking into his eyes, he murmured, "Tyra," in a weakened voice, beaming as he talked to her for what would be the very last time.

For all those positive events, I thank God and the judge who intervened and made it possible to spend time with my own child -- the precious being that God blessed me with, and chose for me to oversee.

Violence Begets Heartache
What was difficult to understand was the untruthful depiction of my character that was being painted.

With all that we had been through, just about anyone would have hated those who tried to ruin what was meant to be. Not me. I had too much faith in God for that. And there was the bigger picture to consider – Tyra.

What was difficult to understand was the untruthful depiction of my character that was being painted. Here I was a Black man with no criminal record, a Christian gentleman who was well raised from a functional home. Yet, I was accused of being everything from abusive to a serial killer.

In those trying times there were also accusations that I was allegedly a *low down, no good Black man* who was a threat to kill my own child. All of these attacks were launched to render me an unfit father.

Unfortunately, there was more. While trying to pick up my child in front of the church for only our second court-appointed visitation, I was nearly beaten to the ground by two men I didn't know. With my daughter nearby, her mother looked on from a half a block away.

Thank God Tyra didn't see any violence or have to witness her father doing something unpleasant to someone. A gentleman from my church, who I asked to ride with me, came to my rescue and broke up the altercation. Anticipating that this would happen, we filmed it all. I later discovered that the gentlemen who accosted me were asked to do so.

In the end, I knew I acted responsibly. I gave a darn about what my daughter saw that day. I cared about her physical and emotional well being, and how the events could have adversely affected her spirit.

I Cried and Prayed Every Night
As a father, I stayed and fought with every ounce of weight, every bead of sweat, every dollar, every second, and all the energy my poor heart could produce.

More attempts were made to keep my daughter and me apart. From restraining orders to a request to raise child support payments, which were already doubled, I experienced it all. I cried and prayed every night. Thankfully, God responded and the judge dismissed the case and cut my child support in half.

I never thought it would be so hard to be a father to my own child. I never imagined that someone from my own race and hometown would try to sabotage that relationship. But it happened; two Black people standing in court making fools of ourselves, disgracing our race and what our ancestors built and stood for.

As a father, I stayed and fought with every ounce of weight, every bead of sweat, every dollar, every second, and all the energy my poor heart could produce.

I Never Had to Fight Like This
Even when I was in the Navy at war against Libya, I never had to fight like this.

Today I am a proud Black father who is loved by a little person that the world tells me to call, *my daughter.* Together we co-host my television show. I read poetry to her, and pry her off of me when it's time to go to school because she doesn't want to leave her daddy. I cook for her and feed her snacks as she smiles and pretends she's going to bite me. I take her to church every Sunday. We skate, swim, run, shop, pray and play together until we fall out.

I don't hate my daughter's mother. In fact, I love her! *Why?* She is a Black woman, and is still my daughter's mother. I am a Christian, and last but not least, she made me value fatherhood and cherish it even more because of the pain I've endured.

Even when I was in the Navy at war against Libya, I never had to fight like this. I'm not glad that this drama happened, but we're both parents and always will be. Based on the end result, it was a good experience for me.

Bottom line is that I am able to enjoy having my daughter in my arms because I didn't give up. I hung in there and WON! Not only for me, but for fathers all around the world who really want the role, and seek to nurture and raise their children.

My name is Terry Moore. This is my story, and it will be until, as my father did a few years ago ... I take my last breath.

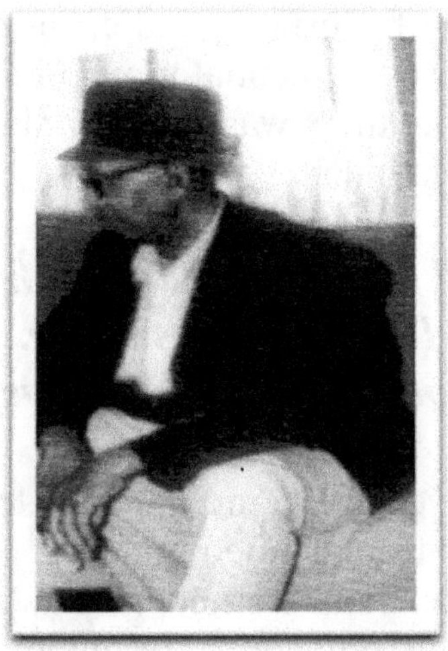

Author's father and role model.

A Portrait of Perseverance

Joean Wright
(as told to Joslyn Gaines Vanderpool)

An Uneasy Road
My story, my life have not been an easy road.

Terre Haute, Indiana is where I grew up in a two-story house. I have six siblings, all older than me, except for a baby sister. Those are the simple facts; however, my story, as my life have not been an easy road. Complications, devastating heartaches, and tragedy have been pervasive; but there was also beauty and examples of integrity, strength, love and perseverance against the greatest obstacles.

My experiences, though sometimes tragic, have made me a strong Black woman of substance and endurance. For that, I credit my late father, who was influential to who I am. I don't know how he did what he did, but there was no other alternative than to do so because he loved us so much.

As sorrow and grief lay heavy on his heart, he raised us, working 8-10 hour shifts a day. When he came home he cooked, cleaned and dispensed love.

In my formative years my mother took care of us and maintained the home front, while my father, who had no more than a second grade education, worked as a well known contractor around town with the skills to build anything from houses and major buildings to funeral homes. His other profession was as a reverend.

My father was born in Arkansas, and had straight hair, hazel eyes and looked as if he was partly Native American, but, he definitely was a strong Black man, who was always there for us. Daddy was so serious about our well-being that he carried a secret to his grave that was too powerful to reveal. It had something to do with the government stripping him of his birthright and real name. He stayed true to his word and never elaborated on the details. My father would only divulge that it was best not to say anything because *he wanted to protect his family at all costs.*

<u>Tragedy for Two Little Girls, and a Daddy Too</u>
"She's in God's hands now."

When my mother was pregnant with my little sister, the doctors had to take the baby early because my mother was dying and she knew it. While on her death bed she told me, "Take care of your baby sister and your daddy. Never split up." Even though I was only 12 years old, I was determined to honor my Mama's wish.

"I'm going to do that, Mama," I said, trying hard to hold back tears. I never wanted her to see me cry, so I'd go outside on the back porch and weep alone. Shortly thereafter, when my sister was just a new born, my mother passed away from breast cancer.

With tears rolling down his face, my father grieved for Mama, saying, "She's in God's hands now." Then he vowed that he'd always be there for me and my baby sister. And Daddy was. He didn't allow any women in our home over his kids. As sorrow and grief lay heavy on his heart, he raised us, working 8-10 hour shifts a day. When he came home he cooked, cleaned and dispensed love.

Daddy tried to maintain as normal a life for us as possible. On Sundays we went to church as a family. However, I'll strongly reiterate that ours wasn't an easy road. I didn't mention that my baby sister struggled with some severe medical conditions. Little Melody was deaf and developmentally handicapped, but that didn't change our love for her or Daddy's desire to nurture and do the best he could for us. We were always his first priority until I was 17, and my life was upended again.

Another Door Closes
I was his "Muffin," and loved him so much because he was a great dad.

For five years after my mother's death, it was Daddy, me and my little sister. All of my other siblings had their own lives; so it was just the three of us surviving together. Through it all, Daddy remained a single father, never remarrying.

My whole world collapsed when my father died of a stroke in his sleep. I was his "Muffin," and loved him so much because he was a great dad. I would have to navigate through life without my beloved father.

I had sole responsibility for taking care of Melody. Where once there had been three, now it was two. In essence, we were all alone. Although I was still a teenager on the verge of womanhood, it was apparent that I would never have a childhood.

Just the Two of Us, and the Lessons Daddy Imparted
After my father's death I wasn't going to let anybody split us up; so the only person who knew about our situation was my best friend.

Without my parents guidance, I would have to remember the lessons and skills I was taught, because the circumstances I faced would require all that I was, and all that I had, in order for me and my baby sister to make it.

I never forgot what my mother said on her death bed and worked hard to raise my sister as if she was my own, but I knew in my heart that she always had a yearning for our mother. Even though I tried to fill the role, I was not even an adult myself.

After my father's death I wasn't going to let anybody split us up; so the only person who knew about our situation was my best friend. There was no social worker, or court intervention to separate or make Melody and I wards of the state.

In order to survive I went to work, received welfare, and immediately applied for my father's Social Security and Veteran's benefits for my sister. When I was told I was eligible too, I didn't care about myself, only that Melody was taken care of.

My efforts drew praise from officials at the VA and Social Security office, but I still had work to do. Undaunted, I went to court to seek help in getting an operation for my little sister to improve her hearing and speech problems. When I stood before the judge to request the medical treatment Melody needed, he was impressed by my level of maturity and my love for my sister. But to me, it was about family. Nothing could stop me from doing what my parents would have done if they were in my shoes.

Today Melody is doing fine. She has a job and a life of her own. As my mother had hoped, we stayed together by maintaining the same determination and faith as my father, whose singular mission had always been to "protect us at all costs." My journey of heartache and triumph continues, but like my Dad, I am a portrait of perseverance.

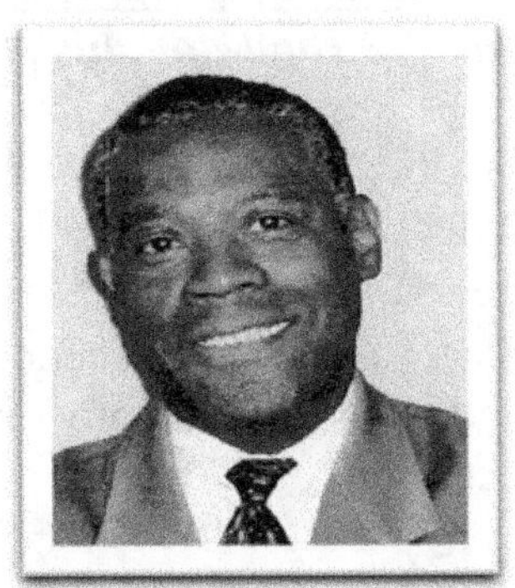

*Author's father, an **African American**
first, Mr. Terry Lee Williams.*

M y Father, My Everything

Allison Anderson

It's a Good Life
***Since Alzheimer's disease runs on my father's side of the
family, I hope it passes us by because he's lived a good life and it
would be horrible if he forgets a minute of it.***

My dad just got back from Tibet on Tuesday. He's always
going to far away places and coming back with wonderful tales
about his journey. Being that he is so descriptive my Dad can
always tell of some major risk taking adventure. I don't see how he
remembers it all. Since Alzheimer's disease runs on my father's
side of the family, I hope it passes us by because he's lived a good
life and it would be horrible if he forgets a minute of it.

<u>Daddy's Shadow</u>
I was his road-dog, his shadow.

My parents divorced when I was a year old. I lived with my daddy until I got married in 1991 and returned for a while after I divorced in 2000. I grew up in a home of love, and can't remember a time when Daddy hasn't been there to encourage me, and tell me how I make him proud. His love has covered me in security and wrapped me in comfort.

I can't remember ever missing a mother because my father's been all that I've ever wanted or needed.

I kid about it a lot, but I truly believe my dad wanted a boy because I didn't play with Barbie dolls, Easy Bake ovens, or stuffed animals. Occasionally I wore ribbons and bows, but mostly I had a softball mitt, a bat, jeans, Chuck Taylor's, marbles, footballs and soccer balls. I hung out with my dad and his friends on camping, fishing, hiking, skiing and road trips. I'd play pick-up softball games with them on Sundays. I also helped change brakes on my dad's three Karmann Ghias. I was his road-dog, his shadow.

<u>Don't be a Spectator…Be a Player</u>
With the philosophy that life is to be lived, not watched from the sidelines, my Dad's mantra is …"Don't be a spectator in life...be a player."

I was born on an Indian reservation in Utah where my father raised me while holding a part-time job and attending Weber State to pursue a degree in Political Science. At 21, Daddy was a young Black father who had sole custody of a small child.

In a sense, we grew up together. So I experienced a lot of things he probably would have never exposed me to had he been older. Every journey Daddy went on, I experienced too. With the philosophy that life is to be lived, not watched from the sidelines, my dad's mantra is …"Don't be a spectator in life...be a player."

When it came to me, Daddy was a little excessive, but his was a learning experience. Although he had nine brothers and sisters, Daddy counted on no one when it came to my well-being. Thus, he never worked far from where I attended school because he wanted to be there should anything ever happen.

My Daddy: An African American First
In high school I was surprised to open a history book and see my dad's name in black and white.

I never really understood the hype behind being Terry Lee William's daughter. He was just my daddy, my protector, and now my best friend. It wasn't until I was a young adult that I saw him as something more than just my play-partner, pain reliever, money tree, and boo-boo fixer. He was a part of history.

In high school I was surprised to open a history book and see my dad's name in black in white. Granted, it was just a paragraph or two, but who opens a history book in class and reads about their living father?

Heavily into politics, my father was committed to the making of laws, righting injustices to those in need, and advocating for his revolutionary ideas to be implemented. In 1982, my father won an historic election in which he became the first African American member of the Utah State Senate. This achievement marked the first and highest ranking of an African American to an elected position in the state. My father sponsored social justice legislation, including the bill creating the Martin Luther King Jr. State Holiday.

He's All I Ever Needed
Someone once asked me why I don't talk about my mother. My response was I don't have a story to tell.

From my first words and first steps, to my marriage, my divorce, and even now, my father has always been there for me. I received an email from him this morning letting me know that he enjoyed his trip and can't wait to visit me again.

Someone once asked me why I don't talk about my mother. My response was I don't have a story to tell. All of my Mother's Day accolades have always gone to the only mother I have... my father. We have this relationship that could never be explained. I can't remember ever missing a mother because my father's been all that I've ever wanted or needed. His love has covered me in security and wrapped me in comfort. I have always been proud of him, and proud to be his daughter.

<u>Better Than the Best</u>
I most remember my father's love for me.

Memories of my father are abundant. He did so much for me, from holding my little hands and letting me dance on his feet to appreciating my art projects. Everything I learned like riding a bike, making my bed, or ironing shirts, Daddy was there to lovingly teach me. I remember him in the park, looking up at the sky while listening to my girlish seven year old chatter; and stopping at a mountain roadside to let me pick wild flowers.

My father was there in the delivery room, and babysat my oldest son. He picked me up in the middle of the night after an argument with my husband. When we divorced, Daddy was there to tell me that, "There is a reason for everything," and "Stay true to yourself."

I sit here today remembering the things Daddy believes in, and where he came from. I envision the way he plays piano flourishes at the beginning of a song, his baritone singing voice, his kindness, the way he runs his hands through his hair when he's tired, or calmly explains that "yelling," isn't necessary to make a point.

When I first moved to New York City, I expressed to my father that maybe I had made a horrible mistake. I didn't believe that I could possibly possess the courage or strength to live 3000 miles away from everything and everyone I had ever known.

My dad words were so empowering, that I had to re-read them.

"There is no way that it could be a 'wrong' decision. God may have brought you to NY to take you to Carolina, or NY may be your home - only you can plumb the depths of your inner person to discern the voice that leads you. Decisions are not financial, political, or cultural - they are always spiritual at their core. Of course, ANY decision you make will be successful if you fully commit to throwing your heart and soul into the venture. I am a witness that the Universe honors any intentional decision and rises up to be a partner in your ambitions."

When he visited for Father's Day, I remember Daddy's hug and being so happy to be around him and sad to see him go. Most memorable about my father is the love he has for me. He is better than the best and more than that! My father is everything that could be, would be, and is.

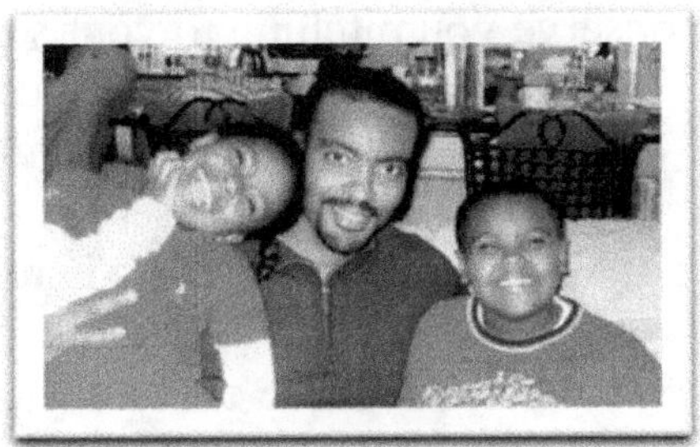

Happy family: Father, James center, with Pumpkin on the left and Ro on the right.

All the Little Things

To James, The Man I Love

Jeanine Lewis

I am fortunate to know a father who isn't afraid to show love to his children. "James, your job is extremely difficult and as much as you worry, they are going to be fine and I am here to help you as I observe all the things you do."

It's the little things that I observe you do --
you do right by your children
At every practice, during every recital,
cheering at every game,
I observe you there
No court papers, no judge, or jury
tells you when to be there, but you are
I observe you buying all the necessities
for your Pumpkin

She will remember one day
I observe you pitching to your son, Ro
He will be a great man one day
They are better people because
of the father I observe
It never occurs to you the heroics
I observe you do, but heroism is
what I observe every day,
every day I observe you
I observe how you listen
You know all their friends
(and their parents)
their interests, their allergies,
and their teachers
You know when their tests and what
projects are due
I observe all the hugs, all the kisses,
and all the love you generously
bestow on them
They will remember the little things
You ask, "who loves you?"
Pumpkin enthusiastically replies,
"Daddy loves me!"
You ask, "Every day?"
And she says "All day!"
I observe traditions that
will stay with them always
I observe you teach Ro
honor and integrity
The private talks you have while
we are in the park
The sideline coaching you do
while at football practice,
The pep talks before school begins,
I observe how your bond
will eventually shape him as a man

I am proud of what I observe,
when I observe you
I observe you going through
flash cards of math problems
I observe you making your famous baked chicken
and watching their faces light up with delight!
As we pray over the meal
you have prepared,
I observe you holding their hands
and hoping their lives will be better
Separation is hard,
but you make loving your children look easy
I observe your dedication in letting your children know
that you are there for them
They have not lost a father,
but inherited another home
I observe hardships you face
being such an involved parent
This is truly a man's work
You are an exemplary example
of a full time father
I observe you
You are there when they are hurting
You are there rain or shine
I observe you there,
doing all the little things,
each and every time

Songs and Sonnets for My Father

The Secret of Hollows

In Memory of Those Who Perished

Joslyn Gaines Vanderpool

Listening beneath the cricket's wing, the moans of Black women
rise up from the massive bowels of the Mississippi,
the broad muddy orifice stirring gently with black blood
and hardship to form a watery grave for their fathers, sons,
husbands...stolen away, away in the grip of mid-summer nights
at the height of their splendor, nights fractured by the putrid scent
of hatred for those, Black like us

Through the mask of southern gentility, death drips venomously
from the succulent nectar of magnolia trees with ancient limbs
bent from Black bodies dangling --

And I can still feel my father's quiet rage amassing like a firestorm,
scorching fields across Georgia with tens of thousands of
Black men, tired vessels -- worn from cotton, public humiliation,
Jim Crow degradation, rolling out of the mouths of those entrapped
in their family's legacy of hate

Some men perished -- as all things black, eventually do,
but voices linger, whispering secrets of our beloved's demise --
secrets singeing the stillness of hollows, open to retrieve
them and scatter truths, just as days of judgement are
set to arrive...

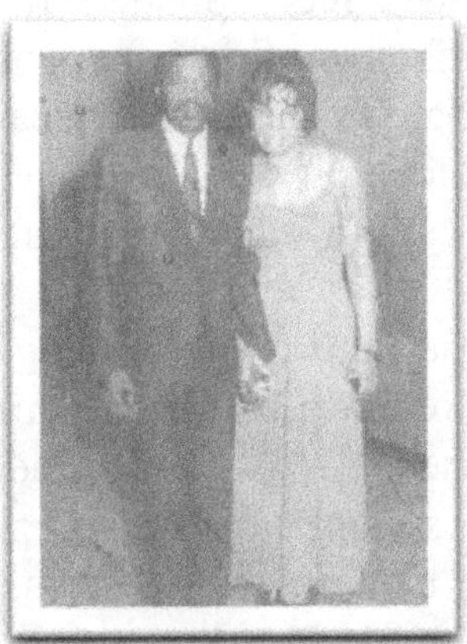

Author's parents, Mr. and Mrs. Art Williams.

A Love Letter to My Father

Rod Williams

As I told you before you went to Heaven, "every day I live, the more I appreciate, admire and am in awe of what you did – particularly for a Black man during the '60s and '70s."

I love you Dad, and I wanted to write to thank-you for the many wonderful things you did – particularly your outstanding daily display of manhood and wisdom.

Thank you for getting up every morning well before daylight to go and provide for your family. Your care, concern, and watchful eye were felt and touched every aspect of my life. As I told you before you went on to Heaven, "everyday I live, the more I appreciate, admire and am in awe of what you did – particularly for a Black man during the '60s and '70s."

I'll never forget your support or the fact that you never settled for what had already been accomplished. Instead you pushed me to the next level. I remember my first paper route and how you got up before dawn on Sunday to drive me because the paper was too heavy for my bike. Since you were still tired from the previous six days of work, we almost ran into a tree when you fell asleep at the wheel.

How can I forget the time while playing football when I busted my head on the concrete walk way. I remember your saltshaker shoes never touched the steps as you leaped from the porch, glided to where I was laying, scooped me up and rushed me to the nearest hospital. You had to be concerned when the motorcycle police officer pulled you over for speeding (particularly since the Watts riot started with a police officer pulling over a motorist not too far from where we were). Instead of a riot, the officer provided a police escort to the hospital.

As I became a father, I always remembered the smile on the faces of my children when they saw you because they knew you would walk them to the candy store. As was your style and your signature move, you gave them a lot more than sweets, you included a good dose of wisdom too.

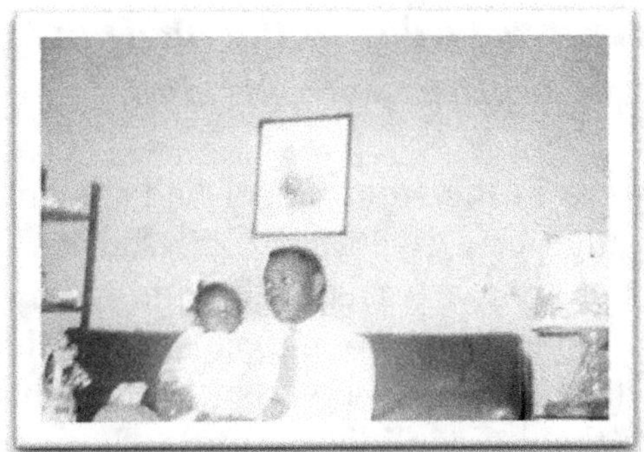

Author with her April Love and father, Mr. Morris Lee Gaines.

April Love

Francene Weatherspoon

<u>The Trip that Almost Never Was</u>
I could barely see through the front window for the rain.
To me, it seemed like the sky was crying.

Although it was fifty years ago, I remember it as though it were yesterday….the beginning of my love affair with my dad.

It was almost the trip that *never was*. I wanted to go with Daddy to take my favorite uncle to the train station. Mom had said earlier that day, "It's raining cats and dogs." So she really tried to get me to stay home but with Dad's coaxing and my insistence that I wouldn't catch a cold if she'd just let me go, Mom couldn't help but relent. So on that cold and rainy day in December 1957 my dad, uncle, and I piled into our big Buick.

***Although it was fifty years ago, I remember it as
though it were yesterday….the beginning of my love
affair with my dad.***

The men were in the front, and I had the entire back seat to
myself. It was huge to a five year old. Dad had warmed up the
engine so it was pretty toasty inside. I could barely see through the
front window for the rain. To me, it seemed like the sky was
crying. The rhythm of the wipers kept time with the crooning of
the balladeer on the radio, sliding effortlessly over the front glass
from opposite ends of the window toward the metal strip in the
center. The wipers temporarily stopped and then on some unknown
signal, started their rotation all over again.

Unforgettable Melody, Unforgettable Memory
***I was focused on the song on the radio. It was something
about "April love being for the very young and a wishing star."***

I don't really remember the details of the murmured adult
conversation. I was focused on the song on the radio. It was
something about "April love being for the very young and a
wishing star." I still remember parts of the melody. It was a
beautiful song. Years later I discovered that it was a number one
hit for Pat Boone in December 1957.

Before long, we reached our destination. My handsome Uncle
Junior was sharp in his uniform as a member of the United States
Army. He kissed me, shook hands with my dad, gathered his bags
and got out of the car in the rain! Somehow the closing of the car
door brought the song to an end.

At Last…Just Daddy and Me
***Instinctively, I knew that anytime I was with my dad I was
safe.***

"Do you want to ride in the front seat?" Dad asked.

At last it was my opportunity. I finally had my dad all to myself. So I lumbered over the top of the seat from the back, plopping down squarely in the front beside him. My big, handsome dad always smelled good; not in a *perfumy* way; but crisp and clean. He sat so tall in the driver's seat. Instinctively, I knew that anytime I was with my dad I was safe.

I could hear the swish of the water beneath our tires as Daddy navigated our big car through those rainy streets. He and I talked about whatever a five year old could think of, which included thousands of questions. But, whatever the conversation, as many years have passed, it tickled my daddy and made him laugh.

My daddy was my *April Love,* and though like the song, he's "slipped right through my fingers," leaving to join the angels…he's never left my heart.

I love you Daddy.

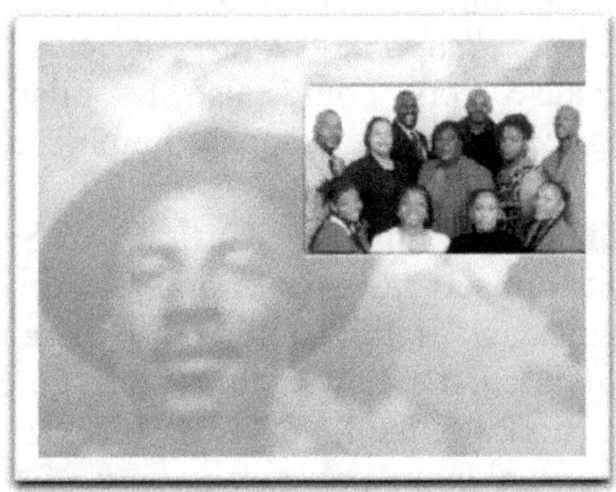

Family patriarch Mr. Curtis Coats Sr. with the Coats Singers inset.

A Man of Quiet Determination

Theris Coats

From the Fields of East Texas to the California Coast
There were no jobs to speak of in the rural areas of Texas farmlands. The dream of employment in the shipyards of California that supported the WWII war effort, beckoned.

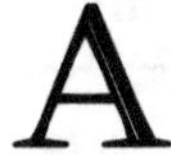here is a contemporary piece of jazz music that came to mind as I sat down to attempt creating this narrative. The song is a tune that began with the floating melody and lyrics, "If there was ever a man who was generous, gracious, and good," and was titled: *Song for My Father.*

During our years growing up with a stern, authoritative disciplinarian, my father often taught lessons of practicality and common sense, versus having fun and chasing after the things of childhood. He also was somewhat demanding in enforcing education, work ethics, and a dedicated adherence to religious principles.

As one of 16 siblings, I was not alone in sometimes seeing our dad, or *Pops, as we called him,* as overly serious. Not that his love wasn't felt, because Pops could also be hilariously amusing, extremely caring, concerned, graciously humble, and wise beyond imagining.

A man of quiet determination, Curtis Coats Sr., who was born in 1914, taught himself to speak and read several different languages (Spanish and Italian) with only the aid of books and recorded tape instructions. It was that same quiet determination that led my father to leave the fields of East Texas in the early '40s in pursuit of a better, more prosperous way of life for his wife, Gradie and their growing family of then, five children.

There were no jobs to speak of in the rural areas of Texas farmlands. The dream of employment in the shipyards of California that supported the WWII war effort, beckoned. Pops succeeded in moving the family to San Francisco, California and securing one of those jobs. Once again, it was quiet determination, nurturing guidance, and spiritual direction that my father used to instruct and motivate the family.

<u>The Locomotive That Could</u>

Slowly, cautiously he creeps along in great anticipation of the open track through the countryside where he opens the throttle, and delights in the unencumbered progression of his charge.

Looking back now, memories of my father's will and his way creates a picture that I can best describe as being like a locomotive pulling a long line of loaded box cars through a town crossing. Slowly, cautiously, he creeps along in great anticipation of the open track through the countryside, where he opens the throttle, and delights in the unencumbered progression of his charge.

If asked what emotion I most feel when my heart embraces the memory of my dad, I can truly say, above the missing, and the ache of loss, I feel pride.

After the shipyards, my father was employed at the San Francisco education department, while nurturing his rather large family, which grew to include an astounding nine sons and eight daughters. Still Pops found the time and energy to go about establishing congregations of the Church of Christ in the San Francisco Bay Area; a ministerial work that he continued well after his retirement from the secular workforce. During this time, he helped form The Coats Singers in 1969, a gospel group that recorded two records. The latest album is titled, *Our Father's Dream*.

Eventually, failing health dictated a throttling back of the old, worn locomotive heart. My father's years of working in the shipyards contributed to his death in 1982 of asbestos poisoning.

To all who were blessed to have shared his presence, I think if they were asked the question, "What characteristic would most describe this Black father, this husband, this man of God, this person whose intelligence was far greater than what one would expect to encounter in someone whose formal education did not continue much past high school?" I believe that most would simply say, *humility*.

If asked what emotion I most feel when my heart embraces the memory of my dad, I can truly say, above the missing, and the ache of loss, I feel pride. Pride in the fact that, as the song goes; "If there was ever a man who was generous, gracious, and good," it was my dad -- the Man!

<u>A Grandchild Remembers</u>
"Growing up in a large family, favoritism really can't be avoided, but I remember him never making any one kid more special than the other...."

Dad had 54 grandchildren and one remembers him, *"preaching forcefully and sometimes humorously with props, charts, and funny stories. I remember his singing voice was strong and when I sat next to him I could almost feel it. I remember waiting patiently to get the last sip of his coffee or him piling my mother and all of us in his car to give us a ride home after night service.*

Okay, I remember when we got locked in the fenced area at the Uptown Church of Christ and we all had to jump over the fence; even Grandmother. I think you were there too Uncle Theris. Anyway, Grandmother and me were telling Granddaddy how we had to climb the fence, and he said, "You too, Gradie?"

"Yeah," she said.

"It's a wonder the fence didn't break," and she was so mad, but she couldn't help but laugh. That was funny too.

Growing up in a large family, favoritism really can't be avoided, but I remember him never making any one kid more special than the other. We all got tickled, we all got our socks taken off and our feet bitten, even when we ran through the house screaming. Now that I think about it, he's like all of you (uncles) wrapped up in one."

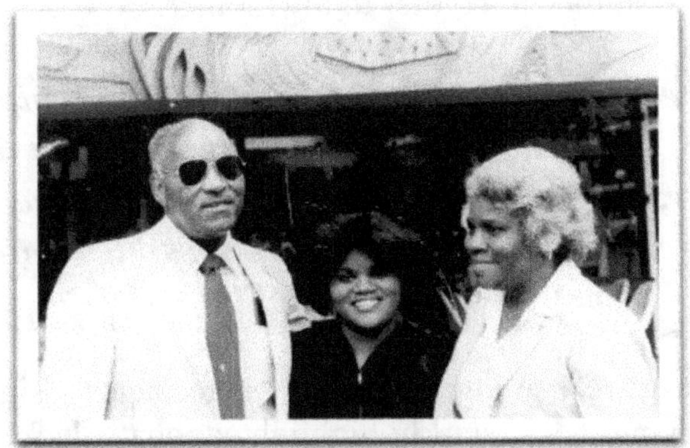

Author center with parents, Mr. and Mrs. Morris L. Gaines.
Graduation UC Berkeley, June 1982.

Beautiful Just Beautiful

A Memoir of Love for my Father

Joslyn Gaines Vanderpool

<u>Farewell Sweet Prince</u>
Before my father's death, preparations were already in place
for his funeral.

Brilliant sunlight flooded the Georgia sky on a clear April afternoon in 2002. The sound of crackling gun fire rang out resoundingly, landing against a few wispy clouds. The marksmen aimed their rifles toward the heavens each time they heard the command, "Pull!"

Before the gun salute, a military detail surrounded my father's flag draped coffin. Moving in sync, they lifted it to a place of prominence. When the service was near the end, the flag was folded in perfect angles with pinpoint precision before it was passed from soldier-to-soldier to my mother.

Eventually, my father gained friendships from soldiers of all hues, most critically in Korea during the war, where the color of a man's skin became inconsequential in the face of possible death on the battle field.

As we were leaving, an unknown teenager's singular action was so moving that it starkly highlighted what Black men like my father had been missing, but so much deserved. It was something my father would have done himself: pay homage to the life of a Black man.

Grazing his brow with his fingertips in a solid, dignified salute, the young man stood solemnly holding his tribute well after my father's coffin was lowered into the red earth of the once segregated cemetery, just a few blocks where he ascended seven plus decades before. The acknowledgement was an enormous gift for my father, a man of faith, distinction and honor.

Before my father's death, preparations were in place for his funeral. The elegant black suit that hung behind my mother's bedroom door was tailored to grace his six-foot frame; the tie, adorned with African flourishes of gold, was dignified, befitting a king. The honor guard at Moody Air Force Base had been contacted and the obituary was nearly completed.

Only weeks before Daddy's death, word came through a thin, firm whisper over the phone, "I think you better come. The doctors don't think your father is going to make it."

"Okay, Mama. I'll be there," I replied hesitantly – unnerved that a significant loss was eminent.

It Was a Wonderful Life
This time we knew that our Dad's journey to Heaven was destined.

The tone of the brief conversation with my mother was hauntingly similar to one we had eight years earlier when we feared it might be Daddy's last Christmas. Our entire family, including my sister, our husbands and my two nephews traveled across the country in 1994 for a most treasured gathering. Although Dad usually tipped the scale at a solid 200 pounds, he was alarmingly frail, but still filled with incredible optimism.

We took walks with Dad in his lovely neighborhood of large homes and sprawling lawns that were light years away from the small shotgun house he grew up in. Daddy tried his best to move in his confident stride.

In subsequent days we put on our Sunday best for a final family portrait. And that Christmas Eve we all watched *It's a Wonderful Life*. Daddy provided lively commentary on actors he remembered from afternoons spent in the *Colored* section of the Albany movie theater back in the '30s and '40s. Everything about the visit was *wonderful* except the pall that hung over us.

When everyone was asleep, my sister and I held hands and cried in front of the fireplace, certain that our beloved daddy – the first man that had ever loved us, was leaving us. Miraculously; however, he survived for eight more years before Mama's fateful call. This time we knew Dad's journey to Heaven was destined. There would be no more miracles. So we quietly prayed for him to be released from his pain, and began the grieving process.

The Last Reunion
*As we encircled Dad in the tiny room of the nursing home,
it would be just us again; our tiny circle reunited.*

When my sister and I arrived in Georgia for our final visit with our father, we cherished our special time together. As we encircled Dad in the tiny room of his nursing home, it would be just us again; a re-creation of our little nuclear family that began in 1959 – Daddy and his three girls: Mama, Fran and I. Or as Daddy would say, "Ruthie J., Prima Donna and Jozzie Baby," his respective nicknames for us.

This homecoming would be different. Our father's wide wonderful smile drooped; his eyes, which had always been alight with hope, harbored little, just a small flicker of light shone for a few minutes when he saw us enter the room. His once jubilant spirit revealed that he had taken many emotional journeys with his illness and had grown weary.

A series of strokes had diminished Daddy's ability to speak fluidly. So what he couldn't say in words, came through the cores of his beautiful, deep brown eyes which conveyed *he was really ecstatic to see us, but he was tired. They further revealed that he didn't want to leave because he loved us. Although he promised to be there if we needed him, the decision was out of his hands. It was time to exit and he was going to miss us more than life itself.*

As I stepped deeper into the room, I hugged my father tightly, savoring being in his presence. Despite trying mightily to sit up at attention, which was customary of a military man, our mighty fortress was slumped in his chair with a fuzzy stuffed rabbit and pillows anchoring his fragile body. He knew, we all knew, that this would be our last official time together on earth.

Daddy's smile returned when we sang, *My Guy, Mr. Sandman, "In the sweet by and by, we shall meet at the beautiful shore...., and amazing grace how sweet the sound,"* words his once melodic voice carried with velvety richness and clarity.

My sister and I rubbed Dad's tired hands – hands that had guided us on our first bike rides, held us through disappointments, and embraced us when we were triumphant.

I'd never seen my father cry, but his eyes teared up because we were saying good-bye. This meeting signified that he wouldn't be there like he always had been. Since Daddy couldn't stay with us, he tried valiantly to stay strong for us to the very end.

Imagining the Possibilities of Our Promise
*He was unequivocally the most positive
man I have ever met.*

Senegalese in size, height, nobility and gait, my father entered the world through the assured hands of Easter Green, a midwife who delivered Black babies, including my mother in a corner of southwest Georgia in the 1920s because the only hospital in town was designated for White patrons. Arriving on May 19, 1927, two days before Charles Lindbergh made his transatlantic flight, Daddy would have a few challenges.

Shortly after giving birth, my dad's mother succumbed to an unknown illness. Dad was fatherless by default, but never displayed any ill-will toward the man he saw only occasionally. So it was a team of loving aunts that doted on him, and a young woman named, Lula that would adopt him as her son and cherish him for a lifetime.

Although Daddy's was an uncertain beginning, he didn't allow anything to negate his ascent. He was unequivocally the most positive man I have ever met. He never stopped encouraging my sister and me to dream and imagine the possibilities of our promise, as he had as a young boy playing stickball and hoping for a shot with the Negro Baseball Leagues.

Despite Jim Crow mandates, the Great Depression, the second World War and other hardships, my parents carved out a secure existence of cultural pride, educational achievement, love, and faith that they bestowed on their daughters like rivulets of gold, making us the women that we are today.

Dad had a razor sharp mind, finishing high school early at 16. Afterward, due to limited opportunities he worked in a factory doing mindless work in Detroit before attending Albany State. Realizing that his dream to become a dentist was too distant to secure, and certain the military would draft him anyway, he completed two years of college and enlisted in the segregated United States Army Air Corps in 1946. Two years later the military was integrated. Being a first, he and other men of his race, were the unsung Jackie Robinsons who had to endure the onslaught of racial attacks and slurs.

Eventually, my father gained friendships from soldiers of all hues, most critically in Korea during the war, where the color of a man's skin became inconsequential in the face of possible death on the battle field.

Never one to complain, Daddy always gravitated toward what was positive. What he recalled about his experience during those years was the kindness of the Korean people he met as well as the natural beauty of the exotic country. Seeing the whole picture was the hallmark of my father. He unfailingly related to the incredible depth of the human spirit, regardless of race, creed, Nationality or color. Sometimes I wondered how he stayed so collected in the face of inequities that were always on the horizon, but he did ....well, for the most part, anyway.

The Day When All Hell Broke Loose
He had always handled difficult situations with diplomacy, but a line had been crossed, and he was still a man after all; and a very decent one at that.

Dad taught my sister and I about acceptance, but it wasn't in the mere words he spoke. It was through his actions that he demonstrated his respect for others. That's why what happened when he was 23, was a story for the ages; a real shocker that was so explosive that I didn't learn about it until I was in my mid-twenties.

In June 1950, my parents were newly married, and primed for a long and happy union that would last nearly 52 years. Dad had been in the service for about five years and my mother had just received a bachelor's degree from Albany State. Everything was idyllic until the day when all hell literally broke loose at the local Department of Motor Vehicles where my father had taken my Uncle Jesse to get his license.

After waiting outside patiently for hours to be called, my father and uncle, both in military dress, quietly witnessed White patrons being served who had arrived well after them. Consequently my father respectfully walked inside, removed his cap and asked the trooper manning the counter, "Excuse me sir, when will it be our turn? We've been waiting a long time."

"Get outta here, *Nigger*!!!" the trooper retorted, red faced and seething with anger. The words did not sit well with a man who was serving his country and had been inundated with inexplicable hatred since birth. Thus, Dad's reaction was swift and sure. With the full magnitude of twenty plus years of racial distress roiling inside of him, my father sent the trooper reeling, unleashing a solid punch that knocked him back.

Daddy always handled difficult situations with diplomacy, but a line had been crossed, and he was still a man after all; and a very decent one at that. No matter, Daddy was whisked to jail in 1950s Georgia -- his fate unknown.

Uncle Jesse caught a cab to tell Daddy's frightened bride about what happened. Mom refused to enter that jail, and stood outside beneath my father's cell as he explained, "I even took off my hat in respect, and still was treated that way."

My mom feared that my father would be stripped of his military career, and worse, his life. The family scrambled to find help, but the NAACP couldn't assist; so they turned to a White friend of the family whose son was a lawyer. Daddy was freed right away, the trooper was relieved of his duties, and the memory of that day was stowed away for decades.

The incident and how Daddy dealt with it gave me more insight into the complexities that made up my father. Nothing could diminish the love I had for him. I was proud of him, and he still was beautiful and totally whole to me.

<u>Threescore and 10</u>
Even though I was unfamiliar with the ninetieth Psalms, verse 10, or what threescore and 10 meant, I clearly knew that my father was reflecting about his mortality.

When my father reached his seventieth spring, he quietly proclaimed that, "I'm threescore and 10. Do you know what that means?"

Even though I was unfamiliar with the ninetieth Psalms, verse 10, or what threescore and 10 meant, I clearly knew that my father was reflecting about his mortality. In looking up the verse the other day for this memoir, I saw that my father had written it on the fourth page of his Bible. *"The days of our years are threescore years and ten; and if by reason of strength they be fourscore years, yet is their strength, labor and sorrow; for it is soon cut off, and we fly away."* And so it came to past. Almost five years after reaching that significant milestone, Daddy flew away.

A Man of His Generation
One's character and moral fabric stood for something.

Dad belonged to what has been termed the *Greatest Generation*. To him, a man's word was his bond. A firm handshake and direct eye contact was good enough. One's character and moral fabric stood for something. Daddy used phrases like, "That's just swell," and loved Glen Miller, Nate King Cole, Carmen McCrae and Charlie Byrd Parker.

My father was also new-age in his way of thinking – sensitive and gentle. He never mindlessly followed anyone, but loved life and was an exuberant participant in the wonder of it all.

Time spent with Dad was memorable. My sister and I basked in the warmth of our father's essence when he took us on drives. The aviator sunglasses he wore were *oh so cool. Oh so California.* With his long arm draped over the steering wheel and whistling *A Theme to a Summer Place*, he gave his signature wave of two-fingers to anyone he passed. Sometimes he would pick up a soldier who needed a lift. Everything felt so safe and secure back then.

If my sister and I begged Daddy for ice cream, we would inevitably get it. He was just that kind of father. Fun, easy-going and firm, he also was a patient teacher. When I couldn't hit the ball in fourth grade, Daddy worked with me until I was the only girl on the boy's team – becoming team captain, and a power hitter who could slam homers with ease and catch anything in left field.

<u>He Was Beautiful</u>
I dream like he dreamt by believing in the possibilities.

I could discuss almost anything with Daddy. Our heart-to-hearts were special because he genuinely cared, and always listened. Through the years we discussed many topics, including racism and our hopes about when, and if it would end in our lifetimes.

My father coveted his role of being a father and a provider. Our parents were mindful of their lives during the Great Depression, and always gave us a middle-class lifestyle. When Dad couldn't find work after 20 honorable years in the service, he went to the base commander and honestly spoke about his need to take care of his family. Within minutes he had so impressed the man with his forthrightness that he was hired immediately.

"Beautiful just beautiful," was my father's favorite phrase, which he would use when he saw an act of human kindness, heard a song he loved or was inspired by God's natural works. For him, a true connection to all humankind was vital to sustaining one's own humanity, which was the principle that most impacted my life.

I miss my father's enormous heart and his incredible embrace, but he lives within me. My face is like his face. I dream like he dreamt by believing in the possibilities. My father was an embodiment of the phrase he so often used. Thus in my world, Morris Lee Gaines will always remain *beautiful just beautiful!*

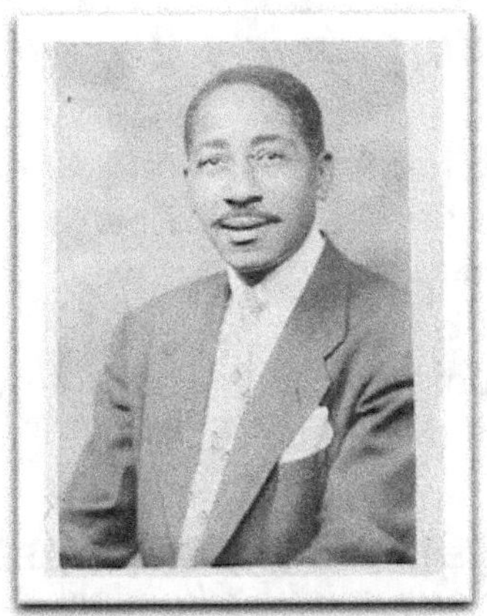

The village chief and author's father, "Buchie."

Song for My Father

Buchie's Song

Raphael Jackson

<u>Advice for a Lifetime</u>
*There was not a place that we traveled
that people of goodwill didn't know my father.*

When I heard Horace Silver's, *Song for my Father*, the music and lyrics of the song said it all for me; and for the man, I called *Dad*. It seemed that the song was written for my father, a gregarious man who was well loved in the community. There was not a place that we traveled that people of goodwill didn't know him. He was always highly spoken of. Even today when I travel or happen to meet people that knew him, he is praised as a wonderful human being.

"Your father was too good of a person to be Black.
He was a White man in a Black man's body."

When I was walking with my son one day, a neighbor said, "Your son should not be like his dad but like his grandfather." It became apparent that my father was someone of special importance in his life. Fortunately, I had the good sense to acknowledge his wisdom, because I did follow my father's every advice, for it has given me guidance, and has lasted a lifetime.

My Father… the Community Activist and Village Chief
Young men from our neighborhood who had fallen on hard times always sought the comfort, wisdom and support of my father who was influential in positively guiding lives.

During the civil rights movement, my father was active in supporting the many drives to assist the Freedom Riders and was an active member in the NAACP. In our particular neighborhood of Brooklyn, Dad also was involved in molding and shaping young men. He organized baseball teams, took all of us to events and most of all, was a leader in civic activities and the Boy Scouts.

Young men from our neighborhood who had fallen on hard times always sought the comfort, wisdom and support of my father who was influential in positively guiding lives. I remember him housing many a young man who had run afoul in their domestic affairs and needed a place to stay for the night.

Many of the immigrant parents of the Caribbean sought Dad's advice on to how to navigate their daily lives in American society in regard to their own children. If a parent refused to let their child become involved in an American activity, it took just one call to Mr. Jackson's house, and his approval mitigated centuries of cultural blockage. In hindsight, Dad was like the village chief and guide.

<u>Thank You, Father</u>

I learned that becoming a responsible person is seeing your involvement in the situation and how you are just as guilty as the one you are accusing.

Not a very talkative person, Dad abhorred foolish talk. He would always analyze conversations that lacked intelligence and foresight, and showed us how illogical the person's reasoning was. Besides his analytical abilities, another quality that my father possessed was his willingness to accept responsibility. He was not a whiner or a victim. When I came home feeling wronged or slighted he would always ask me, "What did you do to warrant this reaction?"

At the time I wanted my father to support me blindly. I wanted him to take my side without hesitation, but I learned that becoming a responsible person is seeing your involvement in the situation and how you are just as guilty as the one you are accusing. You are not totally innocent. This lesson is one of the most important I've been given in life. It has assisted me throughout my career.

At my father's funeral, of all of the praise spoken about him, one strange and bitter comment came from a relative who grew up with him.

"Your father was too good of a person to be Black. He was a White man in a Black man's body."

Years later, I came to understand the sentiments of the relative who equated goodness and kindness with persons, whom were other than Black. I know that many people still believe the mythology that Blacks are not inherently good; that if goodness emanates from a person of my ethnicity, it is a learned behavior from another group. In essence, since my dad embodied the goodness, he could not have been a Black man, according to this theory, but his grace and goodness live on, and were revealed in his many actions throughout his life.

To my father, I give thanks, because from him I learned to be a man, take responsibility for my life and my actions, and do things for myself without waiting on others' approval or assistance.

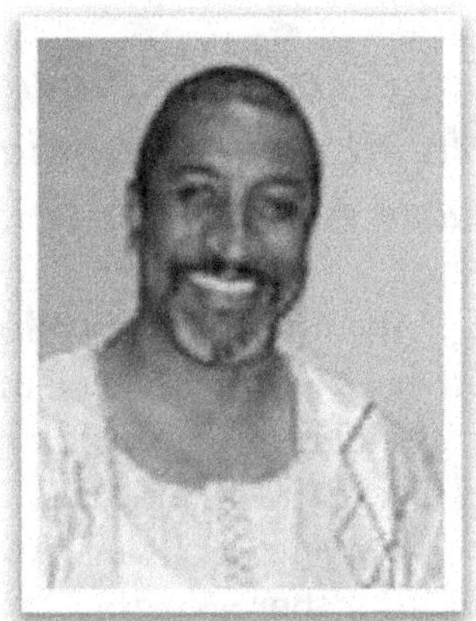

The Spirit of My Father Incarnate

Joslyn Gaines Vanderpool

I have known Jeri Marshall, for 15 years going on 16. We are teased about being a work couple, but he is more than that. Something about him reminds me of my late, great father, Morris Lee Gaines, who passed away less than a year after I started my new position. As I write this memoir, I believe I know why Jeri assumed a vaunted position in my life.

We both attained our positions as outreach specialists at a local community college at the same time, and learned that the hiring committee decided to select two candidates, instead of the one position that was originally advertised. When I have been uncertain, Jeri has been the strategist, and I suppose I have done the same, acting as his compass from time-to-time. Due to who we are, both of us have a lot of individuals who come to us for advice, support, and affirmation. We often talk to students and individuals as a team. Promoting their essence, we assure them to

live in the light because that is what we are called to do, as well
as live life in the same way.

***Jeri loves my father, talks of him and has dreams
about him, yet, he never met him in the flesh, only
through pictures, and remembrances I share with him.***

Straight from the University of New Mexico where I was an
admissions officer and early outreach specialist, I was back at the
community college I attended in California in 1977, but now as a
member of the staff. I heard from Jeri, that there was buzz about
me, the woman from New Mexico, via Howard University, and
UC Berkeley, etc. So, there were myths and mysteries
surrounding who I was, and the same held true about Jeri, for
me. When I met him, I didn't know what to expect. Our first
impression of each other was a bit, well – rough. I saw him as an
angry black man, and he thought that I was a bit angry too, but oh
my, were we both right, but also wrong!

Over time we found that our spirits, belief systems and our
concern about those who'd entered our lives were in sync. We
were virtually in alignment with one another. Life, the value of
others, and staying true to our hearts by choosing to thrive with
purpose and joy in our journeys has been the walk we've
adopted. And knowing that, has brought a certain peace to me, as
if my own father were being channeled through Jeri, who serves
as a reminder that the spirit of Dad has never left because, Jeri
loves my father, talks of him and has dreams about him, yet, he
never met him in the flesh, only through pictures, and
remembrances I share with him.

He calls me the nicknames my father gave me like "Private
Pete", which I hadn't revealed to him. It is uncanny, but his
intuition is real and right. I know from the core that my father
lives in my heart and he planted a legacy that guides me daily,
but Jeri too, mirrors my dad's beautiful and omnipotent spirit.

Our friendship has deepened and the respect we have for one another is untouched, despite our constant and comical insults, there is an unbreakable bond. We have also had some very impassioned disagreements that have resulted in hurt and misunderstandings, but neither of us has held on to it, because the bridge of friendship that we have cultivated will not break.

On more occasion than one, we have some people really believing we are a couple because we spar so much, but it's all in fun. Jeri has revealed that I, as his friend, am a "real keeper" and to me, he will remain in my life forever too. We have faced too much together not to remain connected.

Life Altering Events Forge a Deeper Bond

Scarcely seven months into the job, life-altering events touched both of our lives. The first was the death of his beloved, Grandmother. And then, not long afterward, my father died which was cataclysmic for me. Although Jeri thought I handled his death well, it was tough because my mom, sister and dad were my world for 43 years, and my sister, Fran and I had lost the first man who had ever loved us. Undoubtedly, my father was a massive force in my development because he conducted his life with love. It was simply his way.

The following year, Jeri's brother was killed in Iraq during the war and at the time in 2003, he was the oldest soldier to die, at age 50. Very close in age, Jeri's brother Johnnie was a military man through and through, dying for what he believed in. The day before Johnnie's death, we were walking on campus when Jeri experienced a sharp, piercing pain in his back and then calf. There was no explanation for why it happened, but I witnessed it and saw him writhe in pain.

The next day I was sitting in the office and a call came in from Jeri's mother. Her voice was calm, but had a tinge of worry when I told her, Jeri was out of the office. She asked that he call home, immediately. Before he could get settled at his desk, I told him to call his mom. Information about his brother was sketchy at the time, but the next day, I saw Jeri with sunglasses on, but it was very overcast.

I lightly joked about him trying to look cool, but I knew instinctively that there was more to the story. When he uttered, "Johnnie's not coming back," we embraced as tears rolled from beneath his sunglasses.

In Jeri, after getting to know him, I saw a beautiful sensitivity, mixed with masculinity, like Dad. Raised with 3 brothers and six sisters, I can see as the middle child Jeri was used to compromise and making others content. He was the mediator and doer, often sacrificing his happiness for others.

Like my own father, Jeri has two daughters and I could see the care and passion he has for his family. His girls mean everything to him. Just like my sister and I, who meant everything to our father. Gentle, and fair, both Jeri and Dad are mighty fortresses, but you could see they were not robotic disciplinarians. Both lean in to talk to you and ask intelligent questions, but have the trademark compassion, where you know you are loved, and safe too.

They protected their children and dispensed life lasting lessons. When there was no work to be found after my father retired from the Air Force, Dad sold vacuums and did whatever he could to provide. Jeri revealed that there was a time he sold vacuums too to make ends meet. Most important they were after their children's hearts and would readjust the world for us.

A Quest to Be Alive and Free

Being free and alive was what each man loved. As I've mentioned in a previous story, my dad, gloried in life and saw beauty everywhere, and used to say, "Beautiful, just beautiful," about anything that moved him. Jeri also knows it is essential to be free, traveling, gaining experiences, pouring into, retrieving and replenishing the earth with all that you are.

The times in which my father, and Jeri's father lived, were unkind to black men – still are, but there was nowhere for them to go. No marches, no public outrage allowed, no legal remedy, only internalized pain. Lynching was condoned, slights were overt, discrimination was unchecked, *"Boy and Nigger"* were acceptable nouns and brutality was constant with no condemnation.

Despite the pain and barriers, both of our fathers pivoted to survive, but never lost who they were and made a strong mark with their families. They desperately strived to protect us, but there would be times they couldn't so they try to prepare us for what was to come. Jeri knows and relates to their struggle and grieves their heartache, as he seeks to maneuver through the heavy, suffocating cloak of racism that still persist.

Gentle but Strong

Diplomacy was my father's trademark. Always a gentleman, always coming with a sincere heart. When I was 22 in 1981, I created Appreciation books for both my mom and dad, which had been stored away in a hope chest. They were filled with my thoughts and memories about them and how much I loved them. I found a card to place in the book which was the very essence of my father: gentle, but strong, and then on another page, I wrote that I hoped to find a man in my life akin to my father. Fortunately, I did in 1987 when I married my husband Peter, who is the gentlest, kindness man I know. He too adored my father, and my father adored him. Then Jeri came along and personified many of the traits of Dad. My brother-in-law also speaks positively about my father being a great man and gentleman.

I will never forget that and the love expressed for my father with Jeri quipping, "I love the man." That sentiment continues to breathe life into me. I knew I was truly blessed.

I laugh about Jeri and how he manages his money. My father didn't mess around when it came to his money either. In truth, he would give you what he had, but not as easily as my mother, who gave without any hesitation. Jeri gives too, but doesn't like folks to be late when it comes to his MONEY!

One afternoon, I said to Jeri, "Today is my dad's birthday," as we were walking to the cafeteria to get a cup of coffee. After Jeri got his coffee, he asked for two cups of water, and balanced them back to a courtyard near our office. He said he wanted to honor my father with a ritual where we returned water to the earth. So we found a small koi pond, and stated our remembrances. I will never forget that and the love expressed for my father with Jeri quipping, "I love the man." That sentiment continues to breathe life into me. I knew I was truly blessed.

The other day, I asked Jeri about why he references and admires Dad, and he explained the similarities they have as fathers. Jeri always tells me that my father is telling him that I should listen to him, which makes me throw my head back and release a throaty laugh. Pure fiction! What I do know is they were maligned with a core of strong, opinionated women, who ran the show. All my dad, Jeri and Peter want is peace and quiet and an assurance they are important in a majority of women, but they never really win and I suspect they are not really that upset about it because they love their families.

So despite my father leaving this physical life 15 years ago, I am reminded of him through my own memories, and the admiration he still receives from others who help assure his legacy is intact by how they emulate some of his ways. They cherish the man for what he brought and left for those who knew him directly and indirectly, and oh it has been quite a lasting treasure.

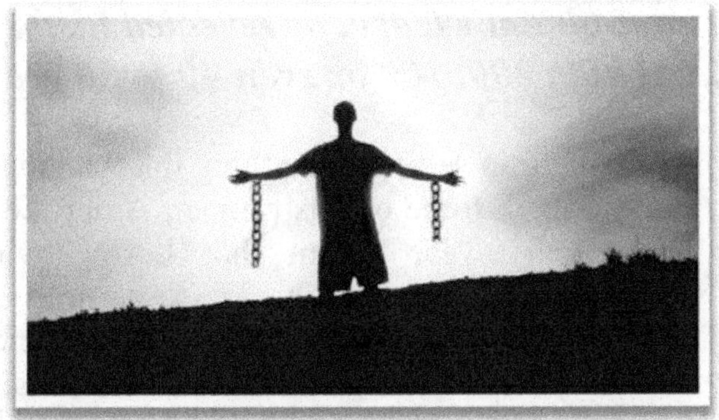

Legacy Leaving Dream — A Slave's Story on the Periphery of Revival

Joslyn Gaines Vanderpool and Vicki Sherman

I learned about Larry Sherman from his wife, Vicki, who I have worked with for several years at a local community college, where her husband was a professor. She shared that Larry was trying to bring the story of Archy Lee, who was the subject of a fugitive slave trial in California in the 1850s, to the masses through film or a documentary. What inspired Larry to get involved in film making, and particularly developing this project was his love of the story, but on a deeper level it was to let people know that the Civil War was alive and well in California and he was fervently determined to reveal that Archy was a 19-year-old political pawn whose struggle went to highest levels of California state government. He wanted to show how Archy was used and caught between the debate of whether he was a slave or a free man?

> *As is the case with many black men's lives, there is*
> *also not enough knowledge, or revealed history about*
> *their plight 400, 200, 100 or even 40 to 50 years ago.*

Larry had gone far in setting everything up. Although, he was the center and the main force of this project, Archy Lee was the catalyst. It was a five-year dream that Larry lovingly and persistently nurtured. Unfortunately, Larry's time on earth eclipsed his dream of leaving Archy Lee's legacy behind on film, where it could impact a new generation and live on through eternity. He had several dedicated individuals on board with the project and had even touched bases with Sony television and had formulated a plan for distribution and marketing, if someone would just say, "Yes."

After Larry died, there were boxes of files containing his dream about retelling the story of Archy Lee. Vicki came to me in 2013 after his death and gave me her husband's papers and file because, as she said, she, "didn't want to throw him or his dream away." In all honesty, I didn't know what I would do with everything, but in reviewing his documents and notes, which even had a plan to get someone like Morgan Freeman or Denzel Washington to be the narrator, he was destined to elevate Archy's story. So, I held on and discovered through divine intervention, that I could write about Larry and Archy Lee with the sincerest belief that the story would assuredly take wing, rejuvenating Larry's dream and reviving Archy Lee's powerful role in history.

Enslaved—Renewed: The Intersection of Two Men Bond by a Story and a Century

Archy Lee was born into slavery in 1840, a little more than one hundred years before Larry entered the world a free man in 1948 in Las Animas, Colorado. Men of different races, their lives intersected based on a story about the Black man's enslavement.

With a desire to bring Lee's story to life, Larry interviewed the author of Lee's story, which had been largely forgotten.

Although other articles have been written about Archy Lee, there is still not enough information about his significance or California's role in the era of slavery. As is the case with many black men's lives, there is also not enough knowledge, or revealed history about their plight 400, 200, 100 or even 40 to 50 years ago. What is known, however; is that their lives have been fraught with challenges, struggles and injustices that are rarely brought to light. In Archy Lee it is critical to know his story.

As a young man, Archy Lee's slave-owner parceled him out for services by bringing him from a slave state, to a free state, California but when his owner was about to return, Lee escaped and found freedom briefly through the courts and support from and refuge with free African Americans and white anti-slavery proponents.His owner claimed that Archy was his property and the state Supreme Court ruled in his favor, stirring the ire of many who tried to intervene in freeing Archy. Finally, the decision was overturned and he won the right to be a free man, but his life could not have been easy because he died in 1873, roughly 15 years after he was freed in 1858, a life punctuated by peril, conflict and numerous trials.

Tributes for Larry during his memorial service were as beautiful as the day he was publicly acknowledged by family and friends. Songs, stories and memories about the unassuming, gentle man, whose passions for family, life, and Archy Lee, ran as deep as the Colorado soil where he was born. Archy Lee, though technically free, probably wasn't, due to the racial climate of the time.

When Larry suddenly died of heart failure 140 years after Archy Lee's death, it was unexpected. Only a day or so before what would be his last on earth, his beloved wife had mentioned he wasn't feeling well and was experiencing severe back pain and had struggled to enjoy an evening out to dinner with friends. Within days he passed away. His last gesture, however, was very poignant, as he struggled to get to their dresser drawer and retrieve old engagement rings which were soda pop tabs they exchanged with one another in the '70s. It appeared as if he was letting Vicki know he would still be there for her until it was her time to transition to meet him again.

Undoubtedly, Larry adored his wife to whom he had been married for more than 40 years. He also cherished his two children, daughter-in law, grandsons, siblings and parents. It is worth noting that he and Vicki met at a small Christian college in the state of Kansas, the cradle of many fiery battles between those who wanted to deconstruct slavery and others who wanted it to live on. At one point the state was referred to as "Bloody Kansas."

John Brown, a well-known abolitionist from Kansas was so deeply opposed to the institution of slavery that he fought to the bitter end for its demise before being killed for a raid he led in Harpers Ferry, West Virginia. I believe that if Larry had lived during those times, he too, might have been an abolitionist due to his character, and core beliefs of kindness, fairness and love. In his last years he strived to make Archy Lee visible, but fell short of his goal, but what is left of both men is still the vision.

Where to Place a Dream? Not the Final Chapter

Tributes for Larry during his memorial service were as beautiful as the day he was publicly acknowledged by family and friends. Songs, stories and memories about the unassuming, gentle man, whose passions for family, life, and Archy Lee, ran as deep as the Colorado soil where he was born. Archy Lee, though technically free, probably wasn't, due to the racial climate of the time.

At the end of his life, Archy was about 33 years old and reports of how he died varied. His place of death was in Sacramento, California, which is where I mainly grew up and was educated in public schools from 1964 until I graduated from UC Berkeley in 1982. In that span of years, there were no stories in my history books about the Archy Lees of the world, or for that matter, a true, fair and comprehensive representation of history concerning African Americans or other people of color. Lesson plans used by my instructors were devoid of that critical history that needed to be conveyed. So I commend anyone who is dedicated to what Larry was intent on pursuing.

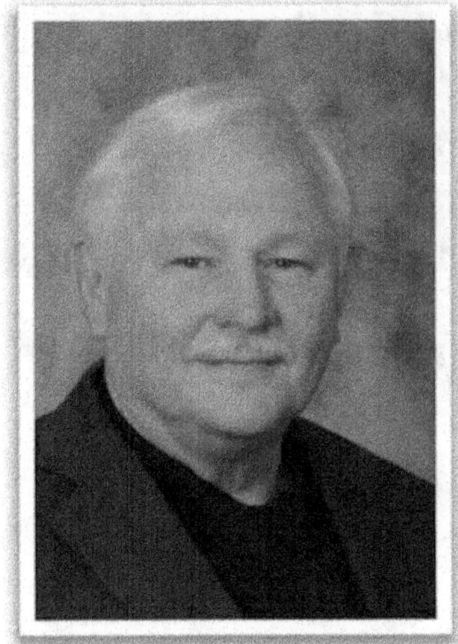

Larry Sherman

In remembering Larry, Vicki wants others to know that he was a "kind, encouraging, caring gentle man who had an amazing sense of humor and who listened to each person's story that he had encountered in life. He believed in each person and their potential." I feel the same, as does Anita McGee Royston, my friend and co-creator of the Brave, Bold and Beautiful Book Series. We know the power and importance of the story, and although Archy Lee and Larry have left this life, their legacies and stories are vital and must be told.

Throughout his sixty plus years on earth, Larry aspired to make a positive impression (as a mentor) in young people's lives. He loved serving as a counselor, leading youth groups, coaching youth sports teams and being in a place of influence for youth. As a man of integrity with a love for English Literature and the classics, he was influenced by many English teachers of his past but foremost, again, it was about the "story".

When I asked Vicki, "What do you want to do to carry on Larry's dream. His legacy?" She paused, looked me directly in the eye and with all sincerity, let her words find their way to my heart, "My hope is that the young men and women who he had influenced would carry on through them. I still hear from people who Larry had influenced. As of yet, nobody has continued Archy Lee's story. (I was hoping you would, Joslyn)."

And so, I am here. The final chapter, is perhaps not completed, as Larry had planned. However, with some help, hope and prayer, our true, authentic histories and respect for humanity, all will finally align with what Archy longed for, and what Larry tried to bring about for a man's life and story that mattered, but still deserves to be freed to land in its rightful and distinguished place in the annals of history.

Color Him Love

Ebony King

Frank Withrow

I invented the traffic light
And the incandescent light bulb, so we can see at night

The first open heart surgery was done by me
I am the man that designed Washington D.C.

I designed the ironing board, refrigerator and baby
carriage, too
I am an Ebony Man, there is nothing I can't do

The shoe as you know it, was designed by me
I even invented the golf tee

Blood plasma was discovered by an Ebony Man
The lubrication system for trains came from my hands

I have proven myself time after time,
As an intelligent human being that has improved mankind

I am a dedicated father, brother, husband and friend
I'll support my family until the end

I've blessed the world with so many good things
I'm a proven mortal, a true Ebony King

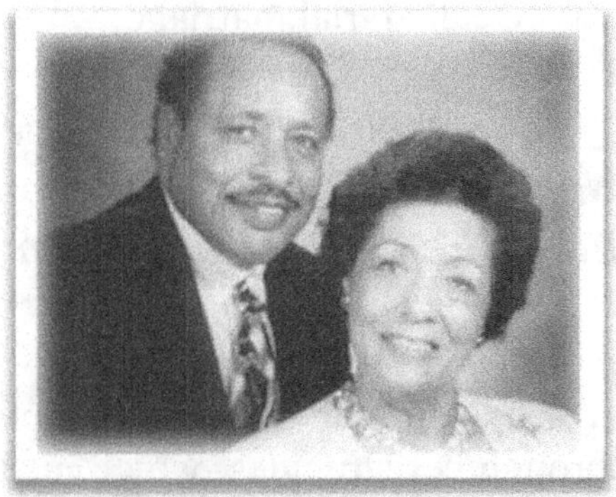

A Life of Divinity and Alleviating the Racial Divide

Apostle Lawrence Campbell

<u>No Shame in the Game</u>

If you really love the person you express it through giving. I give my wife money and never ask what was done with the money. Once you give something it is no longer yours. — Apostle Lawrence Campbell

When I was born in Danville, Virginia, my parents were not married. In those days, the child of this type of union was considered and called illegitimate, which is a word I didn't like because it meant that you did not come into the world the right way. All children are legitimate regardless of how they arrive.

Today times have changed in that respect and can be best described as no shame in the game. If a girl was pregnant and not married it was a shame. Now it's accepted as if it's all right without marriage. Years ago black people were ostracized and considered non-human because they were *shacking up. Today such arrangements are called trial marriage.

I saw my father maybe ten times, when I was stationed in Norfolk. I came to a juke joint he owned, went to the end of the bar and said hello but he didn't recognize me.

I was the only child of Etta Vaughn Campbell, my mother, who reared me through her struggles, which made me appreciate women. Through her I saw the sacrifices a woman will make for a child. As a survivor, she made five dollars per week as a mail carrier. However, my father, George married again and had several children, but I wouldn't see him on a frequent basis.

Pain Equals Manhood

Even though I had a father, I really didn't know him. The black man who most inspired me was Bishop Smallwood Edmond Williams because of his involvement in the Civil Rights sit-ins. However, after completing my education at Phelps Vocational High School and Cortez Peters Business College in Washington, DC, I enlisted in the United States Navy and while stationed in Norfolk, Virginia I saw my father maybe ten times.

I got my Tattoo of a Dagger through a rose, which equals penetration of the heart. Young people think it's a symbol of being cool. It was a customary thing in those days because pain represented manhood.

I came to a juke joint he owned, went to the end of the bar and said "hello" but he didn't recognize me. He did stop though, and we talked. My maternal grandfather, who was a nice man, was there too. We spent lots of time together. When someone asked if he fixed cars I told her, "No. He fixed drinks."

During my stint in the military I got my tattoo of a dagger through a rose, which equals penetration of the heart. Young people think it's a symbol of being cool. It was a customary thing in those days because pain represented manhood.

Love Walked In and Stayed

What I recall about my future wife when I saw her playing half-court basketball in high school, (that's what girls played then) was that she had beautiful legs! And I let my cousin know, that's the girl for me. I actually met her in elementary school and she did become my girlfriend in high school. We lived on opposite sides of the river where there was only one high school for blacks.

The family of the woman I married was so different from mine. But when you care for someone, whatever status you have becomes secondary. They were very prosperous, and she was surrounded by family who knew how to run businesses in the community of Holbrook in North Danville where there were doctors, and lawyers, which was an indication of success. Her father, Elmer Williams, who was already deceased when we married, was the first black man with a successful business and was very involved in civil rights and voting of black people in the '30s and '40s.

In July 1953, my wife and I started Bible Way Church in a vacant lot on White Street where we lived in the projects and walked to church services every night. God's heaven was our roof and his stars were our chandeliers and an old Victrola was my lectern. A man gave me some old wood and I dug holes and built pews for the people to sit on.

By working in the day at Memorial Hospital in Danville, scrubbing floors, cleaning blinds and taking out bedpans, I was able to save enough money to buy a beat up 1946 green Dodge with a broken driver's seat for $75. I used a stick to prop it up.

The heater didn't work and we had to use blankets to keep warm. Even though it was dilapidated, it beat walking to services every night. On one occasion we had eleven all at one time in that car.

My $25-a-week paycheck covered the $19-a-month rent on a 3-bedroom apartment, other necessities and the occasional treat. I'd get paid on Thursdays, and the first thing I'd do is go home and pick up my wife; we'd go to the supermarket and buy groceries. Then we'd eat at what was called the Danville Dairy and we'd all get a 5-cent cone of ice cream. We thought we were in heaven! Yet even the act of getting ice cream was impacted by segregation.

The Day Martin and the Movement
Came to Danville

There was no escaping or denying that Danville was a divided city before the Civil Rights movement. Despite being "free," blacks were not allowed to go to the same places, get the same jobs or expect the same treatment as whites.

Black people simply did not get, for instance, jobs with the city. Blacks were mostly sharecroppers, seasonal tobacco workers or domestics. The only "professional" blacks in Danville then were three morticians, two doctors (who were only allowed to treat black patients) and the teachers at the black schools.

There was inadequate, sub-par medical treatment at Winslow Hospital, and separate funeral homes. From birth to death, you lived in segregation ... we were always placed in a secondary role.

Black people in Danville were fed up with being treated unfairly. Schools were segregated. White schools got new textbooks, while their used books were given to the black schools. Woolworth's had two lunch counters based on race.

There was inadequate, sub-par medical treatment at Winslow Hospital, and separate funeral homes.

From birth to death, you lived in segregation … we were always placed in a secondary role. Even when the 1954 Supreme Court decision on the Brown v. Board of Education case ruled that school segregation was unconstitutional, desegregation didn't occur in Danville until years later.

The first time Dr. Martin Luther King visited the River City, he couldn't get a room at the Holiday Inn in Danville because of segregation. So we took him to the Holiday Inn in Greensboro, N.C.

When he took off his jacket, there was a gash where a woman had stabbed him.

"This is the price I've paid for my struggle with civil rights," he said. At the time, according to Dr. King, "Hatred toward blacks across the South, Danville was the most brutal example of segregation and resistance to civil rights." And his statement would come to fruition on June 10, 1963.

Before Bloody Sunday…There was Bloody Monday

Apostle Lawrence Campbell was co-founder of the Danville Christian Progressive Association, an affiliate of the Southern Christian Leadership Conference. In 1963 he had been in the ministry for ten years, and segregation was still a cancer on the American south with no promise of heeding or healing the fissure that was separating blacks and whites, equal from unequal, haves from have nots.

Everything erupted in Danville, Virginia on June 10, 1963 in what would be called, "Bloody Mary," which preceded "Bloody Sunday," in Selma, Alabama by two years. The price that was paid for civil rights was high, particularly for his wife, who along with many others, were badly beaten by Danville police officers, and hosed down until they fell down. What is key; however, is that they refused to literally and figuratively stay down.

What was frustrating was that everything we were fighting for was constitutionally ours anyway. When a Methodist and Baptist preacher and I staged a sit-in at the F.W. Woolworth restaurant counter, we were not served due to our race and I was thrown down the steps by a group of angry white people and then jailed for protesting under the John Brown Law. My sentence was six months.

Never went to jail as a boy. I was jailed for protesting during the civil rights movement.

Like Dr. King's strategy, non-violent tactics were employed, but fire hoses were still unfurled, torrents of water knocked down peaceful protesters in prayer, including my wife, as the police wielded their nightsticks to push back peaceful protestors merely praying. The aftermath was bloody but we marched, not because we were bitter and angry, but because we wanted things in this city to be better.

Going Forward, but Looking Back

By 1964 the Civil Rights Act helped to breakdown some barriers, and schools were desegregated by 1970. City leaders, and cooperative newspapers and radio stations, tried to ignore the events of the day. But to improve relations between the races, events in the past can't be ignored.

The way I see it, the key to history is continuity; if you don't like the Civil War or slavery and [ignore it], it's not history. The issue is, what have we learned from it?

June 10, 1963 should be used as a means of continuing understanding between the races. Things have improved, but Danville needs to have some forum where races come together and discuss race relations in the city. We need to prepare for uncertainty in times of peace.

Danville officials did not want the media or people to discuss that infamous night. For many years, they said it didn't happen. Although Danville has come a long way because now we see a black superintendent of schools, a black head of the school board, a black mayor, racism is still there. I wish that were not the case, but it is … it's just more subtle now.

A Guiding Philosophy

The Church is one place where segregation is now more mutually agreed upon than enforced. White people are generally not comfortable worshipping in traditionally black churches, and black people are not generally comfortable worshipping in white churches.

When I'm gone I want to leave this behind: that I have loved people and tried to help people. And I believe you can't let worries of tomorrow cripple your happiness of today.

The church may be further behind than other organizations now and needs to catch up. The church is not a holistic approach to this generation of all different denominations. We get caught up in the dogma and forget how to treat people. The church should reinforce language and words that are relevant to the hereafter.

I try to preach about a practical life. So the church can become one denomination. However, a clear life is not all church. Church is a part of life. How to live with your mistakes is to go to god, not people. They cannot forgive.

In regard to relationships, a woman will do just about anything a man wants if he treats her right. When I'm gone I want to leave this behind: that I have loved people and tried to help people. And I believe you can't let worries of tomorrow cripple your happiness of today.

Apostle Lawrence Campbell and his wife, First Lady and Mother of Bibleway Church, Gloria Campbell, have been dedicated servants central to the global church community and integral figures in the civil rights movement. The small ministry they started in 1953 has grown exponentially over the past 60 plus years and has always been a "house of refuge for the saving of souls, ministering to the homeless, hungry, the needy, the senior citizens, the youth, and those who are forsaken and forgotten in our society." Today some of their programs include a Free Breakfast Program, 24 hour daycare, Free Shoe and Clothing program and a radio ministry, which are only a handful of programs that have been created. Their foot print in Danville's Civil Rights Movement and their efforts to improve community race relations continues.

*Shacking Up – Unmarried couples who are living together.

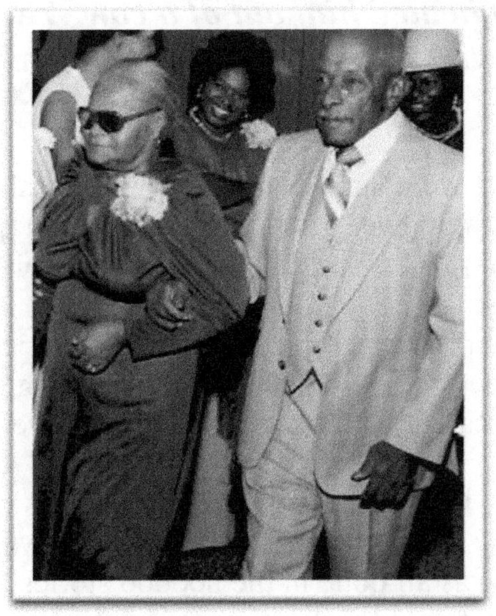

The Griot with his love, Martha.

A Gift for My Grandfather, the Griot

Marcus McGee

Homer Jefferson was my grandfather -- a Griot, a storyteller. Born in Carroll County Mississippi in December 1900, good friends knew him as Homebone. He never learned to read or write, but was known around Greenwood and Avalon for his ability to *spin a yarn*. He'd sit and begin, and whether he was musing about *haints* (spirits), *hoodoo, local affairs, lynching or the Bible, people crowded around for the entertainment. The magic was never in the story itself, but in its telling.

He told stories about lynching and about the time a White man cheated him out of a cow. Yet despite the challenges and injustices of the time, he was never bitter.

The subjects were usually trivial, involving simple folks, but the lessons in them were insightful and often profound. The fantastical *haint* stories bridged the real and spirit worlds with warnings against greed, pride, lust and anger. Many of these involved community ancestors with commentaries provided by goathead sinners, or cats, opossums, panthers, bulls and snakes. Those stories scared us kids to death, but we couldn't help listening.

Hoodooing in Mississippi was as real as medicine, and where medicine and science couldn't provide acceptable explanations, it was all done in the hoodoo stories. He told stories of ceremonies that could make wives never leave husbands, make husbands cheat on wives, put a man in the road, make a person's teeth fall out, let a person speak face-to-face with Beelzebub or cause a painful death.

Grandfather also told of local folk tales in the *Uncle Remus* tradition, stories of bootleggers outsmarting the law, sharecroppers one-upping landowners and Blacks getting the better of Whites. He had a series of stories about a bungling local sheriff whose catch phrase was, "Ev'ry time I see a damn nigga and a dog, I like the dog the best."

He told of being in the town of Money, Mississippi to watch teenager Emmit Teal's bloated body dragged from the river, and a story about Gold-toothed Annie, a *niggah-chasin* hound with a complete set of gold teeth. He told stories about lynching and about the time a White man cheated him out of a cow. Yet despite the challenges and injustices of the times, he was never bitter. Instead, he said he knew plenty of good and bad people, both

Black and White.

My grandfather even had slave stories. I remember one in particular about two women, my great-great grandmother and her sister who were separated at the auction block. After slavery ended, they spent more than ten years trying to find each other. In tragedy, at the moment of their reunion, one sister's petticoats fell against the fire. She fled in panic, causing the fire to consume her.

As Homer was the second of nine children, he started working at 12 or 13 to help pay to raise his siblings. He picked cotton on the plantations and apparently learned to cook along the way, because later in life he accompanied White men on hunting expeditions to specially prepare wild game feasts.

At age 23 he met 21-year-old Martha Liddell and wanted to court her, but she already had a suitor, a young man named John Hurt. Soon thereafter, John, a frugal man, bought a meager sized watermelon for Martha as a token of his affection. Not to be outdone, Homer gave her a much larger watermelon, throwing John's gift to the hogs and his own hat into the ring as a suitor. Homer married Martha two weeks later and John became one of his best friends. Over time, *Mississippi John Hurt* became a world famous guitar player and folk singer, recording six albums and performing on numerous tours.

Homer and Martha had 11 children, seven girls and four boys. My mother, Sora, was their third child and I am the fourth of my parents' seven children. Throughout my life I'd heard talk of my grandfather and his stories. I saw him at occasional family reunions but I didn't get to know him until my early twenties when he moved out to California. By that time I knew I wanted to be a writer, so I was obsessed with stories and eager to listen to him.

I spent hours, days and years listening to my grandfather, fascinated by the way he put it all together: the language, the characterizations, the rhythm, and the magic of storytelling. Some stories made an unambiguous point, while others just flowed languorously, soothing the soul and filling the imagination. I can only hope to have learned something from that great man. The most important lesson he taught me was the final one.

Even at 83, Homer was a vibrant man. He rode a bike, challenged roller coasters and went all over the city by bus. One day he missed his regular stop and got off the bus in a seedy area of town. I'm certain the young man who mugged him had no idea that when he punched my grandfather, knocking him down, he killed my grandfather. My grandfather rose and lived on for six years after the attack, but the better part of his spirit never rose from that blood stained sidewalk. From that day on, he ceased to venture, withdrew and ultimately began to accept his mortality.

He still told his stories, but they were different. It seemed they were more dour and reflective, though he always tempered them with an occasional humorous observation or a witty old saying. I took him to the zoo regularly because he loved watching the animals. He also liked watching *Sanford and Son* and would sit through taped episodes from morning until night, providing commentary for whomever was in earshot.

My sister and I found the John Hurt DVDs at a record store downtown and bought them for Grandfather because he liked listening to best friend John, who was long dead. My Grandmother Martha had passed almost ten years earlier. In fact, all my grandfather's contemporaries were gone. So he'd sit listening to John Hurt all day long, and sometimes I'd sit with him. I had heard the music my whole life, but I had never really paid attention to it. Listening for the first time, I came to the immediate conclusion that many of John Hurt's songs were about death.

Bereft of his former sense of adventure, at 87, my grandfather had finally become an old man. He had drank and smoked since he was a teenager, but he suddenly quit both. I tried to find more positive, upbeat music for him, but he was more at peace with his old best friend's songs. Sitting in silence by the stereo, I'd sometimes ask what he was thinking. "About old friends and fishing," he would answer. On occasion I even got a story.

When I asked, "Why at the end of your life do you seem to

dwell so much on death?" He told me, *"You missed the point of the stories and the songs. Death is the only way to measure life. Death is the final accounting. Ev'ry story that has a beginnin has gotta have an end, or there's no point in tellin it."*

I was at his hospital bed on the night before he died, and when I heard the news the next morning, I understood what he meant. According to African tradition: *As long as there is someone left to tell your story, you will never die.* So this is the gift I give to my grandfather. I have shared the story of his life with you, and in so doing have given him everlasting life.

**Hoodoo: Same as voodoo (religion) misfortune.*
**Beelzebub: Prince of evil spirits, biblically the patron god of Philistines in ancient Palestine*

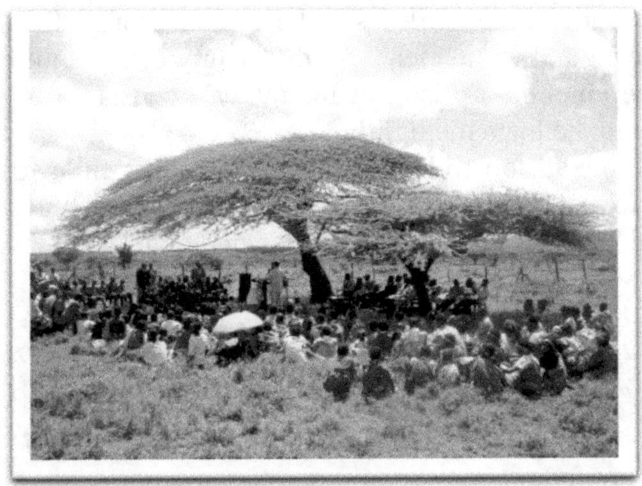

From the Valley of Violence into the Light of Deliverance

Yusuf Salsabil Alkimia

A Damaged Sense of Self-Worth
Within my own community I was belittled by adults and children because of my dark skin and strong African facial features.

There is a little sweet boy that I see in my neighborhood from time-to-time. He is often sad because his father constantly berates him in public. Threats of "knocking him upside his head" are frequent.

When I see this little boy riding his bike alone, we talk and I give him compliments on his inner greatness as well as his present and future abilities. These few words fill him with enthusiasm and excitement. As the beauty of his smile protrudes from the emotional prison of his father's constant destruction of his esteem, he hugs me tightly.

I know all too well the experience of this child for he is the boy that I used to be. My little friend has been dehumanized and belittled so much that his father has undercut his essential worth as a person.

Shaped by my destructive family history, and as an active member of the Crips, a notorious gang, I had become a very violent and angry man.

As happened to me 20 years ago, most of my childhood was emotionally tumultuous. Within my own community I was belittled by adults and children, because of my dark skin and strong African facial features.

On a daily basis I was referred to as an animal akin to an ape or monkey, and I was called, "Joe Lip." These messages sunk in and I began to believe that the comments were true, which destroyed me. As a result, I acquired a damaged sense of self-worth and became severely depressed. When little attempts of attaining achievements failed or setbacks occurred as an adult, my esteem was wounded. All of my difficulties affirmed my belief that I wasn't a human being at all.

<u>Gang Life</u>
I was confused, afraid, and needed someone to make sense out of it all.

I was born in Baton Rogue, Louisiana and grew up in gang activity, drug infestation, and a murderous blood shedding ecosystem. When I was a little boy playing basketball in my neighborhood, I vividly remember a nice guy who was shot no more than a few yards away from me. As he laid there on the court gasping for air, his eyes rolled back in his head while my mother pleaded with him.

"Hold on Jerry! You can make it!" But he didn't. He just laid there and died.

Before the age of 14, I had seen so much death and constant bloodshed within my own family, that the thug life became my way of life. My mother had survived many, many bloody battles against both men and women. She still has buck shot pellets embedded in the back of her legs and arms, which are a reminder of our violent past.

Shaped by my destructive family history, and as an active member of the Crips, a notorious gang, I had become a very violent and angry man. My reality set the course for a life long battle with depression for many years.

Involved with drugs and alcohol, I was trying to relieve the pain of my early childhood experiences, but it resulted in nothing but addiction and more violence. I was confused, afraid, and needed someone to make sense out of it all.

<u>Despair, Discovery, Deliverance</u>
As fathers, we must keep in mind that God doesn't place on us anything we can't handle.

My father, Jessie was a very good religious man, but died all too soon when I was a young boy. So there was no father to turn to until one day when my mother began taking my siblings and me to visit Muhammad Temple in the early '70s. The impact of those experiences didn't come to full fruition until the early 1980s when my mother resumed taking us to the Mosque again. This time, it was in Oakland, California where a powerful, young residing minister of the Most Honorable Elijah Muhammad, emerged from the Nation of Islam.

Known as Billy "X," the young minister who inspired my mother again was none other than the Most Honorable Minister Louis Farrakhan, who would later, at a certain point in my life, become my spiritual father. Minister Farrakhan was the father I much longed and waited for.

For 14 years I strived to live as he said we should. Suddenly things began to make sense to me. I began by the Grace of Allah, to understand the reason for my lifelong affliction with addiction, which had produced lifelong depression.

Through my father, I have come to understand that there is no level of pain that does not give a greater birth, greater understanding of pain, greater reality, or greater peace than the very intensity of pain itself.

As fathers, we must keep in mind that God doesn't place on us anything we can't handle. Therefore, those of us with the most distress are those whom God has prepared with the most capability to handle it. If we knew, and fully embraced this, such brothers could be guides for others out of the mental valley of the shadow of despair.

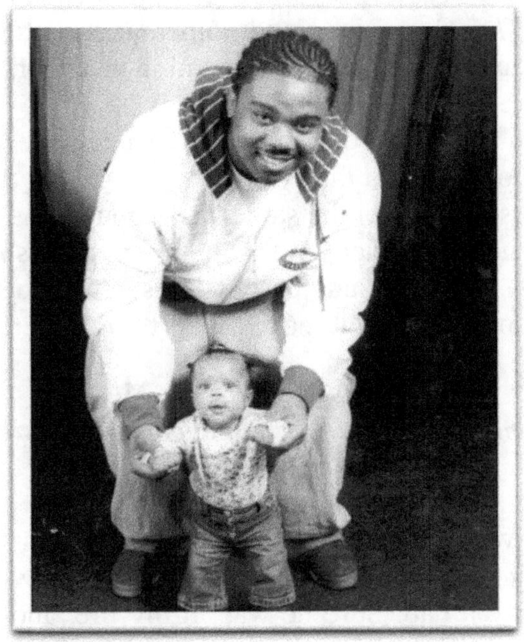

Author and proud father with "The One."

A Blueprint for Fatherhood

Lessons from My Legend

Elias Jackson Webb

<u>Teen Father</u>
Everyone wanted to know was I nervous, scared or was I going to break down and cry, but my answer was simply 'no.'

On June 12, 2007, the greatest day of my life, Taylor Noralee Webb was born. I was only 18 years old at the time. So everyone wanted to know was I nervous, scared or was I going to break down and cry, but my answer to all was simply 'no.' So along came *The One*. My grandmother and aunties asked me, "Elias how do you feel about becoming a father," just a few minutes before my daughter was born.

"I'm not worried about becoming a father because I know what it takes to be a good father."

Months later I feel the same way about being a father. My daughter is getting older and sometimes I wish I had my grandfather to go to for advice but I just think to myself what would my grandpa do and it makes everything better.

<u>Little Respect for Men</u>
By the time I turned nine I had become immune to missing or even wanting a father figure.

When I was younger I didn't have much respect for men. Raised by my mother, it wasn't that I didn't know my father; I just didn't have a dad. Sure he was in my life, and called every Sunday. Sometimes I visited him during the summers, but even when I went to see him he was always at work.

At first it hurt to know that my father put his job before my brothers, and me but by the time I turned nine I had become immune to missing or even wanting a father figure in my life.

The longing I experienced would eventually subside because I sought and found someone else to fill that void in my life. I figured who better could serve as a role model than the man who raised ten of his own children and so many other neighborhood kids, nieces and nephews. This man just happened to be my grandfather.

I watched my grandpa day in and day out just being himself, cracking jokes, watching boxing; and coming to my brothers and cousins football games screaming, "Kill the coach!" because he believed the coach was making bad decisions. It was crazy seeing how people would rally behind him. Even outside of the pulpit where he preached!

<u>Whatever It Takes</u>
Grandfather didn't want his children to know that there wasn't enough food for him to join them.

In every dimension, my grandfather was a great father figure. He did what he had to do to take care of his family, including working multiple jobs. On many evenings he sat in the living room with my grandma while his children ate their dinner because he didn't want them to know that there wasn't enough food for him to join them.

Being a man of God with the determination to take care of his family and make sacrifices were only a few of the tremendous qualities Grandpa possessed. They made him the great father he was, and drew me close to him. There are times when I think about buying myself something new to wear when money is tight because I like to stay up with fashion. But I make the decision to consider my daughter. I can't lie; it makes it easier when I think about what my grandpa sacrificed to provide for his children, that makes me want to live up to the standard that he set for my uncles, cousins and brothers. My grandfather was a legend who deeply enriched my life, giving me the blueprint to father and love my child.

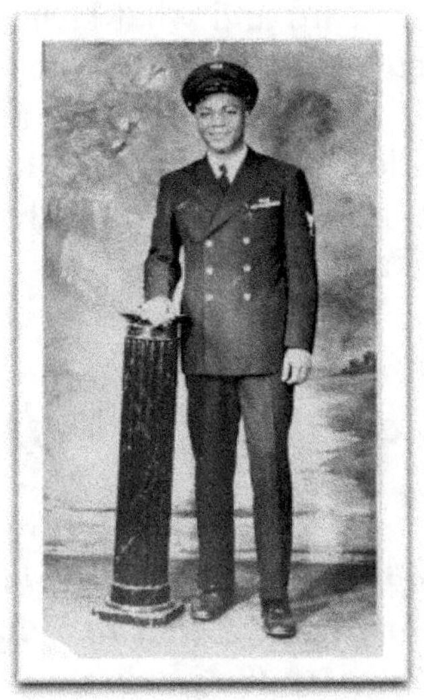

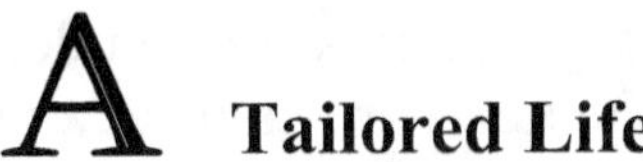

Daddy in Naval uniform looking like a million bucks.

A Tailored Life

Rodney Snell

<u>A Minor Alteration</u>
When he had one daughter away at college, a son about to enter the military and his remaining children of school age, even the accident of my teenaged mother didn't derail Daddy's dream.

My grandfather passed away in 2003 at the age of 78 after secretly living with cancer for seven years. It was my privilege to deliver remarks at his service, which was not difficult as there was so much to say about the man who raised me in the absence of my own father. *Daddy*, as we called grandfather, was known as a great father, but not the best husband.

Between what I'd heard and what I knew, I was able to craft something that reflected the feelings of my entire family in my eulogy. I realized my own creative skills as I quickly patterned something true that allowed him to retain his dignity. At the end of the day; however, he was a loving father, and the man who continues to influence and guide me.

I was blessed to have entered Daddy's life at a time when he was considered well off for a Negro.

A Country Playboy
It was easy to imagine him a country playboy, who once was given the option by local authorities to either enter the service, or go on the chain gang.

On the wall of our den for most of my childhood, was a professional portrait of Daddy in Naval dress. Standing beside a white pedestal, he was flashing a million dollar smile. As a teen, he distilled and distributed corn liquor called *Buck,* which also became his nickname. It was easy to imagine him a country playboy, who once was given the option by local authorities to either enter the service, or go on the chain gang.

Daddy's complexion was known as *red-boned.* It was a smooth, ruddy, light-brown color that can only be derived from Native American ancestry, with a bit of slaveholder mixed in for good measure. In his day, it was a favored boyfriend complexion to many girls in the South. With two such girls, Daddy fathered a pair of daughters. I believe both women had equal opportunity of becoming his wife.

An Unconditional Love
He selected the mother who was best suited to care for him and his children, and a friend who would stand by and support him, even if he was wrong.

The woman Daddy chose was less sophisticated and educated than he. She was from a family of hard working sharecroppers, and was trustworthy, and trusting. To me, the choice painted him as an opportunist who married my grandmother to use her siblings who were in a position to help him. Her sisters had moved north and done well financially. They could provide shelter to Daddy's small family while he established himself.

I couldn't see how love guided Daddy's choice, as he was a constant philanderer, which caused grief throughout his marriage. But over time, I have grown to believe love was a great factor.

Daddy chose a girl who waited upon his return from his tour of duty. He selected the mother who was best suited to care for him and his children -- a friend who would stand by and support him, even if he was wrong. She was the woman, who after 58 not very blissful years would carefully bathe him on the morning he drew his final breath. He chose the one who loved him unconditionally.

Daddy Sews Up A Dream
He was living the dream that was born while he was barefooted and dirt poor in depression-era segregated Georgia.

I was blessed to have entered Daddy's life at a time when he was considered well off for a *Negro*. Daddy owned property in a predominately White neighborhood, was self-employed as a tailor, and drove a new car every four years. He was living the dream that was born while he was barefooted and dirt poor in depression-era, segregated Georgia.

When he had one daughter away at college, a son about to enter the military and his remaining children of school age, even the accident of my teenaged mother didn't derail Daddy's dream. He simply made a minor alteration for my inclusion.

Keeping Him in Stitches
Folks would come in just to shoot the breeze while Daddy worked, usually with his back to them. No one ever

doubted he was listening.

Daddy was consistent in his habits. He was usually at work, church, a lodge function or en route to one or the other. On a typical weekday he would leave the house early enough to drop me off at school on time. I never had to walk or take the bus unless I chose to. He would then head to his shop and spend the day measuring, cutting and sewing for customers who patronized him as much for his affable nature, as his skill with a needle.

Folks would come in just to shoot the breeze while Daddy worked, usually with his back to them. No one ever doubted he was listening. When it was appropriate, he would turn his head, peer over his glasses that always were perched dangerously close to falling off his nose, and offer commentary. You could always tell if he was amused. Even if he stifled his chuckle, his shoulders would move up and down indicating that he was tickled. Sometimes it was easier to read his back than his face.

Daddy usually worked late and then attended a lodge function, choir rehearsal or some other church meeting. Since church was as much Daddy's home as our house, he got nearly as much rest there as at home.

While Daddy was ushering, he remained alert, but as soon as he sat down, his chin would hit his chest. Even in the choir loft where he sang baritone between song selections, he could be heard snoring in the back.

<u>From Broke Down to Locked Up—A Road Story</u>
I couldn't have been anymore than three years old, but I can distinctly remember hearing one of our jailers say, "Put this little Nigger over there with his daddy."

Daddy loved to see his children happy. We always had birthday envelopes and ridiculously extravagant Christmases. Even when he would pack us up in the car and haul us to Georgia, Christmas day never suffered. Somehow gifts came along too and we never rode less than seven or eight to a car.

After all, children were not considered full passengers, especially before the days of safety seats.

Our road trips were infamous. We have been everything from broke down to locked-up. Daddy was *King* of the short cut. In the days before the Interstate cut a quick path through the East, we used to ride along Route 301, a journey that seemed to take days.

Back in the early 1970s, our entire three-car caravan was stopped for speeding in South Hill, Virginia. My cousin, Kizmo was piloting the lead car and those following might have gotten away clean, but Uncle Buck pulled behind to make sure his nephew was alright.

The trooper surmised that all the cars must have been speeding and led us off to a little jail. We were even placed in holding cells due to the number of us. I couldn't have been anymore than three years old, but I can distinctly remember hearing one of our jailers say, "Put this little Nigger over there with his daddy." At that age, I looked so much like my cousin Frankie, that they must have assumed he was my father.

The Civil Rights Act had passed, smoke was still rising from rioting in cities across the country and everyone was visibly upset, but not Daddy. After negotiating with the *good ol' boys*, the funds to expedite our release appeared courtesy of my grandmother's sister, who always traveled with exorbitant amounts of cash.

<u>Family Man</u>
When he was happy, there was no making his joy.

Daddy enjoyed being surrounded by family and loved when the house and yard were packed to capacity. He wanted to share with everyone. Even if empty-handed, he was glad to see folks come. Our idea of family has never been bound by what was traditional. There was always some character at our house with which we shared no blood.

Marital problems aside, Daddy remained a father who provided shelter and support to his family. When he was happy there was no making his joy. I'm proud to be responsible for at least two of those moments; the day I acknowledged his influence in my graduation speech when I received my A.A. degree. And the day I marched across the stage of Boston's Wang Center to receive my B.A. from Emerson College.

I didn't expect Daddy to make the trip for the commencement ceremony, but not only did he come, he arranged a delegation of family members that I didn't expect to be in attendance. In those moments, I realized that Daddy also tailored a dream for me.

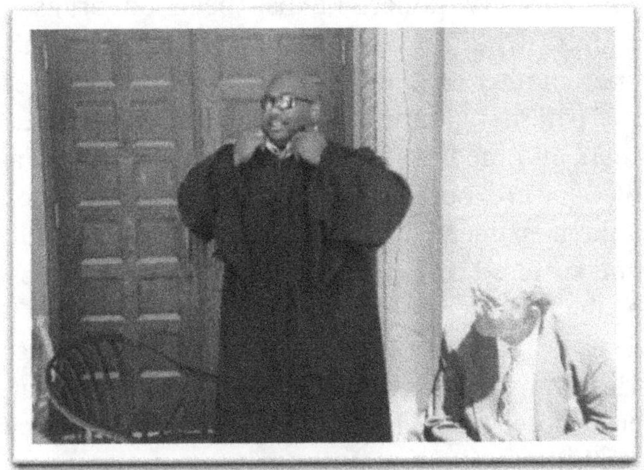

Author's God given father on the left, standing.

A God Given Father of My Own

Marcus Kellam

In Pursuit of a Family
My brothers and I were in and out of adult group homes for years….

My life had been in constant flux since I was five. My brothers and I were in and out of adult group homes for years because my mother has a mental disease called schizophrenia for which she suffered years of depression. Due to her inability to care for us, we were taken away from her.

We soon ran out of options being that we were Black teenaged males and most foster homes wouldn't take us.

In regard to my father, he has been on drugs since I can remember and a deadbeat dad for even longer than that. So I never had a proper mother and father household, so to speak. In their absence, my paternal grandmother stepped in and cared for my two older brothers and me until she suddenly passed away at 72. While the rest of us were outside playing basketball one evening, she choked in the apartment. From the age of 12 my grandmother had smoked, and suffered from upper respiratory problems.

Once again, my brothers and I moved in with my father's sister and her daughter. Broken-hearted from her mother's untimely death, my aunt soon buckled under the pressure and had a nervous breakdown. She died within a year of our grandmother's death of a debilitating terminal illness.

Finally a Father
When I finally aged out of the group home, I, like most children in the system, had no place to go and little preparation for survival.

My father continued to be nonexistent. Although I see my mother from time-to-time, I have no contact with him. I am now twenty-two years of age and had been in foster and group homes since I was fourteen, which has been a difficult journey. When my oldest brother was of age, he decided to live with my father, but my other brother and I ended up in a three month receiving home where we were introduced to group home living. Unfortunately, because the placement was temporary, we soon ran out of options being that we were Black teenaged males and most foster homes wouldn't take us. So we took a risk to be together by moving in with a couple, which was a big mistake. They couldn't stand us, and we resented them. So we left after only a short period of time.

After all of the problems we had with previous group and foster homes, my brother and I were finally placed in the Girls and Boys Homes of North Carolina where we would stay until we graduated from high school.

When I was 19 I met a man who worked at the group home named, George Bowers. With a lot in common, we formed a bond that I've never had with any male figure in my life. It was the first time since my aunt died that I felt like someone truly believed in me and what I could accomplish. He's given me the focus and purpose I once didn't have.

<u>I Love You Pop!</u>
***After receiving his foster parenting license, George
came to my rescue again...***

When I finally aged out of the group home, I, like most children in the system, had no place to go and little preparation for survival. After receiving his foster parenting license, George came to my rescue again, welcoming me to live with him with open arms.

Now I live on my own and can attribute almost all that I've learned about being a responsible, independent adult, through the living testimony that embodies George Bowers. He has mentored and encouraged me to attain a higher education, which I am diligently pursuing.

George has many honorary sons just like me who he's helped and been a father to. Through the ministry that God has given him, he aspires to run a group home of his own to advocate for, and mentor young adults.

I love this man, who I call, Pop! He is an inspiration to me, and most significantly, my very own God given father.

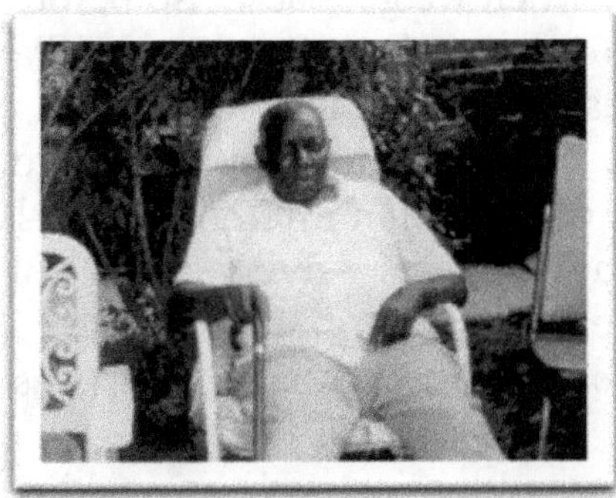

"Pa"

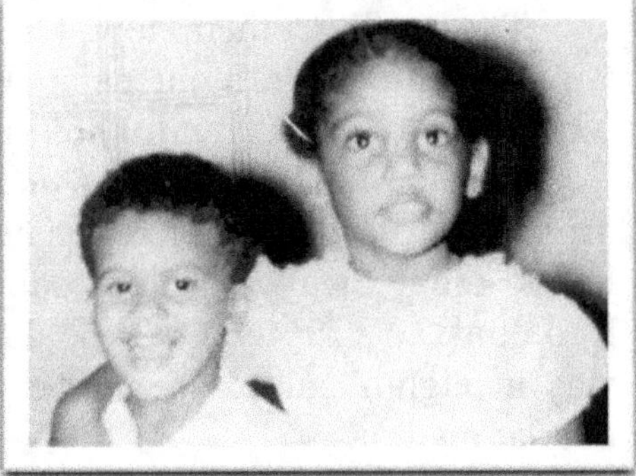

Brother, Zooey, and author.

Never Really Got to Know Daddy

Virginia Lathan

Never really got to know Daddy. I was about three or so when he and Mommy split up. But I do know he and Mommy used to fuss and fight a lot. I remember the police coming sometimes. I'd get so upset when that happened that I'd call Grandmother to come get Zooey (my little brother) and me.

Of course Grandmother would have to wait until Pa (my step-grandfather) got home. Pa worked hard at a steel mill and would always be tired and sore when he got home. He just wanted to eat and go to bed.

I was so happy Glenda finally got to see my daddy because I always saw hers. He lived with her family.

But as soon as he got in the house, Grandmother would say, "Ben, the kids called. Della and Martin are fighting again. The kids want to come out here, so after you finish eating, we better get them."

"No, we'll get them now. I'll eat when we get back." So before we were able to grab our pajamas for good, Grandmother and Pa were there to take us out to their house, where we felt safe.

Never really got to know Daddy. But I do remember he used to drink a lot of whiskey, and because of that, Mommy, Zooey and I had to move away from him one day. But every five years or so, he'd come to visit us. Once he came to see Zooey and me when I was in eighth grade. Glenda, my best girlfriend back then, was over at my house.

Daddy spent some time playing and teasing with us, making us laugh. I was so happy Glenda finally got to see my daddy because I always saw hers because he lived with her family. Anyway, Daddy must have spent the night somewhere in the neighborhood because the next day when Glenda and I were walking home, I saw him again.

Aunt GG told me a story about how he scored higher than all the other students in the state on a math test when they were in high school someplace in Louisiana. The school superintendent was so shocked that a "Colored" boy did so well on that test that he went to the school to meet Daddy.

Daddy was sitting barefooted and shirtless under a shade tree with some red-eyed, bad smelling men. Whiskey bottles were at their feet and Daddy was slumped over the back of his chair. His mouth hung open, allowing the odor of stale whiskey to escape as he snored. I was crushed because that's not the way my daddy was supposed to be.

"Look, there's your father," Glenda said.

"No he's not!" I said defensively, blinking hard to hold back tears.

Glenda looked puzzled. "I thought you told me that's your father?"

"Well he's not. Not really."

I was too hurt and deceived to try to explain things to her, so I just hung my head as Glenda and I walked by him.

"I'm going to take the short cut home," I said to Glenda, knowing she had to go a different way. When we parted, I ran fast. Tears streamed down my cheeks even faster than I was moving. When I got home, Pa was sitting on the porch. It was his day off from work. He didn't ask me any questions about why I was so upset, but when the ice cream truck drove by, he got me some.

Never really got to know Daddy. Aunt GG told me a story about how he scored higher than all the other students in the state on a math test when they were in high school someplace in Louisiana. The school superintendent was so shocked that a *Colored* boy did so well on that test that he went to the school to meet Daddy.

Pa, on the other hand, couldn't do that well on math tests, or any kind of written test for that matter. He couldn't even read or write. He signed his name with an "X." But he could drive. He used to take Zooey and me to the library.

"Ben," Grandmother would say, "the kids want to go to the library, but they can't take any more books out until their fines are paid."

Pa would say, "I'll take care of that when we get there." Then he'd say to us, "Now, if you kids stay in there too long, I'm not going to bring you back next week."

"Okay," one of us would say, as we darted off to the children's section.

But Pa couldn't take us back the next week anyway. He only had one weekend off a month, so our books were always overdue. However, Pa would always pay the fines.

Never really got to know Daddy. I didn't even know Daddy had died until Aunt GG called after he was already in the grave. He was 55. Now when Pa died, that was something else. He had been sick for a long time -- bedridden for over 15 years. In fact, he hung on so long that people just thought somehow he was going to outlive everybody in the family.

In his last year of life I started having dreams about Pa walking. Before I realized I was dreaming, I'd be shocked that he had gotten out of bed and was all dressed up in a khaki hat and brown and green sports jacket.

One night when I had one of those dreams, I asked him, "Pa, what are you doing out of bed? You could fall and get hurt!"

He just headed down the steps and said, "It's time for me to go."

"But Pa, does Grandmother know you're out of bed?"

"She'll know in a little while."

"But Pa, she may be upset that you got up."

I tried to get him to go back to bed, but my pleas were in vain. Pa was determined. He was leaving.

"Pa, why'd you let me see you leaving?"

He smiled. "Cause even though you're my granddaughter, I've always loved you more like a daughter, Sissy, and a daughter needs to know what's happening with her pa."

"Thank you, Pa," I said beginning to release him. "Just be careful going down those steps."

He squeezed my hand. "Don't worry. I'll be going down them in a little while." As I felt him let go of my hand, I watched as he ascended.

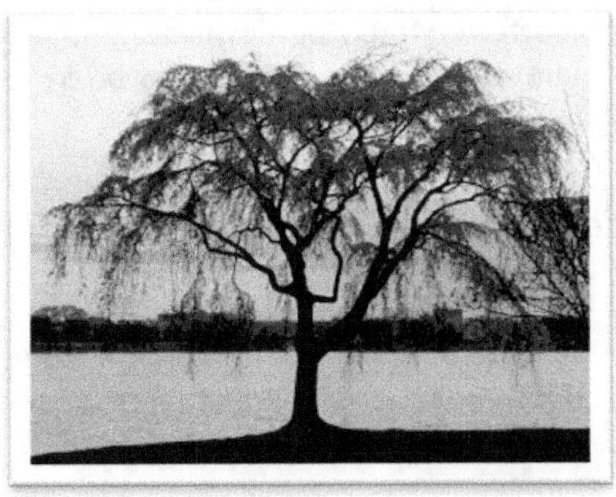

From Fury to Faith and Forgiveness

Pastor Dale Miles

<u>Devastating Dysfunction</u>
As a child, my father's rage and violence was a significant, emotional event that I was ill equipped to cope with.

In my family life was hard. As the youngest of five children, I was raised in a very dysfunctional home. At the age of six, I was exposed to the continual abuse of my mother by my father, which lasted for fifteen years. There was nothing worse than witnessing the jealousy, envy and hate that my father exhibited towards her.

I never knew or heard of generational curses. However, what I did know was that I would never abuse my wife. Even though I didn't inherit the curse that had consumed my father, I was afflicted by a spirit of anger and self-abuse; and I began to develop a strong hatred for him. As a child, my father's rage and violence was a significant, emotional event that I was ill-equipped to cope with. The after effects would be devastating and leave a lifelong struggle to reclaim my spirit and restore my broken soul.

Over time, I learned that you don't wake up and become mad all of a sudden, something has to contribute to one's fury.

Mama, Why Did It Take So Long?
I realized that my father had broken her spirit and she would never be the same.

The love that I had for my father diminished because the love I had for my mother outweighed any other feelings. Many times I tried to help her only to be knocked down in my attempts. No matter what I did, it was never enough for my father. He would always degrade me, and tell me that I needed to be like my oldest brother who was gifted, well liked and smart. He was considered most likely to succeed in high school. Growing up in his shadow was hard.

After fifteen years of torment, my mother finally retaliated against my father when he threw an apple at her, leaving an imprint on her chest that is still visible. She in turn, grabbed a knife and skillet and went after him.

"Mama, why did it take all of those years to defend yourself?" I asked her. Then I realized that my father had broken her spirit and she would never be the same.

You Can Run, but You Can't Hide -- A Man Addicted
I know now that I was running from my problems, unaware that I had to confront my demons.

It was tragic to have a father that never expressed any feelings of love for me. So at the age of 17 I made up my mind to join the U.S. Army. My parents knew nothing of this decision until the recruiter arrived at our front door. I know now that I was running from my problems, unaware that I had to confront my demons. Over time I learned that you don't wake up and become mad all of a sudden, something has to contribute to one's fury.

It was the fall of 1976, and I took any drug that was out there to try to negate my pain. The use of hash, cocaine, marijuana, acid, and alcohol was my solution to resolving my problems. For the next three years that I was stationed in Germany, I just abused my body. No matter how high I got, I still carried my issues inside of me, which inevitably multiplied, because I was unfamiliar with spiritual warfare. I understand now that I was destined to become one of God's spokespersons.

In my first year in the service, I never called home. But by lashing out at my father, I was only hurting my mother who had to contact the Red Cross just to locate me and implore that I call home. My commander had to even get involved. He pushed me to at least, get in touch with my family, and tell them that I was alive and doing fine.

<u>Don't Make Me a Widow</u>
My wife pulled me to the side and begged me not to make her a widow.

When I arrived in Ft. Jackson, South Carolina, I met my wife Ernestine Vanlue. We dated for all of three months and then married. She too was in Germany when the Holy Spirit told her that her husband would be in Ft. Jackson. I wed this wonderful woman without her knowing that I had emotional baggage and demons that I battled daily.

After one year of marriage my son Dale Jr. was born. The second year Santino arrived. For the next seven years I was on the run and refused to return home to see my parents. I had made a decision that if I did go home, my plan was to jump my father and inflict the same pain he had delivered to my mother.

When my wife would ask, "Why don't we go home to meet your family?" My response was always the same. I gave her no answer at all.

In 1985 we resided at Ft. Monroe, Virginia, and I was still drinking and drugging. My wife pulled me to the side and begged me to not make her a widow. Her own father died from alcoholism, and she didn't want our family to meet the same fate.

New Generation, Same Curse
My boy's would always ask their mother why I was so angry and crazy.

After years of running and being tormented, the spirit of my father was upon me. Even though I kept my vow and didn't abuse my wife, I channeled my anger toward my children. My boy's would always ask their mother why I was so angry and crazy.

I would snap at my children at any given moment. I had an anger problem that I didn't know how to conquer until the fall of 1985 when I began my journey to transforming my life.

My wife and I joined Antioch Baptist Church in Hampton, Virginia where I sat Sunday after Sunday, not acknowledging I was still sick. The next few years the spirit of my father overwhelmed me and I began to snap at my children again. When they grew up, God had to heal this anger because I was still drinking and trying to medicate my pain.

Three years later I was saved and the Lord released me from all the drugs and alcohol I had relied on. Thankfully, I never had the desire to seek those vices again. For more than 20 years I have been free of them. God delivered me and set me free.

Forgiving Doesn't Mean Forgetting
The pain of my father's legacy would still be embedded in my soul upon our return to Virginia.

Howard V. Booker was our pastor. It was through his teaching that I began to see how sick I really was. He was the one who patiently fed me the Word because of everything I'd been through. It was through him, that I understood I had to forgive my father and myself.

The day of reckoning came when I had to return to the place where my pain began. I gathered my family and went home. For the first time in years, I saw my father and mother. I asked them to forgive me for all of the years I strayed from them, and had allowed my hatred to overtake me, which they did. I told my father, "I forgive you, but I can't forget what you did."

It was apparent that my past still haunted me. All that time I was away, my father, who was a Christian, was the chairman of the deacon board. Everyone loved him, but no one knew the hell that occurred behind the scenes.

<u>Finding a True Father -- Finding Myself</u>
I know the thoughts that I think toward you and they are good and not evil to give you an expected end. Jeremiah 29:11

My birth father was only a sperm donor. Pastor Booker became my mentor -- the only father I knew. When the man that I loved the most died, I mourned this giant for two weeks. His death signified a release of the past and that healing was on the horizon. I soon understood that the seed had to die for the flower to bloom. After his death, I embraced my destiny.

When we opened the doors to Temple of Faith in 1999, I had asked God to give me the ones that no one else wanted. Thus our motto is "To Win The Lost At All Cost!" With only a handful of people as members, the early years were not the easiest, particularly without my mentor to guide and instruct me on what it is to be a pastor. But after quiet reflection, I realized that his lessons had been there all along because he had been training me through all the years.

Men have given to our ministry in multitude. Blessings came from the north, south, east and west. Keeping His word, in season and out, has been a cornerstone of true wealth. Thus, Temple of Faith is flourishing today.

When my birth father passed in 2004, I had to preside over his funeral and burial. Although I had forgiven him, there was no love lost -- no tears shed. I apologized to my mother saying, "I can't fake tears for someone that I didn't know. To me he was a stranger."

Pastor Booker was the man who strengthened, nourished, enriched and loved me. This great man spoke in my life, allowing God to do his work. He prayed for my damaged spirit to be healed. While I flailed in darkness, rudderless without the embrace of the man that brought me in the world, God delivered a true father in Howard V. Booker. Due to his great faith, he redirected my legacy of generational pain to one of renewal and light.

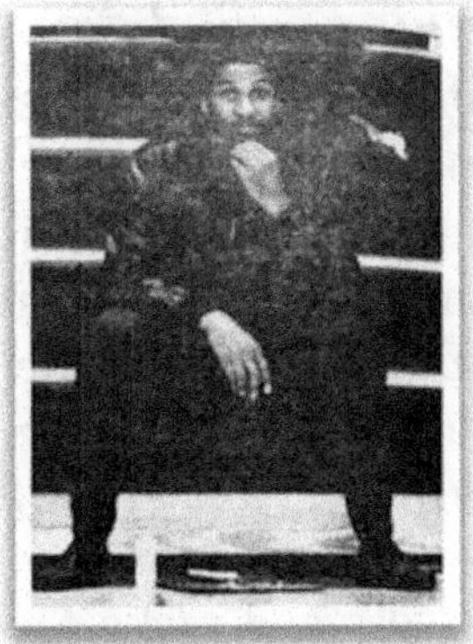

The Surrogate

Jamariah Morris, Gerald Chasten, Jezelle Nelson and Joslyn Gaines Vanderpool

Students flock around Professor Jeri Marshall, or "Marshall" as they affectionately call him. Beaming and bopping with questions after class, following him back to his office as if he were the pied piper of an organized but lively parade of pupils; learning at the knee of the great African scholars and philosophers, eager to quench their thirst for knowledge beyond a textbook often devoid of stories about black geniuses, heroes and heroines. They banter and laugh, exchanging lighthearted barbs because Marshall has a cool persona for an "old gee" some might say.

There is no room to play when young men and women of our particular hue are dying (being slain) literally on streets or dying a death of non-belief in self. Or dying because they never lived, dying from oppression,

inequity and conditions called poverty of mind, desire, opportunity and need.

What holds his students rapt is the wisdom he dispenses, but also his way of listening, schooling, preaching, teaching and engaging is impacting. Recognizing their strengths, and their fears he admonishes and pushes them to dive deeper into their soul to discover their brilliance and know their own history.

Jeri implores his students to dance with their destiny, push forward into their greatness and make a difference in the world. There is no room to play when young men and women of our particular hue are dying (being slain) literally on streets or dying a death of non-belief in self. Or dying because they never lived, dying from oppression, inequity and conditions called poverty of mind, desire, opportunity and need. Jeri has explicitly told me he works with this group, the youth of today in helping them redirect and restore dreams and helps those who never dreamed learn to do so.

What is very clear about Marshall is that he fills a critical void for women and men who come to him for what they are missing. There is a hunger, daddy hunger that he fills to an extent.

Jeri reads his students and is concerned when he feels someone is slipping through the cracks. Genuine, hardworking and loving, he fights every day to keep them leaning in and inspired to ask the tough questions, analyze their thoughts, question the ifs and whys of life, and learn to love who they are and become centered in their universe, not self-centered.

Professor Invested in Pupil Equals Hope for Success

After applying for several counseling positions, Jeri landed an adjunct teaching position a few years ago, which I secretly believed was more attuned to who he is. That first semester was challenging, but through the years I have seen a seasoned, confident sage and elder who is deeply dedicated to helping his students see what he sees in them. He hopes one day to have an Umoja Institute or University based on the principles of the program.

What is very clear about Marshall is that he fills a critical void for women and men who come to him for what they are missing. There is a hunger, daddy hunger that he fills to an extent. He provides a certain stability and consciousness and he shows that they matter. He doesn't fear being vulnerable. Some students have fathers who can't relate, are not there, are missing, or have died, and in "Marshall," they've found a surrogate. I see students stopping to speak to him, get a dose of fatherly advice or acknowledgement that they get an opportunity to connect to someone who really cares. Several times a week students stop by and ask, is Marshall here? When he is, they light up and gather around his desk.

Mr. Marshall is greatly selfless with a very high spirit personality that makes your day every time he enters a room, and he always carries good vibes with a big red heart. I really from the bottom of my heart thank him for all he has done for me and I will forever and always be grateful."

Young men smile when Marshall admonishes them to use their common sense. Female students like having a male figure take interest in their challenges. According to Gerald, a budding entrepreneur and business major, Mr. Marshall was at first just another professor. "When I first met Mr. Marshall I really didn't think much about him besides he is another African American male but as soon as he told me stories about his mistakes and what he did to correct those mistakes he became something greater. To me Mr. Marshall is a mentor because he teaches me how to read people's body language and he has explained many times to me how I should open myself in my writing and in person. And yes, on many occasions he has told me how I should act on a college campus instead of acting like a high school student, which when I look back at it now I say thank you."

Jamariah Morris, a member of the esteemed drumline and a bright young student, lost her father as a small child, and remembers trying to get her father to wake up at his funeral after a tragic death. When she said, "Get up daddy, all these people came here to see you." Everyone fell apart, but she has held his precious memory all of her young life. In Mr. Marshall, she found someone to listen, and states, "Mr. Marshall will be a part of my life for forever. Ever since the day I met him he was an amazing person. He has always been helpful and open hearted about others. Mr. Marshall is greatly selfless with a very high spirit personality that makes your day every time he enters a room, and he always carries good vibes with a big red heart. I really from the bottom of my heart thank him for all he has done for me and I will forever and always be grateful."

Jezelle Nelson is a student who has defied great odds to pursue an education, something that she once thought was not even within her grasp until she had a chance encounter that would propel her to where she is today. In her own words, Jezelle explains her first impression of Professor Marshall. "In 2013 I was diagnosed with breast cancer. After undergoing a double mastectomy and reconstruction I decided to fulfill my dream of getting my college degree. In the Fall of 2014 I met Jeri Marshall. My initial impression of him was that he was just another Black man acting like he cares but, he is just doing his job. After going through the Umoja-Sakhu Community classes I learned to value Mr. Marshall and his dedication to making sure his students were successful. After graduating from ARC, with honors, I transferred to Howard University, in Washington DC. Prior to meeting Mr. Marshall, Howard was just a dream. He has truly helped me to realize a dream that I never thought would come to fruition. The world needs more men like Mr. Marshall. He has been an integral part of my success. I am blessed to know him."

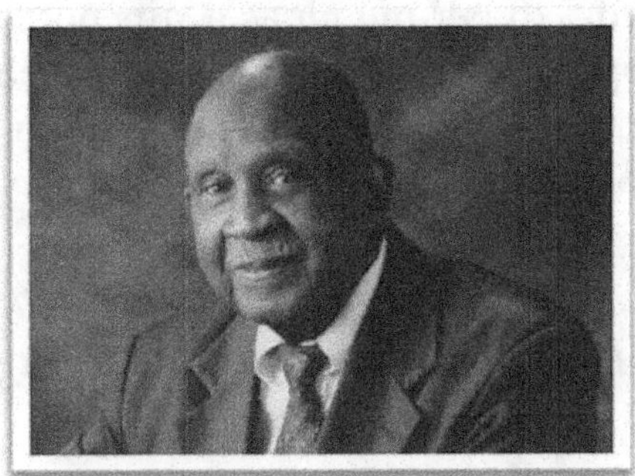

Mission Possible

Lolita Blackman

<u>Building a Dream with a Bit of Luck and a Strong Belief Self</u>

Herb Blackman Jr.'s approach to life was that of an engineer - anything could be achieved if you believed in yourself, worked hard and took advantage of any little piece of luck that came your way. He used this approach to become an engineer at a time when there was no such thing as a black engineer in segregated America. Unable to attend the State University in Kentucky, and there being no school that blacks could attend where they could study engineering, Herb discovered a well-kept secret, which was that the state would pay his tuition to a school in the North to study engineering. So, he chose Howard University – the premier black university in the country. He then had to figure out how to eat and have pocket money, since he was only given funds for tuition.

At 135 lbs., he was too light to play football, not tall enough to play basketball, and not speedy enough to sprint, but he had stamina, so he competed in long distance running. This earned him the right to eat at the athletes' dining table. He joined ROTC because he earned $20 per month as a stipend. He worked nights as a telephone operator in a hotel so that he could study, since very few calls came in at night and sold Watkins products door-to-door, as well as Christmas cards.

Corporate America was now searching for black engineers. His problem became deciding which offer to take.

By using his bit of luck, he graduated as a civil engineer. However, no one would hire a black engineer, and he refused to work at any drafting job that anyone who studied high school drafting could do. So, he picked strawberries, laid railroad ties, painted houses and did any other job that he could for a year after graduating until he finally got a job with the Bureau of Reclamation in Denver, CO as an engineer. After working there for six months, he was drafted into the Air Force as a second lieutenant and sent to Wright Patterson Air Force Base in Dayton, Ohio where he met his wife Lolita Harley who was working there.

If at First You Don't Succeed

It was love at first sight for Herb and Lolita, and they were married in less than a year of their first encounter in 1952. Herb's next move was to apply to the Air Force to attend Purdue University to earn a Master's degree in Civil Engineering. He was accepted, and received his degree in 1954. After serving his "payback" time in Nagoya, Japan, Herb, and "Lo," (short for Lolita), had a baby girl who they named Nicola. When they returned to the United States, they were free to leave the Air Force.

Once again, Herb tried to get a civilian job as an engineer, but was unsuccessful. He then decided to stay in the Air Force and take advantage of any advanced training programs in engineering available. During this time, he earned his professional engineering certification. His next Air Force assignment took his family to Colorado, where another baby girl, Rene' was born. Through the years his other Air Force assignments took him to Alaska, Montana, Ohio, England, Vietnam, and finally South Dakota where his last assignment before retiring from the Air Force was to build underground missile sites.

By using his bit of luck, he graduated as a civil engineer. However, no one would hire a black engineer, and he refused to work at any drafting job that anyone who studied high school drafting could do.

Corporate America was now searching for black engineers. His problem became deciding which offer to take. He went with Ford Motor Company. While working at Ford, Herb could see that the personal computer was going to bring big changes to engineering, so he went back to college to study Computer Aided Design (CAD) and Computer Aided Manufacturing (CAM).

In 1984, he retired from Ford and moved to San Diego because of its wonderful weather. Now 57 years old, he was facing age discrimination, but luck struck again! He applied for a job at a company that had just bought a multimillion dollar computer system that the company engineers did not know how to use. When Herb listed his CAD/CAM training on his application, he was hired on the spot. He worked there for twelve enjoyable years before retiring for the last time.

The last years of Herb's life were spent encouraging young people to consider engineering as an occupation. He started a tutoring program at his church to help students improve their math skills. In addition, he hired young people to do work around his house, paying them the minimum wage to encourage them to develop a good work ethic.

In sum, Herb Blackman Jr. exemplified the term Engineer as – belief in your abilities, hard work, and recognizing and being prepared to take advantage of any luck that comes your way, which is what he did in building a successful career and life.

A Father's Day Promise
Petri Hawkins-Byrd

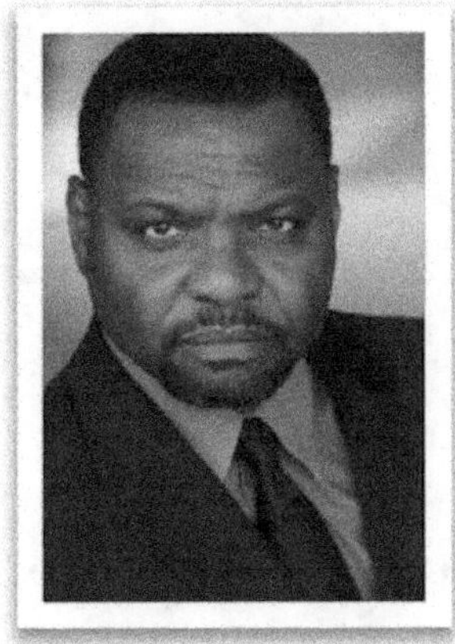

Well folks, as you can tell by now, I didn't make it to this illustrious event this Father's Day. However, I do have a legitimate excuse for my absence. I am busy keeping a promise; to be a good dad.

You see, my youngest daughter, Darcy, was a preemie, born May 28th, 1994 at 28 weeks. She was 1 lb. 14 oz. She fit right in the palm of my hand. Fell in love with her the day I met her. For the next 3 months after she was born, it was touch and go. One June morning we got a call that she might not make it through the day. I began to weep and got down on my knees and made a deal with God. "If you lend her to me," I said "I promise to give You a return on your investment. I promise she will honor You all the days of her life"

Well, yesterday I was back in a hospital room with my baby, bargaining with God again as she battled pneumonia. And again, just like 15 years earlier, I got the best of the bargain. To paraphrase Linus in "A Charlie Brown Christmas," That's what Father's Day is all about, Charlie Brown!"

God bless all the daddies who have bargained with God and upheld their part of the bargain. Happy Father's Day, gentlemen.

EPILOGUE

A FINAL WORD

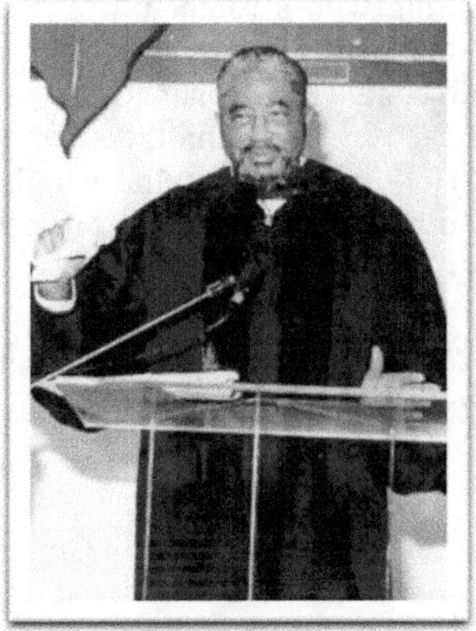

My father acknowledging the Father of all fathers.

His Way

Anita Royston

Real Men, Real Daddies

***Now, we can tell…no SHOUT out to the world the stories
about our wonderful Dads!***

As the co-creator of the Brave, Bold and Beautiful book series, I am blessed to know Joslyn. And most fortunate to have a friend who understands my ways because she too, as you know by now, is a Daddy's Girl.

While we were both attending a meeting at a local college, the facilitator was sharing with a room full of professionals from all stratums of life, the reason there are fewer African Americans coming to the university. He explained that it is due to children who are mostly raised by single mothers and that Black men are absentee fathers. He went on for some length of time espousing that children raised without their fathers are not doing as well and that Black men don't care, etc.

Though my father did many things to help those in his presence, what His Way truly connotes is that he lived his life the way his heavenly Father ordained.

When all was said and done and the meeting was ending, I found myself in somewhat of a emotional fog. As people were leaving, I stood by the desk motionless. I noticed three other Black women still there, seemingly as mystified as I. Finally, I broke the silence

"Was that your experience?" I asked aloud, laying it out there for anyone to answer.

"My daddy was not like that," one of the women said. "My dad was there for me," another one added, shaking her head. The third woman said, "My dad was always with us and never deserted us."

Our initial shock gave way to our truths, as we all piped in and began sharing similar stories about these brave, bold and beautiful men that we all still called Daddy. Cloteal, who is a colleague, was one of the women who joined us in conversation. Her father passed on several years before. Joslyn's father died in 2002; and my Dad had only been gone less than a year. So you can imagine the pain we were feeling hearing such negative statements about the men we adored. Our friend, Shelia whose father is still living, also took each statement by the facilitator personally.

In the spring of 1957, when word came that my father's name had been moved up on the list of hate groups such as the Klan, he had to depart in a hurry to avoid certain death.

Oh, I am not delusional and neither are my sister friends. We all know that there are a lot of absentee fathers for one reason or another, but we also know there are a heck of a lot of Black daddies who are there every day for their children. Joslyn mentioned that she was thinking of writing a book about Black fathers. I had thought of doing the same thing so when she called me and said she was ready and would be honored if I would co-author with her, I was thrilled. Now, we can tell…no SHOUT out to the world the stories about our wonderful Dads!

To see the stories that came our way and currently fill this book is the icing on the cake which is already sweet! This is our way of providing a rare depiction of Black fatherhood. Like all things in life there is a negative and a positive perspective. Since scant attention has been paid to what is right about Black fathers, we chose to look at those men who we identified with -- the type of fathers we know exist and are real to us.

I know there are many more stories that are similar to ours that will be shared in subsequent volumes of this series, but I wanted to introduce my daddy too. My earthly father helped those in his presence as his heavenly Father ordained; Thus His way was in every action, every breath, every word, and deed my father performed. I hope to convey how much this beautiful man touched my heart and everyone that entered his life.

<u>Leaving Mississippi</u>
Daddy had to leave the Hospitality State, which had been everything but that to people of African descent.

You might have read a little about my dad already. My brother, Jerome called him his hero, my sister, Jackie wrote that he was the man who could deliver smiles, and Alberta, who is the tenth and youngest child, referred to him as big, strong, and honorable. Dad meant so much to us, and we cherished him dearly. What I learned from my dad has empowered me to this day.

Daddy was born May 5, 1930 in Avalon, Mississippi to Rev. Mack Clarence and Caroline McGee. He was the youngest of four sons until he was 17, and his brother Calvin was born. Of the five sons, Daddy and Calvin were the two who followed in their father's footsteps and became preachers of the Gospel of Jesus Christ.

Living his life according to what he believed to be right in the eyes of God, and in the best interest of the people who possessed a lesser voice, was the way my Dad existed. He knew that the treatment of his people was unjustified and said so. Due to his outspokenness; however, Daddy had to leave the Hospitality State, which had been everything but that to many, if not most people of African descent.

In the spring of 1957, when word came that my father's name had been moved up on the list of hate groups such as the Ku Klux Klan, he had to depart in a hurry to avoid bodily harm or death. Although my mother was about to deliver their fourth child, she understood the grave consequences that would occur if her beloved husband stayed. So together they quickly conspired for Daddy to leave a few days later and she and the four of us children would join him later. Imagine, traveling with a new born half way across the country.

One of my earliest memories was riding a train from Mississippi to California to join Daddy. We moved to Mather Air Force Base with my uncle Richard and Aunt Sora until we found a place in downtown Sacramento. Later we moved to the River Oaks Housing Projects. My dad was in the Army Reserves, and also worked at Antonita's restaurant as a waiter. He wore uniforms and tuxedos…wow!

<u>When I Grow Up, I'm Going to Marry My Daddy!!!</u>
In essence, we thought that all men were going to be good, like our daddy.

I thought my daddy was the best looking man I had ever seen, and as a young girl I vowed to marry him when I grew up. I've heard that girls marry men who remind them of their dad. My parents were in love for 55 years, and happily married for almost 53 of them. Shortly before their 53rd Anniversary, my father took leave for his homegoing celebration.

People often ask me, "If your parents were happily married for all those years why have their daughters had such difficult times with relationships? Three of us divorced, two remarried, and one never married. Anyway, my answer to that question is easy, "We only saw respect and unconditional love at home regarding how our father treated and loved our mother." In essence, we thought that all men were good, like our daddy. Inevitably, we got into relationships without asking the right questions. We treated all men as if they had our best interest at heart.

Since daddy left, I have gained more understanding. I realize that I had never done the leave and cleave that is outlined in the Bible. I have always had my dad as a backup. If my husband couldn't, wouldn't or didn't, I called my dad. And he could, would and did with expedience and a smile.

I feel for children who don't have fathers at home. I thank God for the men who step up and take in children they did not create and provide a healthy environment filled with good solid teachings of values, morals, and how to be a man. All are principles that can be taught by a woman, except the last one, which is so essential that it cries for a man's direction to model it to their sons.

For almost 13 years I was married, and to that union four children were born. I lived as a divorced single mom for 10 years before meeting my second husband, Steven. Divorce was not something I understood and it was a scary time in the beginning. I made sure my children spent time in the homes of relatives and friends who were happily married so that they could experience what I was unable to provide.

Had I not grown up in a household where there were rules and defined roles, I don't think I would or could have known what was missing. I also believe that my children would have suffered more than they did by not having their father in the home during those formative adolescent years. Reading my son, Clarence's story, Fathering While Falling Out of Love, I had to sit back and fight the tears until I tired of fighting them and just let them flow. I had no idea that the pain went as deeply as it apparently did from the marital unrest he and our other children experienced.

The Last Days, Would Be His Best Days
The climber gets a better view of the mountain from
a distance. The more time that passes the more
clearly I see life as it really is. --Kalil Gibran

In his earlier days, my dad wasn't well thought of by some male ministers because he allowed women in the pulpit at his church. He wasn't afraid to have a woman teach him what he needed to know. As a matter of fact, he said that the Word came first through a woman. What sane theologian can dispute that?

When my father was at the end of his journey, one of the ministers acknowledged that because of this great man, he had ordained 30 women. My father's unwavering conviction and teaching in regard to women led more men to leave the old ways of the past behind and embrace the role that God called both genders to do: spread the good Word to the masses that Christ was born, lived , died and rose again for their salvation.

Daddy agreed with scripture believing that his last days would be his best days. Mama said that he once asked her, "What do you think people would say about me when I'm gone?"

Well, daddy suffered a stroke in 1999 which slowed him down quite a bit and in 2006 after more health problems he lost his ability to speak. The beauty of daddy not being able to speak was that he was able to hear what everyone had to say about how he had affected their lives without interrupting, as he otherwise would, with humble inferences such as "It is all to the glory or it wasn't me but the Lord isms."

I remember the last time I saw him laugh. It was a silent body riveting laugh that I was accustomed to, though without the booming sounds of joy attached. What sent my Dad into convulsions of laughter was my comment that, "lots of churches would be closed on Sunday." Using his eyes and shoulder gestures as language, he asked, Why?

"Because Sunday is Christmas," I replied. He looked at me as if to say, *That's nuts!!!* His shoulders shook up and down, and I could hear his howling laughter in my mind the way he used to laugh when something just didn't make sense. Then he looked like he was trying to say, *They just don't know any better.*

Unfortunately it was no laughing matter when the last days drew near for Daddy. Ministers came from near and far as we kept a 24/7 vigil around his hospice bed once he came home. On December 27, 2006, Daddy went into the hospital. As a family, we decided to pray, let go and accept God's plan for him.

We put up signs in his room to make sure the healthcare workers understood that he was more than a patient. He was a family man and a child of God. When the doctors said he would be going to a convalescent home we let it be known that that was not an option. There were enough of us to provide around the clock care. On that Saturday evening at 6:46pm, Daddy transitioned from this life to forever. Word of his passing brought fellow pastors, friends and family from near and far.

Somehow I thought Daddy would always be here. We had just lost the one man on this earth whom loved us unconditionally. The pain of his physical absence will always be in my heart. Yet, all in all I was, and am blessed to have had a loving father, doting grandfather and uncles. To this day I depend on my Uncle Freddie (my mother's brother) to visit me on my birthdays and any other special occasions. But that is what one does for his favorite niece isn't it? Keep vigil, continue to love and nurture, as my father also would have surely done for any child longing for her father's embrace.

In Memoriam – Two Pioneers for Justice in Elevating the Legacy of Black Men

George Rene Francis

June 6, 1896-December 27, 2008

It is with heavy heart that we mourn the loss of Mr. George Rene Francis, whose story, "**A Man of Three Centuries**," appears in both this edition and the first edition of *Our Black Fathers, Brave, Bold and Beautiful.* Known as the oldest man in the world at the time, he was a joy, sage, blessing and treasure to us, his family and the world. When Mr. Francis was anywhere, he could light up the room with his infectious spirit.

In 1896 Mr. Francis was born in New Orleans, Louisiana, and in time befriended the great jazz legend, Louis Armstrong, and as a young school boy, listened to the educator Booker T. Washington when he visited his classroom. After living 112 years and 204 days, he took his final breath of an amazing life on December 27, 2008. In his lifetime 21 men took the oath of office for the United States presidency, but perhaps the most critical, to Mr. Francis was the election of Mr. Barak Obama (The first African American president of the United States), who he proudly voted for.

On being told that Mr. Obama had won, Mr. Francis who was wheel chair bound, commented in an interview with The Associated Press "I felt like jumping up and down," and proudly pronounced, "He is going to give black men a break in the world, and give them a better opportunity to live and make more money." He went on to say, "For people who say voting doesn't matter, I think that's crazy."

Mr. Francis comments are understandable, and his plight like so many other black men is why we continue telling their stories. Living in three centuries, he witnessed major historical events, experienced Jim Crow racism, which was prevalent and legally condoned; saw the fight for Civil Rights, the fall of Apartheid and the day many thought would never come, the election of the first African American president.

In connection to his story, we published a poem that Mr. Francis was known to often recite, **"A Black Man's Plea for Justice."** Sadly, despite progress in the world, the journey to find justice for men of African descent has not been achieved. So, the struggle continues, but Mr. Francis took his place and was a shining star, working for himself, speaking his truth, carving a place in history and leaving a powerful legacy of perseverance. We will miss this brave, bold and beautiful gentleman with the young heart, who attributed his longevity to his loving family. We are so deeply honored by this great American, son of the universe and pioneer for justice, for sharing his story and life, and extend our most heartfelt condolences to his family.

Donald Bailey

August 16, 1939-June 9, 2014

Mr. Don Bailey, was a fireball of energy, who got around town in his little truck, worked in his own company, ***Pulsar Video Productions,*** where he did voiceovers, commercials, and produced projects for the NBA, NASA, the Montel Williams Show and whomever else needed his video production services. He also worked with Ella Fitzgerald and Muhamad Ali to name a few, but he was humble, hardworking and a down to earth gentleman who adored his wife, daughters and grandchildren. He also served his country in the United States Navy; and in our eyes, was truly brave, bold and beautiful!

In deciding to promote *Our Black Fathers: Brave, Bold and Beautiful* we met with Don who at first agreed to assist us but as a business arrangement. Then he came back to us with a heavy heart and said, "I'm sorry," quickly realizing this was about a "mission" that had to be advanced and he very much wanted to be a part of. So, there he was, helping with anything we needed. He passionately stated on more than one occasion, "We have to get these stories out there!" and lent his voice to a commercial about the book and gave us his contacts and tips on how to try to get it to media outlets. He was a genuine "soul" promoter, whose efforts came from his heart. His desire to ensure that black men were recognized and elevated was authentic and heartfelt.

When we embarked on writing the stories, Anita and I were motivated by our own fathers. Even though they brought happiness, stability, strength and love to our lives, we knew that they endured pain and hardship due to racial hatred and discrimination; and we wanted to tell the stories of their, and other men's lives to counter stereotypes typically assigned to men of African descent.

In Don, we knew he had a story too, and it was beautiful, but also had dimensions of pain. His story, **"The Man Who Propelled Me to Soar,"** was a tribute to his father. Don achieved many of his dreams because of his father's support and his own determination. At an event at American River College, Don was asked to read his story about his father, and it happened, suddenly tears flowed down his face because of his father's meaning to his life, and his remembrance of what he endured as a black man during his times.

Don's father was born in 1914 and ironically, Don passed away 100 years later in 2014. I still remember an adopted philosophy that they shared, when faced with racism, that Don included in his story: *If the front door is closed there's always a back door and sometimes it's smarter to open the door slowly rather than try to kick it open."* Not surprisingly, they did open a few doors that resulted in some major successes.

Attending Don's funeral was mind-boggling, I was not sure he was really gone. Yes, his spirit remains, and his emails about the project haven't all been erased (too difficult). At the end, I don't know if he told us this story or we read it somewhere, but as a youth, Don was a boy scout in the South. While shopping for his uniform at a Dillard's store, a white security guard approached him, and told him that the first uniform he touched would be the one he bought because of racial hatred based on the belief that black hands touching anything meant it was ruined. So, fighting back tears, Don gathered up his uniform, and the pain of that event, settled within for a lifetime, but could not stop his ascent to his many accomplishments and his efforts to promote young people with pursuing their dreams.

Like, Mr. Francis, Mr. Bailey left a powerful legacy. We are grateful for their contributions because each were heroes, and self-made men who credited their families for playing substantial roles in their lives. As proud black men, they were assets to not only their race, but to the human race. As with Mr. Francis, Don will be greatly missed for first and foremost, being our friend, as well as for his talents and being one of the biggest catalyst and cheerleaders to the work we are doing on the behalf of our Black fathers. As his father was the wind beneath his wings, Don is the same for us, propelling us to soar, and get the stories out, so Black men won't be forgotten. And so, we will, and are honored to do so.

About The Creators

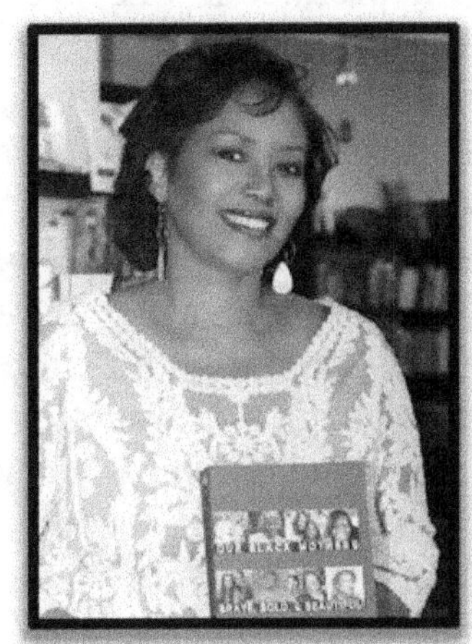

ANITA MCGEE ROYSTON is a writer, publisher and an education consultant who specializes in engaging family and community involvement in public education environments. She has worked with the Sacramento City Unified School District as Parent Advisor. She also worked for the University of California Davis as Early Academic Outreach Programs ("EAOP") Family Programs Coordinator and later with two private think tanks, Linking Education and Economic Development ("LEED") and GEAR-UP!" as Director and Family Programs Coordinator, respectively. In 2002, she was a UC Davis Chancellors Award winner for her multi-lingual, multi-racial work with students and families.

Ms. McGee Royston also served as President of the Del Paso Heights Elementary School District in Sacramento County, California and as a Consultant for North Sacramento's Roberts Family Development Center. An artist at heart, she is one-third of the Lexington, North Carolina Southern Gospel southern gospel trio known as "Pryme Tyme".

Currently an am radio personality with wkby1080.net where she covers weather, music and weekend news, Ms. McGee Royston also hosts a hit Saturday morning women's program entitled THE VIEWPOINT. Anita is a gifted connector of resources-to-needs for social and academic success of families and students.

430

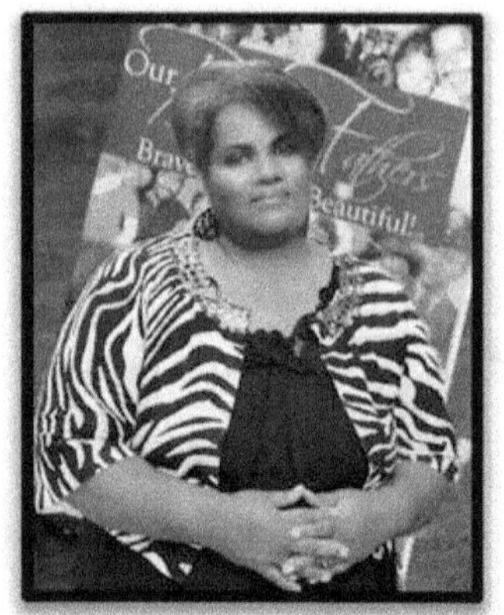

Joslyn Gaines Vanderpool is a motivational speaker, writer, editor, entrepreneur (http://www.cafepress.com/jozzygeestees); and an educational and empowerment specialist. She is married, and the proud mother of an amazing daughter with autism. A graduate of the University of California, Berkeley, she worked for the United States Congress, and wrote for political, educational and non-profit magazines, newsletters, and newspapers. As a staff writer for a national public interest lobby, she covered issues about human rights, poverty, education, Apartheid, nuclear disarmament, and military wars and conflicts.

She has a credit as the principal researcher for two educational documentaries: *Beyond the Dream I and II.* In addition, she has worked at Howard University, University of New Mexico and American River College, where she has helped numerous students attain scholarships. As a career counselor she worked with learning disabled adults

Ms. Gaines Vanderpool has given presentations at many venues, and institutions, and is passionate about imploring others to realize their dreams and acknowledge their beauty, strength and worth. She enthusiastically exults all to live in a positive light and be mindful of how our humanity and capacity to love can break through racism and other societal ills. As co-creator of the *Brave, Bold, Beautiful* Book Series, she is excited that she met Anita McGee Royston and has the opportunity to write again, including the children's books, poetry, memoirs and plays, she had put aside. Most critically, she loves reviewing stories from individuals from every stratum of life; and encourages everyone to begin the process of leaving an intentional legacy so others know that YOU existed and made a positive and impactful contribution to the planet!

About the Authors
Permissions & Acknowledgements

Every effort has been made to secure proper permission/acknowledgment for each story in this work. If an error or omission has been made please accept our apologies and contact Five Sisters Publishing, P.O. Box 233721, Sacramento, CA 95823 so that corrections can be made in future editions.

Permissions to reprint any of the stories from this book must be obtained from the original source. Acknowledgments are listed alphabetically by author's name. Heartfelt thanks to all the contributors who allowed their work to be included in this collection of stories.

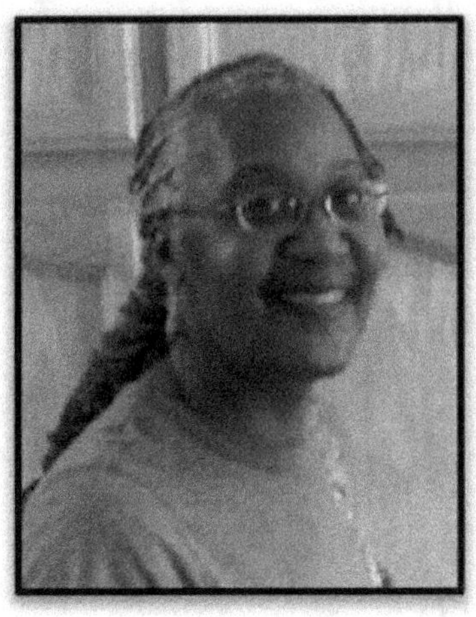

Alfreda Abdul-Ahad
JT Whitman, A Good Man

One of These Days I'm Gonna Get Out of Here

Alfreda Stephens Abdul-Ahad is a military brat, whose father retired from the United States Coast Guard. She has lived from coast to coast, and has always loved reading and writing. She currently resides in northern California, and plans to continue working on other writing projects. JT Whitman, A Good Man copyright 2017 Alfreda Abdul-Ahad. Used by permission. All rights reserved.

Yusaf Salsabil Alkimia
From the Valley of Violence into the Light of Deliverance

"With God's help," and as much time as he has to give, Yusuf Salsabil Alkimia can be found on the streets of the community talking to youth about God and the history of "our people." Whenever he is asked to teach at a school, he makes it a priority. Yusaf reaches out to the homeless, and youth where they are, whether it is on the light rail, the bus or downtown Sacramento. When he finds work in the field of home repair, he tries to balance it with his spiritual work, along with fatherhood. From the Valley of Violence into the Light of Deliverance © 2008 Yusaf Salsabil Alkimia. Used by permission. All rights reserved.

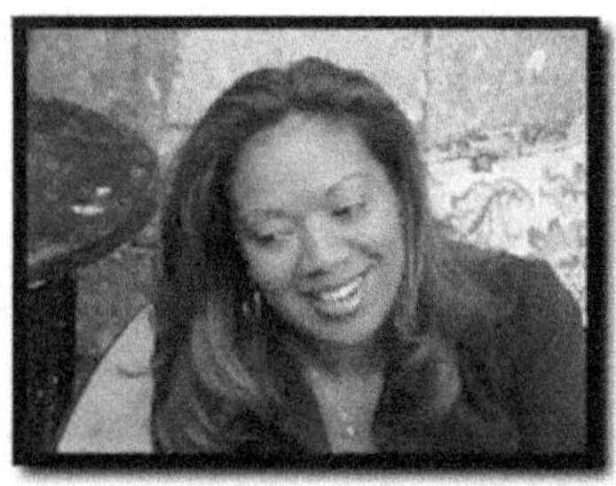

Allison Anderson
My Father, My Everything

Allison Anderson is originally from Oakland, California and moved to New York City in 2004. She currently works in the 3D technology world. Having been in the workforce, Allison decided it was time for a change. She has returned to college and has set about reinventing herself. An avid blogger, Ms. Anderson has turned what started as just another way to practice her writing, into a dedicated passion. My Father, My Everything © 2008 Allison Anderson. Used by permission. All rights reserved.

Sha-Toyia Anderson
A Lasting Legacy: Goodnight Sweet Prince

Sha-Toyia Anderson, is 29 years old and resides in Sacramento California. She currently attends American River College where she is completing her A.S. degree, but will be transferring to Sacramento State University to attain a B.A. in Business Administration. Sha-Toyia professes a love for words, and states, "Writing has always been a passion for me because I love to express myself through writing and letting others read about my life by giving a vivid picture for the mind, which is well worth me putting it in writing rather than telling someone face-to-face. When I was just 8 years old I wrote my first story and I have always loved to rhyme and write poems and sing. My story expresses my struggle and my love towards my family and my upbringing. I want to use my success as a student to help other people and reach out to those who can relate to me and understand the real reason for our purpose on the planet. In the end, we only regret the chances we didn't take and I want to take every chance I get to help change someone's life with my story." A Lasting Legacy: Goodnight Sweet Prince copyright 2017 Sha-Toyia Anderson. Used by permission. All rights reserved.

Donald Bailey
The Man Who Propelled Me to Soar

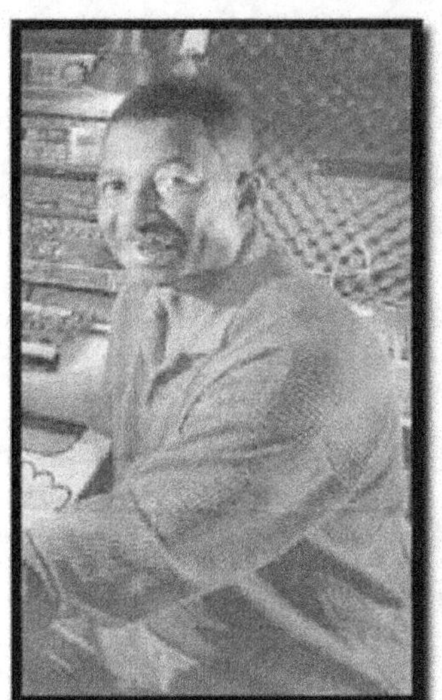

Donald Bailey is the married father of three children. A native of Baltimore, Maryland he graduated from Pepperdine University with a degree in business sciences and has had a wide variety of experiences. He served eight years in naval aviation, 17 years with the Xerox corporation and 25 years as president and CEO of Pulsar Video Productions, which is a small full service production company with a home office in Sacramento, California. He has worked with many notable individuals including Ella Fitzgerald, Bill Cosby and Montel Williams. Pulsar also provides video production services for NASA and the National Basketball Association. Don is always eager to share his experiences with others, especially youth. He can be contacted at www.pulsarvideo@sbcglobal.net. The Man Who Propelled Me to Soar © 2008 Don Bailey. Used by permission. All rights reserved.

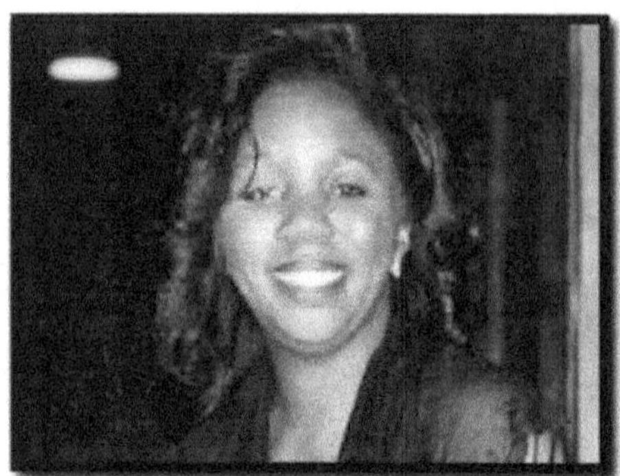

Alberta Barrow

When Heaven Calls

Alberta is a wife and mother of three wonderful daughters. She is a preschool teacher and works part time as a Creative Memories consultant. Alberta truly believes that scrap booking is a fun way to pass stories on from one generation to the next. When Heaven Calls © 2008 Alberta Barrow. Used by permission. All rights reserved.

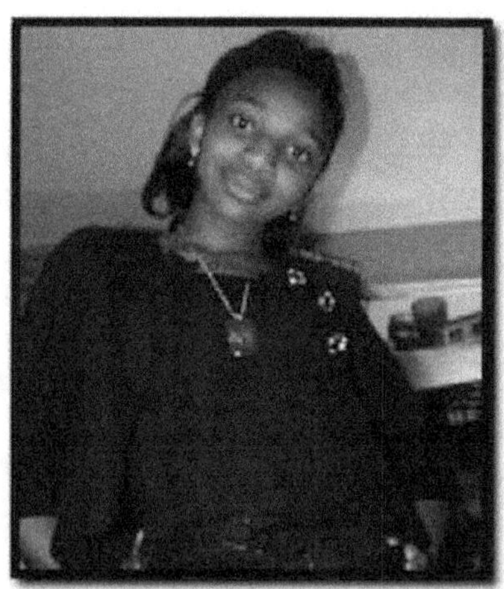

Genesis Barrow
The Guardian that Walks with God

Genesis Elease Barrow was born on April 28, 1995. The eldest of three girls born to Mr. & Mrs. Barrow, she currently resides in Stockton, California and attends Progressive Community Church. As a student at Christa McAuliffe Middle School, she takes Pre-Advanced Placement (AP) courses. Ms. Barrow is interested in art, architecture, music, and hanging out with family and friends. "I am a blossoming branch from a deeply rooted tree. My Grandmother used to sing a song about a tree planted by the water. My family, like the tree is nourished by a supply that is never far from it -- God. My family consists of authors, preachers, lawyers, teachers, actors and comedians -- very distinct branches all from the same tree." The Guardian that Walks with God © 2008. Used by permission. All rights reserved.

Lolita Blackman
Mission Possible

Lolita Blackman graduated with a masters degree in Special Education from Wayne State University.Currently retired, she was happily married to a loving husband, Herbert Blackman Jr., for 58 ½ years; and is the proud mother of two daughters, Nicola Blackman and Rene' McGaugh, and the grandmother of Ryan and Aaron McGaugh. She also has an older sister, June Dumas. For 15 years Ms. Blackman taught Special Education and worked as a counselor in the evenings at an adult school for five years. She has always believed that having an education is important, and helping students with challenges, and taking care of yourself are crucial. Her previous hobbies were sewing, arts and crafts, and upholstering furniture. She loves getting her daily exercise, reading, playing bridge, and doing crossword and word search puzzles. Mission Possible, copyright 2017 Lolita Blackman. Used by permission. All rights reserved.

Ruthie Bolton

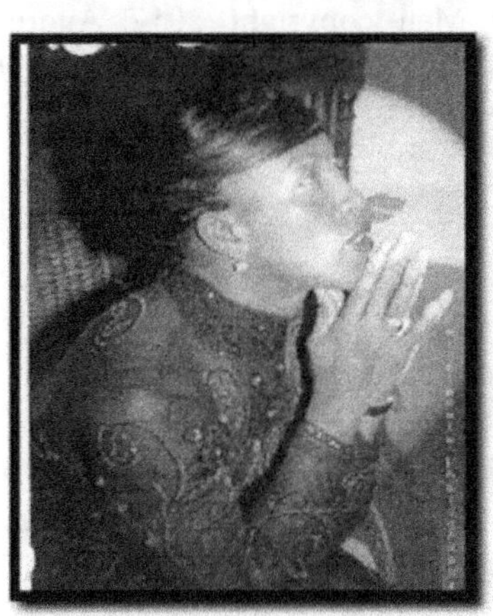

Thanks for the Incredible Ride Dad!

Ruthie Bolton is the sixteenth of 20 children. Inspired by her late parents, Reverend Linwood and Leola Bolton, Ruthie has achieved many of her dreams. She played basketball for the University of Auburn, after previously being rejected. It was her father who freed her spirit and belief in herself through his messages of adopting a positive mental attitude -- principles she would use repeatedly throughout her journey. Not given an invitation to try out for the National U.S. Womens' Basketball Team, she paid her own way, made the squad and defied the odds by leading the team to five World Championship victories, including two gold medals in the 1996 and 2000 Olympics. Ruthie became the U.S. National Team's *Most Valuable Player*. In 1997 when the WNBA was formed, Ruthie Bolton was the cornerstone of the Sacramento Monarchs franchise. A two-time All-Star, she retired in 2004 and thus far, is the only Monarch to have her number retired in Sacramento's Arco Arena. Ruthie is engaged in the community, and loves inspiring youth with the principles her father taught her. She has appeared on the *David Letterman Show, and Regis and Kathy Lee.* And she has been highlighted in *Sports Illustrated* and in a Nike commercial. Thanks for the Incredible Ride Dad! © 2008 Ruthie Bolton. Used by permission. All rights reserved.

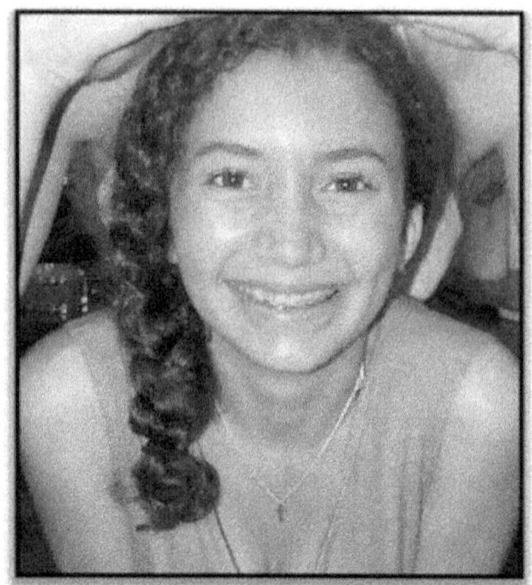

Audrey Booth
The Million Dollar Man
Audrey Booth is a student at Mira Loma High School in Sacramento, California. She was born to Dr. Derrick and Denise Booth, and has an older brother, Derrick Jr., and a younger sister, Dorsey. She loves spending time with her family, reading books and writing stories. The Million Dollar Man copyright 2017 Audrey Booth. Used by permission. All rights reserved.

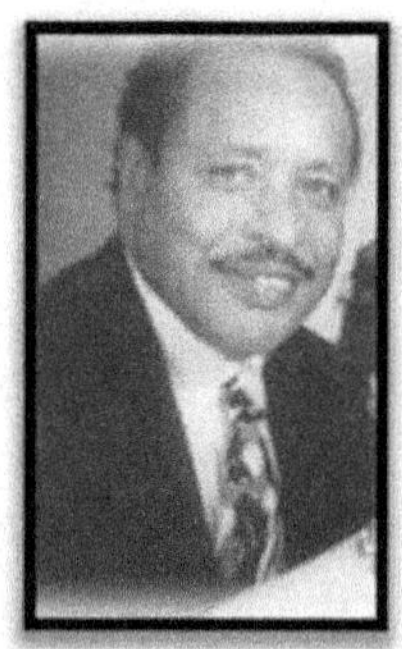

Apostle Lawrence Campbell
A Life of Divinity and Alleviating the Racial Divide
Apostle Lawrence Campbell has an Associate of Arts from Virginia Seminary and College in Lynchburg, Virginia. He received a BS in Psychology from Averett College. In 1988 he was elected to the Danville School Board and in 1991 he was consecrated Apostle by the Board of Bishops. Today he is the Senior Chief Apostle of the International Bible Way Church of Jesus Christ, Inc. and serves on the Executive Board of Bishops and is the Diocesan for the state of Virginia. Currently, he is in the process of writing a book called the Turning Point of Civil Rights, which is all about 1963; and he is considering forming a Race Relation Committee for the city of Danville, VA. Apostle Campbell is the father of five successful children: Allethia, Lawrence Jr, Angela, Philip, Hope. A Life of Divinity and Alleviating the Racial Divide copyright 2017 Lawrence Campbell. Used by permission. All rights reserved.

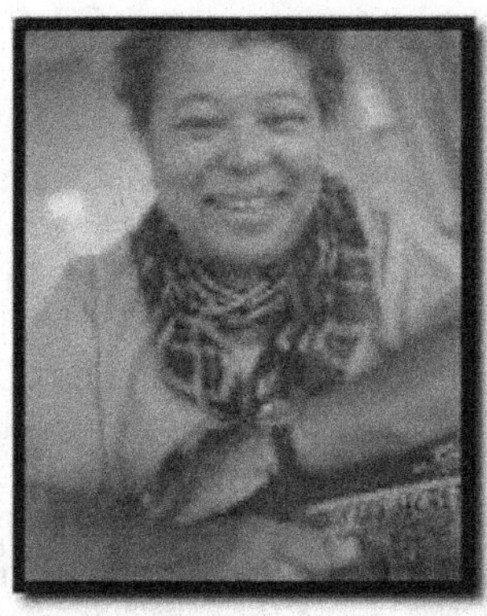

Patricia E. Canterbury

Larger than Life

Patricia E. Canterbury, who is a native of Sacramento, is also an award-winning poet, short story writer, novelist, philanthropist and political scientist. She is the author of *The Secret of St. Gabriel's Tower* and *Carlotta's Secret*. She lives with her husband Richard, and is active in Sisters-In-Crime, Mystery Writers of America, Northern California Publishers and Authors, the Society of Children's Writers and Illustrators and ZICA Creative Arts and Literary Guild. Her website is: www.patmyst.com. Larger than Life © 2008 Patricia E. Canterbury. Used by permission. All rights reserved.

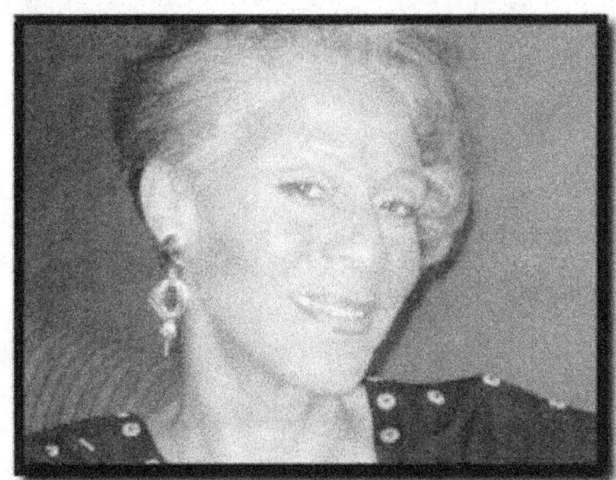

Virginia "Honey" Carter

I Didn't Know

Honey Carter is a San Francisco native who currently lives in Sacramento, California. She is a mother of two and a step-mom to one, a grandmother of five, and a wife. She loves to educate. Honey is a real estate broker with a B.A. in business, and she blends *Ms. V's Spice Is Nice One Step Seasoning*. Her most recent accomplishments include writing a children's book about telling time, which is titled: *What Time Is It?* and *The Many Faces of Big Mama*, which is dedicated to her mother and was recently published. A forty plus runway model, Honey has experienced her twisty twenties, trying thirties, fortified forties and is now in her feisty fifties. She's looking forward to her sexy sixties, sensual seventies, elegant eighties and nice, nasty nineties, but more importantly, she wants to center the century mark on her memories. I Didn't Know © 2008 Virginia "Honey" Carter. Used by permission. All rights reserved.

Gerald Chasten
The Surrogate

Gerald Chasten currently is a student at American River College with plans to become one of the leading CEOs in a fortune 500 company. He loves to run and meet new people and inspire them to "Dive Deep" and share their experiences with him. After graduating from ARC, he plans to attend Sacramento State or the University of Southern California and become a Business Entrepreneurship Graduate. The Surrogate copyright 2017 Gerald Chasten. Used by permission. All rights reserved.

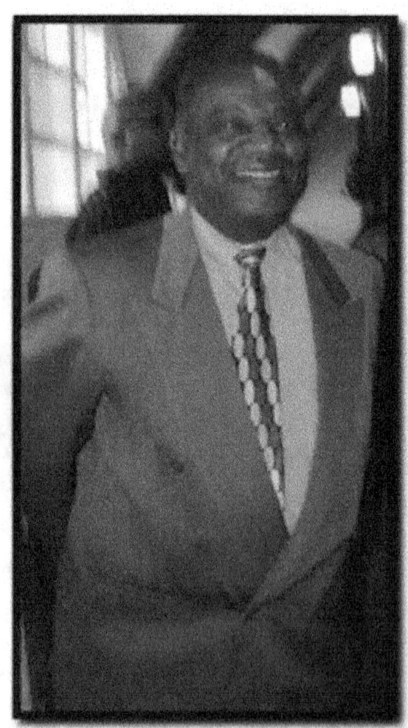

Theris Coats
A Man of Quiet Determination

Theris Coats grew up in San Francisco. He is the eleventh of 17 children of Curtis and Gradie Coats. Early on he discovered a love for music and singing, developing into a Gospel singer at an early age. He sang and performed with 9 of his brothers and sisters in the group, The COATS Singers for more than 35 years. The group traveled as far as Japan and did the music video, *Cry* with Michael Jackson. Theris graduated from Balboa High School and attended San Francisco City College, later graduating from Polly Priest Business College in Oakland, CA. He's been married for more than 25 years and has 4 children. Retired from the State of California, he manages his entertainment business, TLC PRODUCTIONS (www.tlcee-productions.com). He has a deep passion for the Church, his family, music and all children; some of his hobbies include singing, producing, mechanics and writing music. A Man of Quiet Determination © 2008 Theris Coats. Used by permission. All rights reserved.

Lee E. Downing

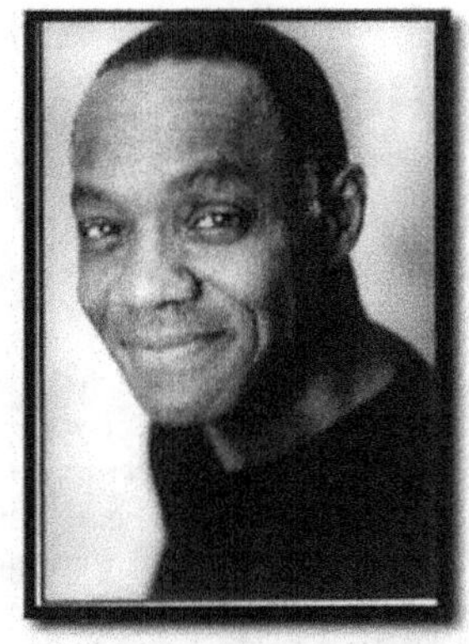

Forgotten Horseman: A Son's Weekend Memoir

Lee Downing was raised in North Canton, Ohio. With a B.A. and M.A. from Central Michigan University, his professional career has spanned a wide range of educational endeavors from, junior high school teacher to college instructor and Student Program and Services administrator for Temple and Penn State universities. Following a liver transplant in 1988, he became actively involved in transplantation education as a volunteer, which led to a new professional career working for an organ procurement agency as a community outreach educator and as a senior product specialist in Immunology for Fujisawa Healthcare, Inc. (Astellas Inc.) He has devoted much of the past 17 years following his transplant to improve organ donor awareness through publishing articles. Lee recently wrote a moving story in remembrance of his father which is a part of this book with the same title. A film and theatrical screenplay adaptation of his book has recently been written by the author and is being reviewed for future development and production. To learn more about these productions, please contact the author at his email address: leedowning8@msn.com. Lee currently resides in North Wales, Pennsylvania, a suburb of Philadelphia. The Forgotten Horseman: A Son's Weekend Memoir © 2006 Lee Downing. Used by permission. All rights reserved.

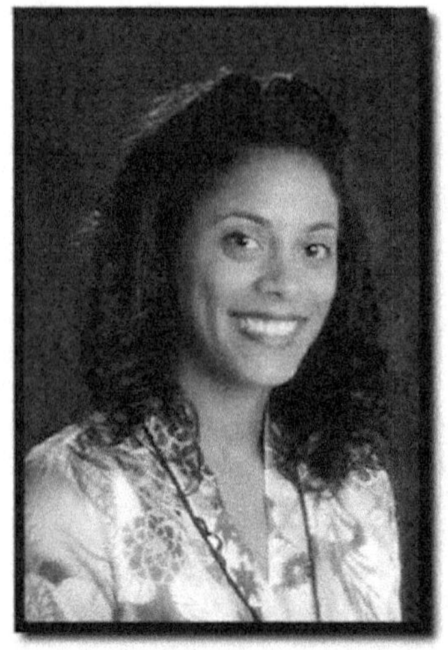

Shelia Duruisseau-Sidqe

The Audacity to Dream

Shelia Duruisseau-Sidqe received a bachelor's degree in social welfare from the University of California, Berkeley and a master's degree in educational administration and policy with an emphasis on outreach and retention from California State University, Sacramento. She recently left the University of California, Davis after 13 years of employment and is currently the director of "Operation: College", a college access program at Hiram Johnson High School in Sacramento. She has over 10 years of experience in counseling, tutoring, mentoring, and developing student support programs. Her interest lies in student equity, access, and eligibility. Shelia is happily married to her husband of 15 years, Rashid Sidqe, and is the proud mother of three daughters. The Audacity to Dream © 2008 Shelia Duruisseau-Sidqe. Used by permission. All rights reserved.

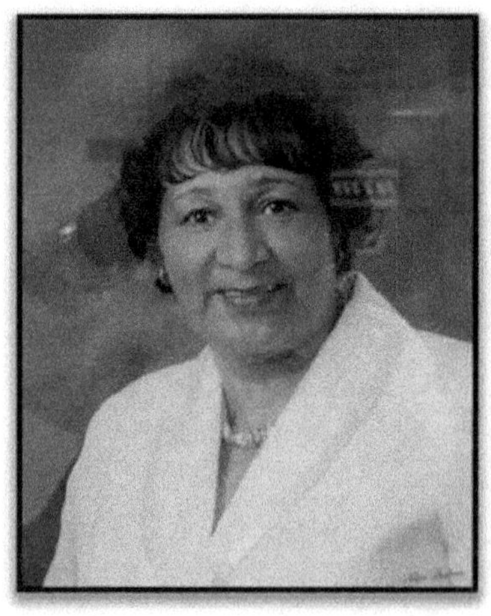

Portia Fitzgerald
The Willie Fitzgerald Story

L. Portia Thompson Fitzgerald, grew up in rural Pittsylvania Co., VA. She is a product of a "one-roomed school house", where she dreamed to someday become a successful elementary school teacher and marry a wonderful, Christian husband. Portia even recorded those exact words in her Senior Memories book as she graduated from Northside High School. Through faith and hard work, her dream came true. She received her B.S. degree in Early Childhood Education from Virginia State University in Petersburg, VA, and later went on to obtain her Masters' Degree from the University of Virginia in Charlottesville, VA. In 1970, she married Willie T. Fitzgerald, who would become not only her husband, but her best friend for life and an awesome role model for their three children along with other neighborhood youth. He emerged to become a strong leader in his church and the community – always aspiring to *"Help someone else along the way and make a difference."* His dreams coincided with her dreams. Portia's story of her Brave, Bold, and Beautiful husband, Willie T. Fitzgerald copyright 2017 Pertia Fitzgerald. Used by permission. All rights reserved.

Roshaun Fowler

My Dad, My Friend, My Hero

Roshaun Fowler is a former Bay Area native and has resided in Sacramento, California for two years. She felt it was her utmost responsibility as a daughter, to share the story of her relationship with her father, her friend and hero. Their relationship was one based on love, respect and being honest with one another. My Dad, My Friend, My Hero copyright 2017 Roshaun Fowler. Used by permission. All rights reserved.

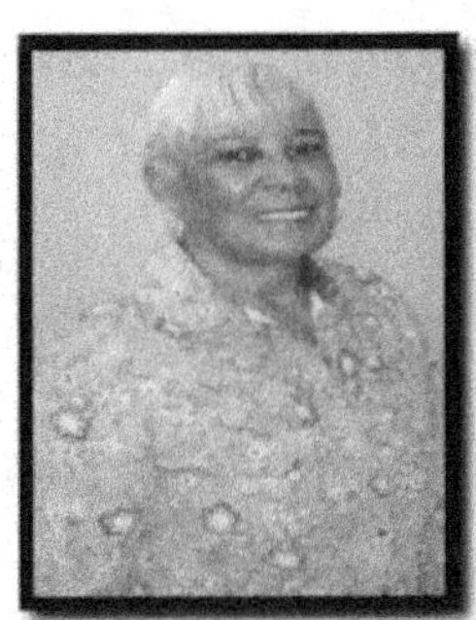

Shirley Francis Wade
A Man of Three Centuries

Shirley Francis Wade was born in New Orleans, Louisiana and lived in the 7th Ward. The youngest of 4 children born to George Rene Francis and Josephine Alcidia Francis, she grew up Catholic. While living in New Orleans, Ms. Wade attended Corpus Christi Catholic Church which had the largest *Colored* congregation in the United States. She moved to Sacramento, CA in 1949 at the time when the city was called *Cow Town* and graduated from Sacramento High School. Ms. Wade is married with four children, six grandchildren and four great grandchildren. She is retired from California state service as the executive secretary to the statewide director of the Office of Administrative Hearings. During her tenure she worked closely with administrative law judges. She continues to be very busy enjoying life with her wonderful family. A Man of Three Centuries © 2008 Shirley Francis Wade. Used by permission. All rights reserved.

442

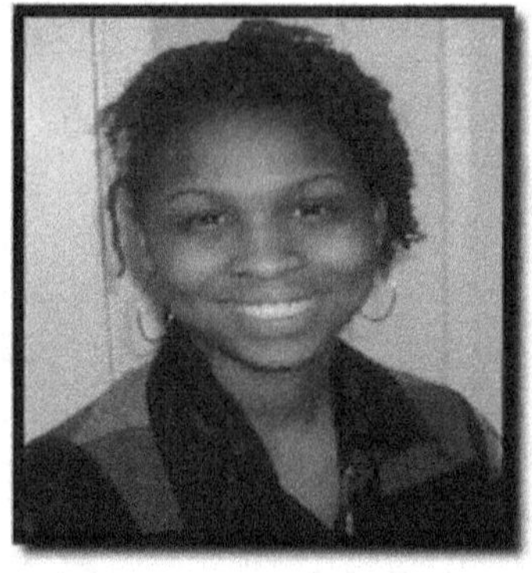

Tracy Gailes

The Man Who Would Never Give Up

Tracy Gailes is a 22 year old college senior. She has gone from nearly dropping out of high school to becoming an honors student at the University of Memphis. She has written and self-published a book of poetry, performed spoken word at numerous events and written various published articles. She has been active in the community for about five years. Tracy is a budding historian and teacher. She mentors youth as a part-time teacher at the Boys and Girls Club and plans to continue mentoring youth through life. The Man Who Never Gave Up © 2008 Tracy Gailes. Used by permission. All rights reserved.

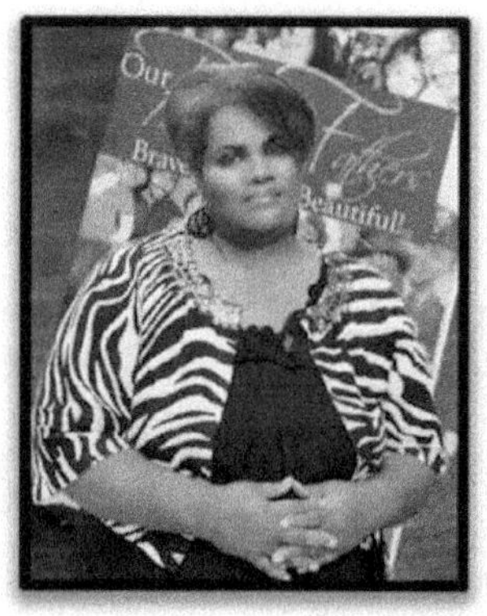

Joslyn Gaines Vanderpool
Our Black Fathers, A Father With No Child to Love, Beautiful Just Beautiful, Spirit of My Father Incarnate, Long Lost but not Forgotten—A Tale of Three Uncles

Joslyn Gaines Vanderpool is married and has a lovely inspiration named Sydney. She was a congressional intern, and writer/editor for political magazines and associations, in Washington DC. Her works have appeared in diverse publications. Joslyn has a B.A. in Political Science from the University of California at Berkeley. She is dedicated to encouraging all of those she encounters to believe in their gifts, abilities and talents. A budding entrepreneur, she has started a line of gifts to inspire. She will continue her work to empower others to pursue their dreams and passions through her unique and powerful motivational presentations and projects that are designed to give individuals an opportunity of expression through words. "Telling one's own truth(s), enlightens and frees!" To contact Joslyn about speaking engagements, and other projects regarding the Brave, Bold and Beautiful series and her line of inspirational gifts, please email her at joslyngaines@comcast.net or contact her at (916)427-3318.

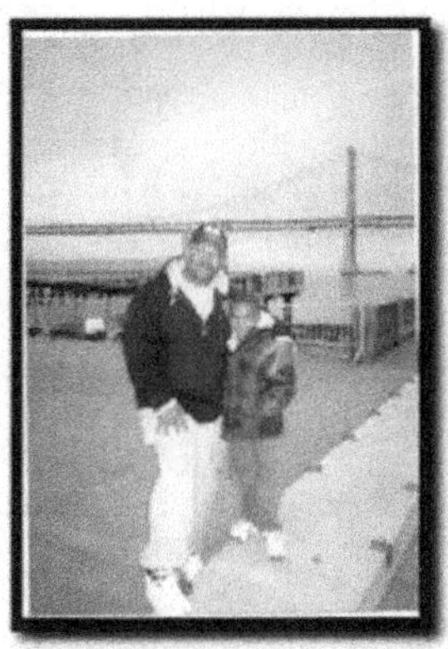

Leon Alexander Gray

I Wanna Go Anywhere You Go!

After working 23 years in the stock brokerage industry, Leon Alexander Gray is currently a business consultant. He also is a freelance writer and musician of the band, LSB (www.lsb13.com). "I'm a short story writer and look one day to have a syndicated column." His work, which mainly is on the subject of family, has been published in newspapers. Presently, he is working on a book about the making of his band who he describes as "a unique group of individuals who have overcome obstacles." Married 19 years to Angela, they have five children: Kisha, who is his stepdaughter and mother to granddaughter, Dymond, and four other children: Danielle, Kristen, Tamera and Jayson. "My love is God and family; my passion is writing; and my mission is to bless others as God has blessed me." I Wanna Go Everywhere you Go! © 2008 Leon Alexander Gray. Used by permission. All rights reserved.

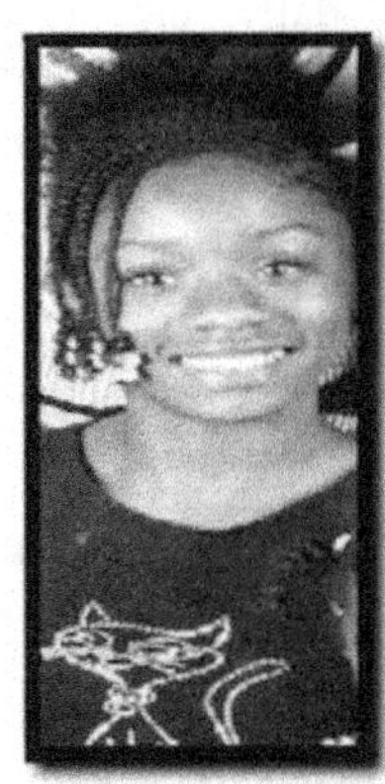

Breanna Griffin

Lucky Girl, Lucky Shoes

Breanna is 12 years old, runs track and plays softball and basketball. She attends Herman Liembach Elementary school in Sacramento, California. Breanna thinks her little brother Isaiah is a good basketball player for four and that her brother Deion is a smart boy. Lucky Girl, Lucky Shoes © 2008 Breanna Griffin. Used by permission. All rights reserved.

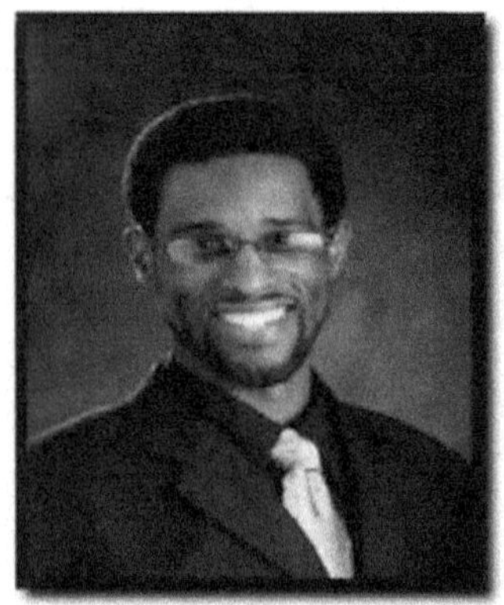

Clarence Griffin

Fathering and Falling Out of Love

Clarence Griffin serves as the director of Community and Local Government Relations for Loyola Marymount University where he is pursing a M.A. He grew up in Sacramento, California, and later worked for the California state assembly. As a child, his mother, who instilled the importance of community activism, took him and his three other siblings canvassing in her quest to become a member of the local school board. His interactions with key policy makers sparked an interest on the impact of state and local government on world affairs. He graduated from Pitzer College with a B.A. in organizational studies. Afterward he served as coordinator for the Pitzer College study abroad program in Zimbabwe. He sits on numerous local boards in Los Angeles including, LAX Coastal Area Chamber of Commerce. Clarence loves spending time with his daughter, Tiyanane and teaching chess at the Baldwin Hills Public Library. Fathering and Falling Out of Love © 2008 Clarence Griffin. Used by permission. All rights reserved.

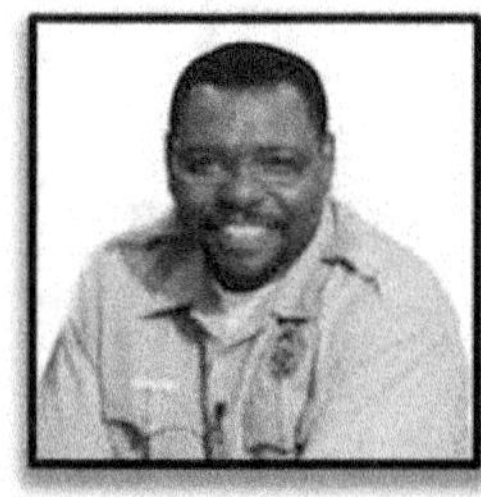

Petri Hawkins-Byrd
Foreword

Foreword by the most well-known bailiff in the world, Petri Hawkins-Byrd, a dedicated husband and father of four, who has served with Judge Judith Sheindlin "Judge Judy" on the highest-rated daily, half-hour, nationally syndicated television program. Foreword copyright 2017 Petri Hawkins-Byrd. Used by permission. All rights reserved.

Beatrice M. Hogg
Mr. Big Wheel

Beatrice M. Hogg was raised in Western Pennsylvania and currently lives in Sacramento, California. She has a M.F.A. in Creative Writing from Antioch University Los Angeles. She facilitates a weekly writing workshop at a local women's homeless shelter. Besides the anthologies *Life Spices from Seasoned Sistahs* and *Amazing Cat Tales*, she has been published in magazines and newspapers such as *Astronomy, Black Issues Book Review, Reminisce and the Sacramento Bee*. She is currently working on a memoir and a novel. Mr. Big Wheel © 2008 Beatrice M. Hogg. Used by permission. All rights reserved.

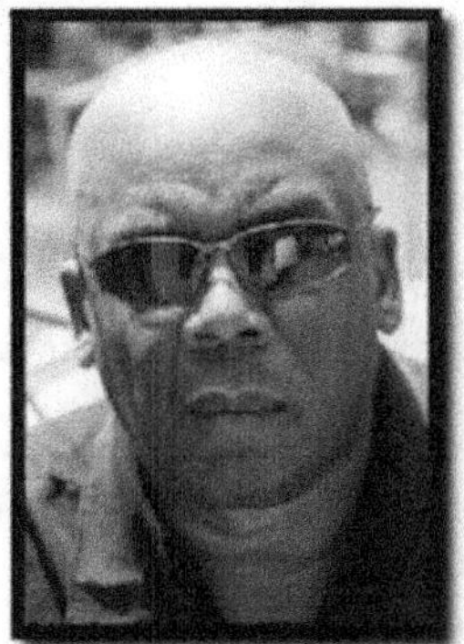

Raphael Jackson
Song for My Father, Song for Buchie

Raphael Jackson is a professor of history at Bethune Cookman University in Daytona Beach, Florida. He hosts the *International Rhythm Train* radio program on WPUL 1590. As a career administrator and educator, he has taught all grades from K-12, in six states and the Caribbean. He is also a photographer, videographer and visual artist. His passions are world languages, painting, drawing and landscape architecture construction. A Song for My Father, Song for Buchie © 2008 Raphael Jackson. Used by permission. All rights reserved.

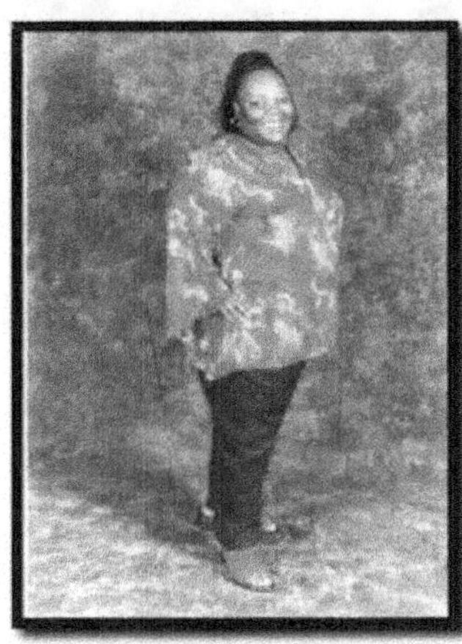

TeChina Jackson
A Black Girl's Dreams Can Come True

TeChina Jackson was born and raised in Chicago, Illinois. In 2007, she graduated with an A.A. degree in Liberal Arts from American River College, in Sacramento, California. Currently she is pursuing her B.A. at Central State University in Wilberforce, Ohio. She is a phenomenal young woman of many talents. Ms. Jackson sings, advocates, serves and ministers. She also is an accomplished and published author of poetry and short essays. Project REHOAT is an outreach she started, which serves as a catalyst to an international initiative called, *"A Million Pencils for Haiti."* Her goal is to change lives for the children of the small impoverished island country, "one pencil at a time," with love. TeChina is "a voice that continues to sound an alarm that will shake and impact nations through her generosity and ability to think outside the box." A Black Girl's Dreams Can Come True © 2008 TeChina Jackson. Used by permission. All rights reserved.

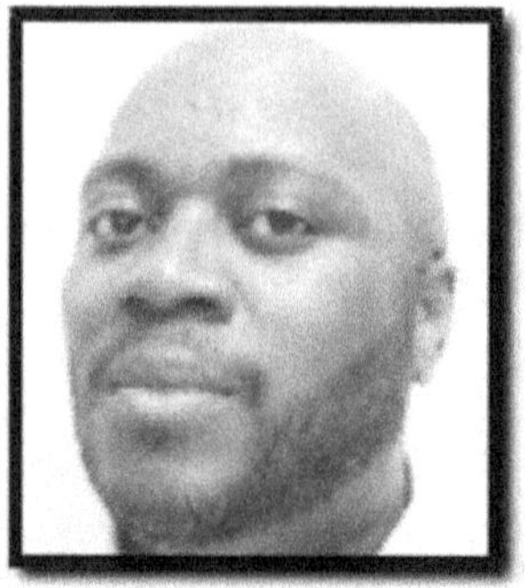

richard jones
Daddy, Do Better

richard jones (rj) is founding editor of BlackMaleAppreciation.com. He is an ordained minister, freelance writer, musician, and IT professional from Detroit, Michigan. He is most proud to be *Daddy* to three of the most wonderful daughters a parent could ever have. Daddy, Do Better © 2008 richard jones. Used by permission. All rights reserved.

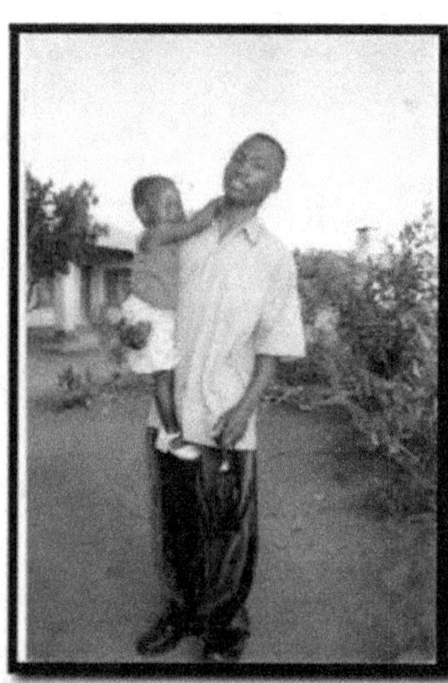

Sam Kalimba
Mtandire's Tinsmith

Sam Kalimba was born in 1980 and is a Malawian budding poet and writer. He is a fireman by profession who works for the Department of Civil Aviation. In addition, he is an ex-seminarian who was sponsored by his brother, Maxwell from his standard six to his leaving the seminary. He is married to Scholastica and is now a "Black father of Theophister and Samson Jr. May the soul of Thomas and Maxwell rest in peace." Mtandire's Tinsmith © 2008 Sam Kalimba. Used by permission. All rights reserved.

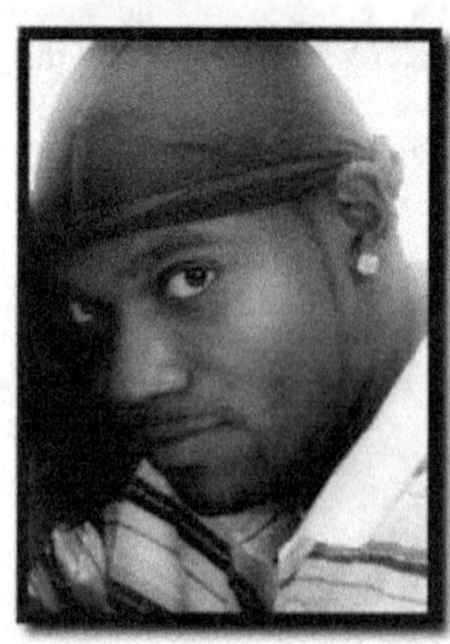

Marcus Kellam
A God Given Father of My Own

Marcus Kellam lives in Wilmington, North Calorina and currently works as a customer account manager at a local store. He is 22 years of age and pursuing his B.A. in Business Management. Marcus enjoys going out to all kinds of events and playing football and basketball with friends. He dreams of one day having his own business and helping unfortunate youth realize their dreams too. A God Given Father of My Own © 2008 Marcus Kellam. Used by permission. All rights reserved.

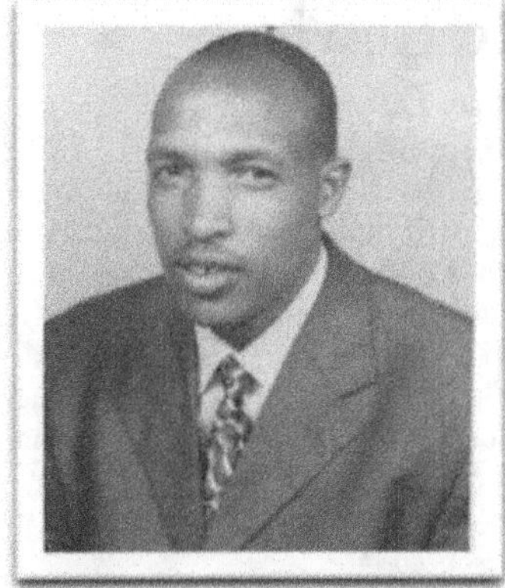

Stephen Ole Kesire
Maasai Fathers, One Man's Mission to Merge Two Cultures

Stephen Ole Kesire was the first Christian leader ordained in Maasailand. A loving father of three, with a fourth child due this summer, he and his wife Leah, work together to minister in their community and bring families together. They wish to honor the positive rituals of the Maasai and merge them with Christian traditions of love for God and one another. Maasai Fathers, One Man's Mission to Merge Two Cultures © 2008 Stephen Ole Kesire. Used by permission. All rights reserved.

Virginia Lathan
I Never Really Got to Know Daddy

Virginia A. Lathan has been writing since childhood. She would write "rough" plays for the children in her neighborhood to perform. "Although, this was before copiers were readily available, so with all the children having to use the same copy of a script, these little productions never took off!" Since then, she's written numerous short stories and nonfiction how-to-books that sell through Curry-Co Publications, her micropublishing company (www.CurryCo.cjb.net). Her most recent undertaking is a suspense-thriller novel that is in the final phases of editing and should be available sometime in 2008. She also writes *stories to be told*, which she and her daughter Angela perform at various venues throughout the Chicago area. (See www.GenuinelyGood.cjb.net) Virginia is a member of ZICA Creative Arts and Literary Guild and ASE: Chicago Association of Black Storytellers. These professional associations are two of the biggest contributors to her continuing to further her writing and storytelling goals. I Never Really Got to Know Daddy © 2008 Virginia Lathan. Used by permission. All rights reserved.

448

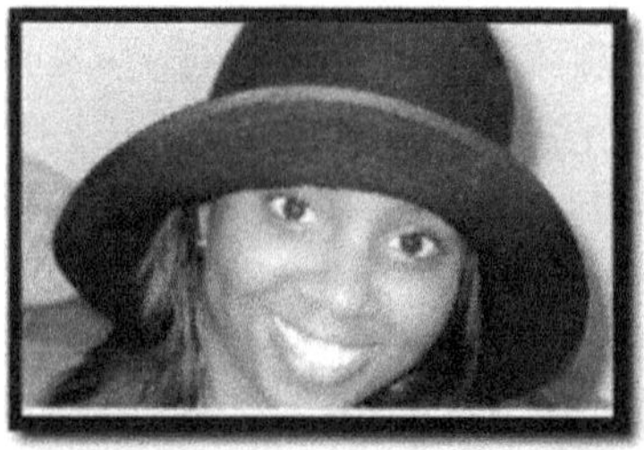

Jeanine Lewis
All the Little Things

Jeanine Lewis was born in Los Angeles, California and moved to eastern Washington after her parents divorce at age nine. She graduated with a B.A. in Philosophy and an Art History minor from the University of Washington in Seattle. During her college years, she studied Italian Renaissance in Florence, Italy. After college, Jeanine interned on Capital Hill for a Washington congressman and landed a staff position in a district office with another congressional member. Currently, Jeanine works for *Lockheed Martin Space Systems* in New Orleans, Louisiana. All the Little Things © 2008. Used by permission. All rights reserved.

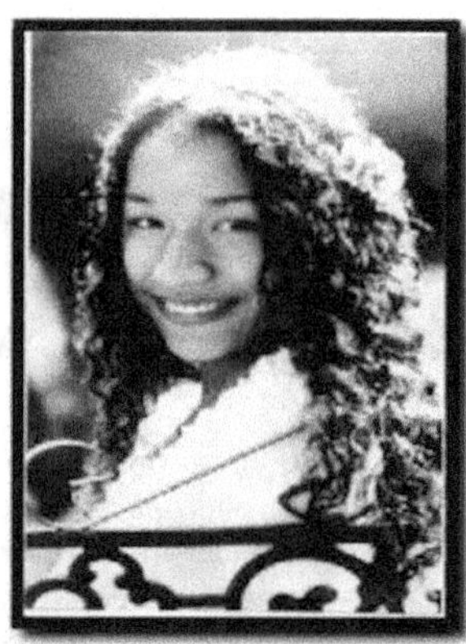

Apple Loveless
To Be Pale in Comparison

Apple Loveless moved to Woodland, California after residing in the Philippines for the first 12 years of her life. She moved just in time to begin Jr. High in the United States. Then Apple graduated from Pioneer High School and entered the University of California at Davis with a handful of scholarship money. Currently she is in her sophomore year and a double major in English and International Relations. To Be Pale in Comparison © 2008 Apple Loveless. Used by permission. All rights reserved.

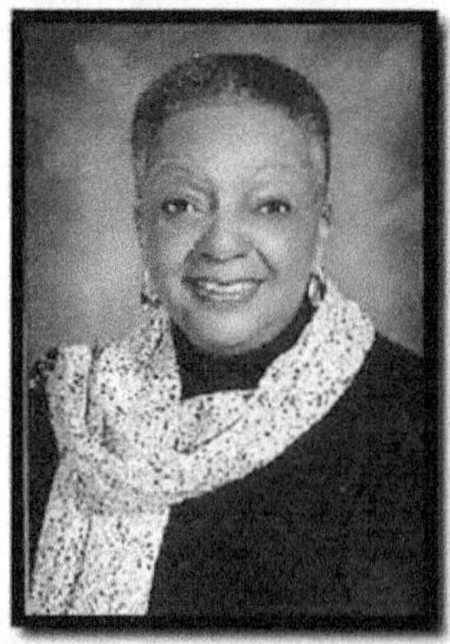

Ethel Mack-Ballard
Daddy-boy

Ethel Mack-Ballard is a retired social worker and freelance writer. She specializes in writing speeches. Her published work includes articles, reviews, short fiction and poetry. She is founder and coordinator of ZICA Creative Arts and Literary Guild. Ethel is a native of Cleveland, Ohio and a graduate of Howard University. She resides in Sacramento, California. Daddy-boy © 2008 Ethel Mack-Ballard. Used by permission. All rights reserved.

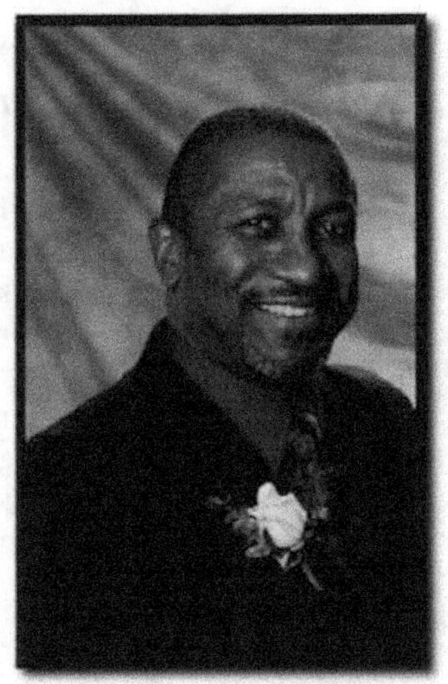

Jeri Marshall
The Tallest Man

Jeri Marshall is happily married to his beautiful wife, Teresa and is the proud father of two daughters. As an ordained youth minister, he is active in his church and community. Jeri holds a B.A. from Sonoma State University and two masters degrees from the University of La Verne, and Oklahoma State University. Currently, he is an outreach specialist at American River College and an adjunct professor who teaches College Success classes with an African American emphasis. A gifted athlete, Jeri played college basketball, and was invited to try-out for the Chicago Bulls in the '70s. An impassioned motivator, he speaks to numerous groups on violence prevention and *anger, fear* and *pain* through his *Alive and Free* seminar, and is widely sought in his community as a speaker and consultant. Jeri will not be deterred in his quest to "encourage and empower people to success in all endeavors." Interested parties can reach him at (916)768-3987 or (916)967-5339. The Tallest Man © 2008 Jeri Marshall. Used by permission. All rights reserved.

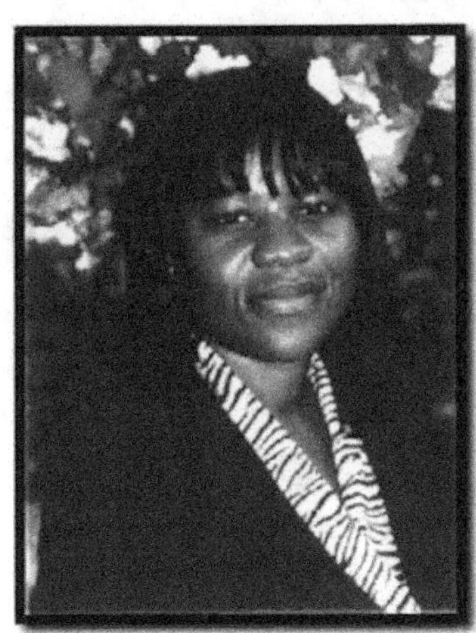

Carol Mattocks
A Well Lit Path to Wisdom

Carolyn Mattocks is a native of Edwards, North Carolina. She is a summa cum laude graduate of North Carolina Central University with a B.A. in History. She also has a M.A. in Public Administration from North Carolina State University. Ms. Mattocks is a burgeoning entrepreneur. In 2007, she created a company called *Historical Inspirations.* The company promotes history through inspirational, motivational, and educational perspectives. Products can be viewed at www.historicalinspirations.net. Her first book was titled, *Essays of W.I.I.T.S.* (Wisdom, Insight, Inspiration, Truth, & Strength) which she self-published in 2002. Ms. Mattocks is honored that her essay was chosen to be included in *Our Black Fathers: Brave, Bold and Beautiful!* She hopes that it will "inspire fathers to understand that the lasting legacy of a father is defined by the wisdom that he leaves within his children." A Well Lit Path to Wisdom © 2008 Carolyn Mattocks. Used by permission. All rights reserved.

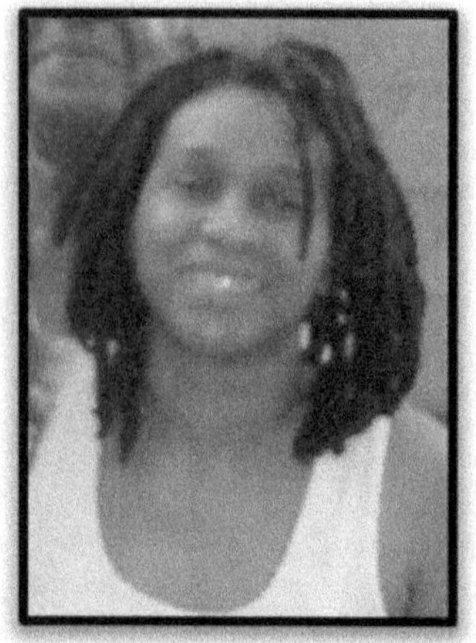

Rene' McGaugh
Herb Blackman Jr. —The Man Who Engineered Love

Rene' McGaugh graduated with a bachelor's of science degree in Mechanical Engineering from California State University, Northridge; and has been working for the federal government for over 26 years. She was born to Herbert Blackman Jr. and Lolita, and has an older sister Nicola Blackman. Happily married to a loving husband, Ronald McGaugh for 31 ½ years, she is also a proud mother of two handsome sons, Ryan and Aaron. She is also proud to have a loving and devoted daughter in-law, OdudBanke ("Banke") who is married to Ryan. She enjoys wine tasting, mud baths, massages, solving super tough Sudoku puzzles, and playing monopoly with her family. Herb Blackman Jr. — The Man Who Engineered Love copyright 2017. Used by permission. All rights reserved.

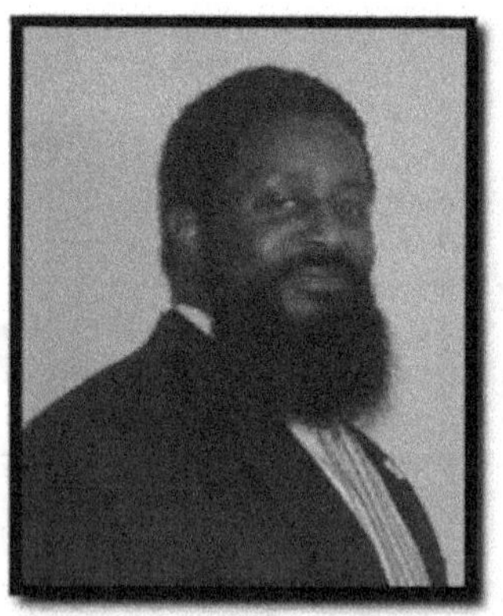

Jerome McGee
A Real Superhero

Dr. Jerome J. McGee Sr. is a married father of four children and one granddaughter and a newly born grandson, Jerome III.

He holds a B.A. and M.A. in Theology, and is a Doctor of Divinity. Dr. McGee has been active in ministry since 1978. U.S. Air Force officials gave him recognition for ordaining and installing a pastor in 1995 in Dhahran, Arabia while pastor of a United States Chapel service. According to records, this was a first ever in the kingdom of Saudi Arabia. In March of 2002, he and his wife, Donna launched Jubilee Training Center, *A Place of New Beginnings*, in the Franklin Villa Community Park in Sacramento, California. Dr. McGee is on the board of directors of Fellowship Covenant Ministries International. He also is the chief executive officer of The McGee Foundation. A Real Superhero © 2008 Jerome McGee. Used by permission. All rights reserved.

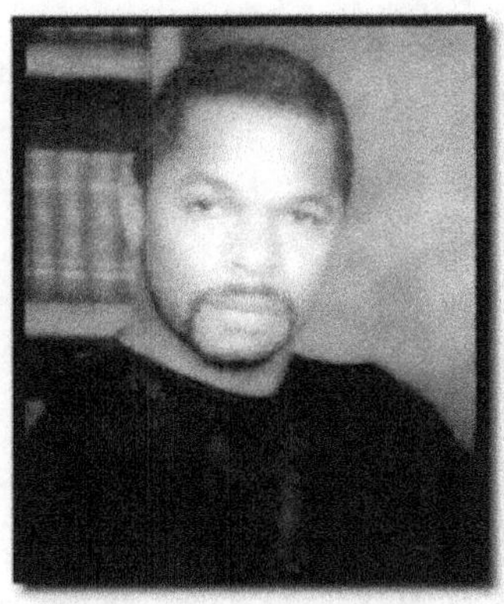

Marcus McGee
A Gift for My Grandfather – the Griot

Marcus McGee is a Northern California based writer and producer. He has directed and produced several plays in the area. He is the author of No More Cheesecake! (stage play); Willie: The Man; The Myth & The Era (biography); Four Stories and Synchronicity (short story collections). And other essays, screenplays and novels. A Gift for My Grandfather – the Griot © 2008 Marcus McGee. Used by permission. All rights reserved.

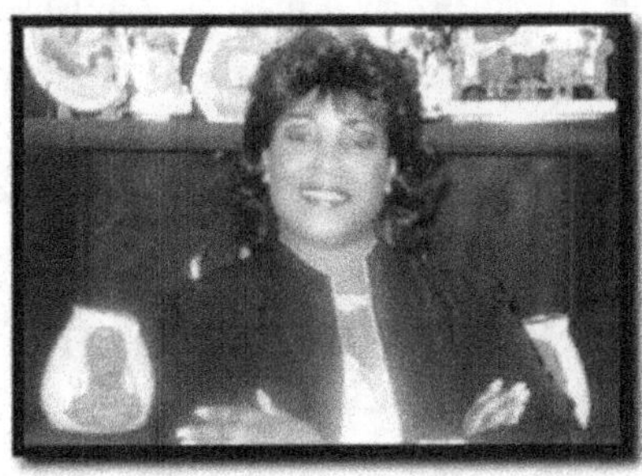

Jona McNair Brown
Peace in the Midst of the Storm
No Barriers Could Stop Henry's Cadence

Jona McNair Brown, a mother, wife, daughter, sister, author and Desert Storm Veteran was born in Lubbock, Texas to wonderful parents: Ret. MSGT, USAF Henry and Katherine McNair Jr. She's married to Lieutenant Ray Brown, and has three children: Tasmaine, Gigi and Dominique and two granddaughters: Dominique LaNya and Sarah. Jona is recognized for being one of the, "Distinguished Servicewomen in American History" at the Women in Military Service Living Memorial, in Arlington, Virginia. In honor of her contributions, her story and photograph are permanently displayed in a computerized database. Currently in her last semester at the University of Phoenix, Jona also is a community liaison at Westwood Heights Elementary School. Her children's book, *The Shade Tree*, debuted at the African American Research Library on December 3, 2005. It can be ordered at www.trafford.com. The curriculum is in print and will be released soon. In March 2007, Trafford, her publishing company featured her as a new author. No Barriers Could Stop Henry's Cadence, Peace in the Midst of the Storm © 2008 Jona McNair Brown. Used by permission. All rights reserved.

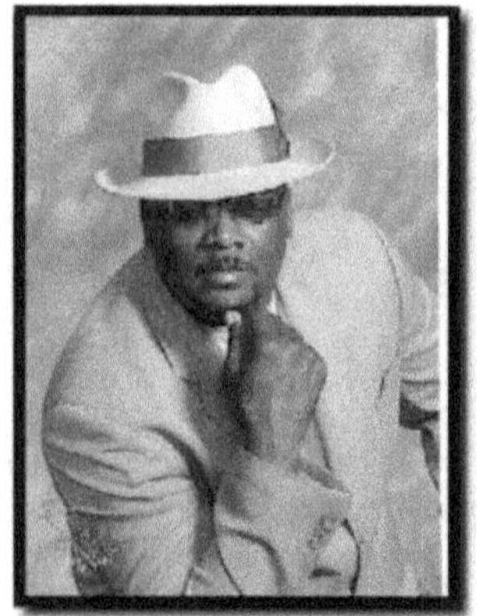

Dale Miles
From Fury to Faith and Forgiveness

Pastor Dale Miles was born on July 7, 1958, in Denham Springs, Louisiana to Joel and Inez Miles. He is the fifth child born of five children. He received his diploma in 1976 and served twelve years in the U.S. Army, ending his career at Fort Monroe in Hampton, Virginia. Mr. Miles attended Boyce Bible College, received a bachelor's degree in Theology from Sacramento Theological Seminary and is presently working on his master's in Christian counseling. He was licensed to preach by the late Rev. Howard V. Booker. He is blessed to have a helpmate and wife in Co-Pastor Rev. Ernestine. They have two children: Dale Jr. and Santino. With confidence in God, Pastor Miles stepped out on *His Will* and *His* Word and left the security of a 20 year government career and moved out into the things God had for him. From Fury to Faith and Forgiveness © 2008 Dale Miles. Used by permission. All rights reserved.

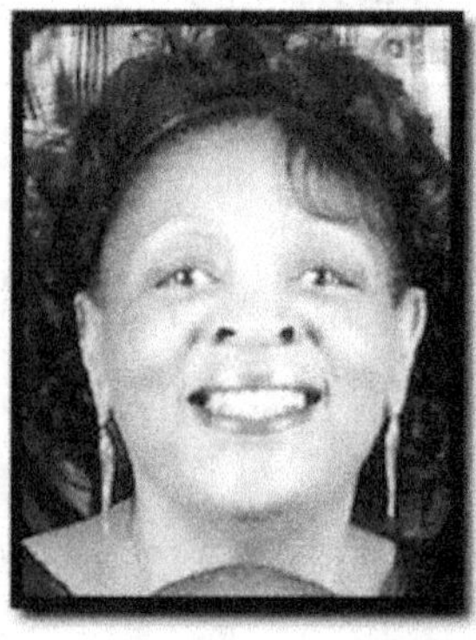

Hortense Mitchell-Brown
What's in a Name?

Hortense Mitchell-Brown was born in Monroe, Louisiana to Ms. Anetha Wade and Mr. Jesse Mitchell. She currently lives in Houston, Texas where four of her five surviving siblings reside. Her other sibling lives in Chicago, Illinois. Recently, her beloved sister passed away. A graduate of Carroll High School and Bish Mathis Institute, Ms. Mitchell-Brown has been married to the same man for 39 years, and has three children and two grandchildren. Over the years she has lived in Portland, Oregon, Oakland, California, Cleveland, Ohio and Chicago, Illinois. She works as a library assistant for an oil company and has served as an administrative assistant and clerk typist for the United States Navy. Ms. Mitchell-Brown enjoys writing, singing, and crocheting. Once a month she attends Mitchell family gatherings to ensure that the same values that her parents instilled in their children, continues through the generations. What's in a Name? © 2008 Hortense Mitchell-Brown. Used by permission. All rights reserved.

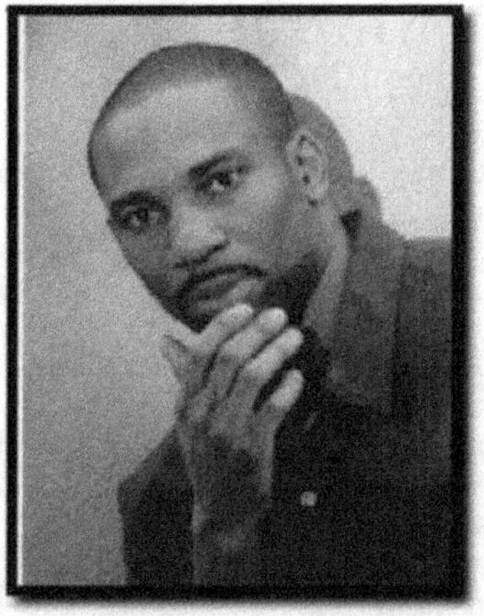

Terry Moore
Father of the Year

Besides being a father, which is Terry Moore's greatest honor, he is founder of *Born 2B Poets*, and *Daddy's Here*. A master poet and spoken word performer, Terry is a twelve time Slam Champion. Some of his other achievements include *2001 Poet of the Year, 2005 Best Male Word Performer, 2002 Nominated Entertainer of the Year, 2004 Los Angeles Black Music Awards* nominee, and *2005 Center for Black Fathers and Families Father of the Year*. In addition to his many awards, Terry is the author of fifteen poetry books and seven spoken word CDs. He has appeared at the world famous *Showtime at the Apollo* and opened for many entertainers, such as CeCe Winans, The Temptations, Philip Bailey of Earth Wind and Fire, Maya Angelou, Iyanla Vanzant, Kirk Franklin, Rick Braun and many more. To find out more about Terry and upcoming events and performances, visit www.mybmsf.com/terrymoore. Father of the Year © 2008 Terry Freeman Moore. Used by permission. All rights reserved.

Jamariah Morris
The Surrogate

Jamariah Morris is a current student at American River College, and a part of the Umoja Sahku Community. Her plan is to attend ARC for two years then transfer to an HBCU. Her major goal is to become an OBGYN/MD in order to help educate women about their bodies and offspring. The Surrogate copyright 2017 Jamariah Morris. Used by permission. All rights reserved.
*HBCU--Historical Black College and Universities

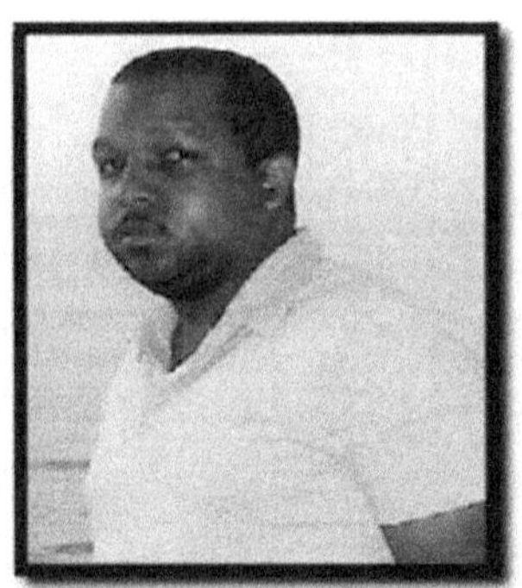

Keith D. Morton
Same Place, Same Face

Keith D. Morton is a 29-year-old father and husband with a career in non-profits that (so far) spans more than a decade. He is an administrative support professional that was lucky enough to progress from part-time receptionist at a mental health clinic to director of operations, Early Childhood programs for the Children's Aid Society in New York City. In addition to his day job, Keith spends his evenings, after reading and social time with the family, blogging and podcasting in collaboration with Malecare Inc. His blog, *African American Dad* (http://fatherdad.com) has a loyal following, as does his *Five Minute Father* podcast show. His wonderful wife Shalawn is a licensed medical social worker and psychotherapist. Their four- year-old son is currently unemployed, but he performs the tasks associated with being a kid very well. Mr. Morton also has three brothers and three best friends who are very supportive. Same Place, Same Face © 2008 Keith D. Morton. Used by permission. All rights reserved.

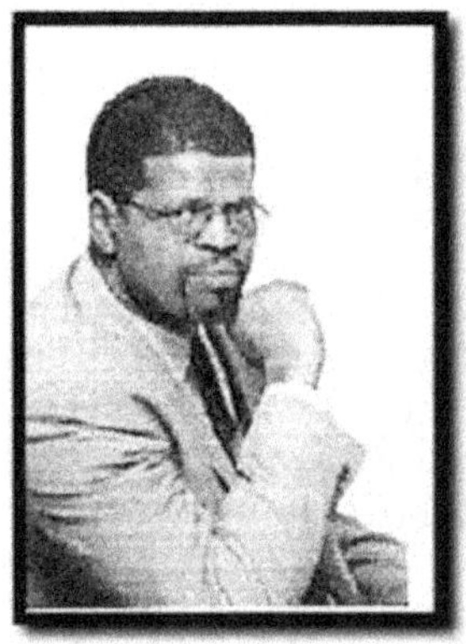

Derrell Roberts

Dad, Daddy and Me

Derrell Roberts is the co-founder of the Robert's Family Development Center that he started with his wife Tina. Based in Sacramento , CA the center's mission and focus is on early childhood and family education, for which much praise is raised for the wonderful services and work the center provides. Mr. Roberts and his wife are "respected community leaders who have proven track records in community-based organizations. Between them they have more than twenty-five years of well-documented community experience and success. They have been executive administrators in some of Sacramento 's most visible non-profit agencies such as: The Birthing Project, St. HOPE Academy and the Salvation Army Community Center. Individually they are uniquely qualified to undertake and succeed in a project of this magnitude." Derrell, in conjunction with his wife and a dedicated team of professionals, continues to impact the community with invaluable knowledge and resources that make a difference in the lives of many individuals. Dad, Daddy and Me © 2008 Derrell Roberts. All rights reserved the following: Used by permission.

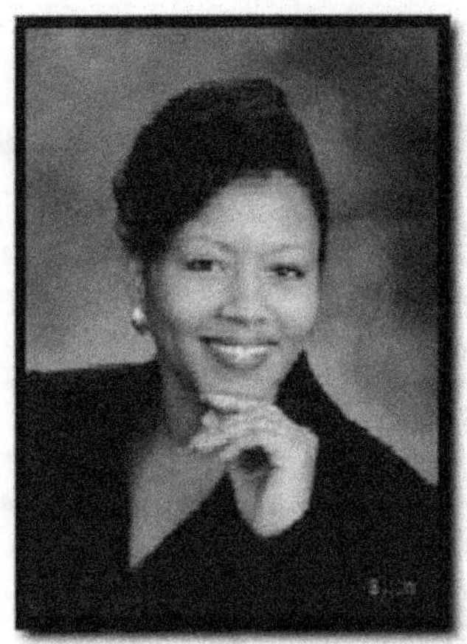

Anita Royston

His Way

Anita Royston is an education consultant specializing in engaging family and community involvement in the educational environment. She has worked for the Sacramento City Unified School District as a Parent Advisor. She has also worked for UC Davis and Linking Education and Economic Development (LEED). A former Del Paso Heights School Board member, she is currently working with the Roberts Family Development Center, the Del Paso Heights School District and GEAR UP. "Ms. Royston is a gifted connector of Resources and needs for the academic and social success of students and families." His Way © 2008 Anita Royston. Used by permission. All rights reserved.

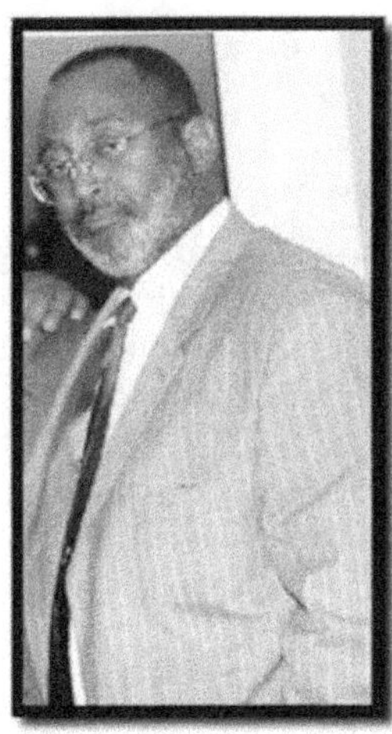

Steven A. Royston
We Are Professionals!

Steven Royston has had a multifaceted legal career since 1981. He's been a trial deputy and did poverty law work with the Legal Aid Society of Alameda County in Oakland, California. He served as an attorney with the Oakland Unified School District; the Sacramento City Unified School District and, later, as General Counsel for the Oakland Unified School District where he acquired in his words "fame or infamy," as the author of the *1996 OUSD Ebonics Resolution.* He currently serves as a law professor at the New College of California School of Law where he was Acting Dean in 2007. The first in his family to graduate from college, Steven holds a B.A. from UCLA, and a J.D. from Western State University College. He is married to Anita, and their blended family consists of Bruce, Clarence, Marsha, Ben, and Kristina. We Are Professionals! © 2008 Steven A. Royston. Used by permission. All rights reserved.

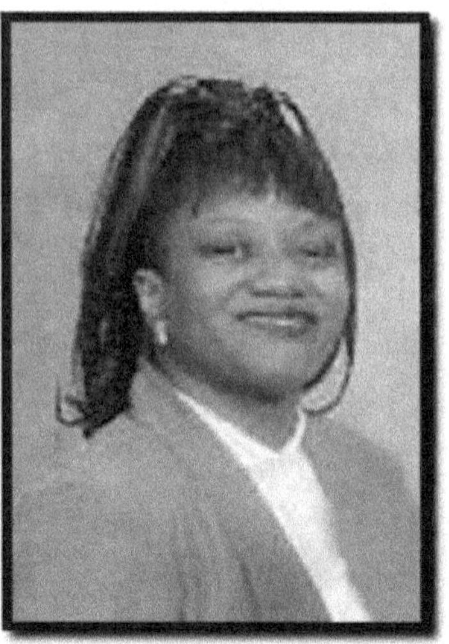

Vanessa Rushing

Tomorrow I'll Be Stronger

Vanessa Rushing has been married for twenty-one years. She and her husband have four gifted and talented children. Mrs. Rushing teaches 6th grade, holds a B.A. and M.Ed. in education, and is pursuing a Doctoral Degree in education. Mrs. Rushing loves to read, sing and spend time with her family. Tomorrow I'll Be Stronger © 2008 Vanessa Rushing. Used by permission. All rights reserved.

Katha Satterfield Redmon and **Karen Satterfield**
The Art of Loving, The Satterfield Way

Katha Satterfield Redmon and Karen Satterfield are sisters who had the great fortune to share a father who was a teacher and loving patriarch who taught many lessons that have stayed with and empowered them throughout their lifetimes. Together they collaborated on sharing memories and penning this loving story about their father. Art Satterfield. The Art of Loving, The Satterfield Way copyright 2017. Used by permission. All rights reserved.

Vicki Sherman
Legacy Leaving—A Slave's Story on the Periphery of Revival

Vicki Sherman is the mother of two adult children and four adorable grandsons who she loves spending time with. She has worked in the field of education for several years in the Career Center at American River College, and other departments on campus. For 42 years she was married to her beloved Larry, before he passed away in 2013. Vicki keeps active through involvement in her church. One role that Vicki truly enjoys is as a leader who teaches small groups of women about the Captivating program which is based on the following message: "Your heart matters more than anything else in all creation. The desires you had as a little girl and the longings you still feel as woman-- they are telling you of the life God created you to live. He offers to come now as the Hero of your story, to rescue your heart and release you to live as a fully alive and feminine woman. A woman who is truly captivating." Legacy Leaving—A Slave's Story on the Periphery of Revival copyright 2017. Used by permission. All rights reserved.

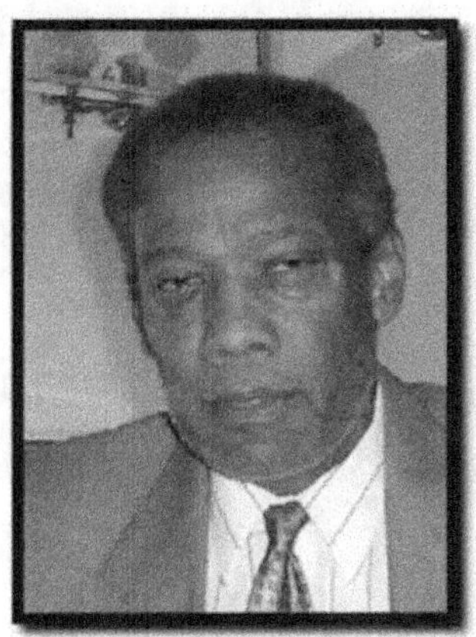

Bernie Siler
Phases of Fatherhood

Lieutenant Colonel Bernard Siler is an attorney with the District of Columbia Office of the Attorney General and on active duty in the Judge Advocate General Corps with the US Army Reserve. He is an adjunct professor, a lecturer, a historian and a Civil War re-enactor who has appeared in the motion pictures, *Glory, Andersonville* and *Tad*. Mr. Siler has written articles for the *Washington Times*, and *Washington Post*. He tried out for several professional football teams in the early 1980s. A man of many achievements, Bernie has a B.A. from the University of Dayton, and a J.D. from the University of Cincinnati. Phases of Fatherhood © 2008 Bernie Siler. Used by permission. All rights reserved.

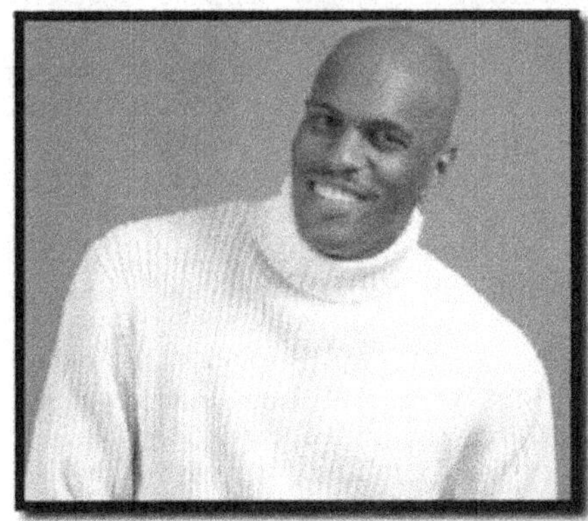

Rodney Snell
A Tailored Life

Rodney Snell is a native of Long Branch, New Jersey. He grew up on the shore surrounded by a large and loving family. He holds a B.A. in Creative Writing from Emerson College in Boston, and has completed credits toward a M.A. in Speech Communication. Rodney is a featured contributor to *Velocity Magazine* and also an accomplished vocalist. Currently, he is compiling a collection of short stories inspired by tales overheard while growing up in a small town and has completed a workshop series for emerging leaders. His story is featured in *The Read-Aloud Handbook* by Jim Trelease. He lives in Brooklyn, New York. A Tailored Life © 2008 Rodney Snell. Used by permission. All rights reserved.

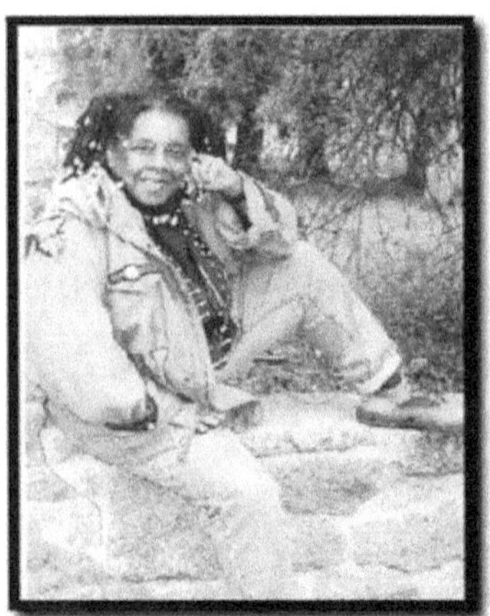

Staajabu
Kindergarten

Staajabu resides in Sicklerville, New Jersey. She is a writer, poet, journalist, graphic artist, administrative assistant, prison rights activist, event coordinator and organizer. Additionally, she is a member in good standing with ZICA Creative Arts and Literary Guild. Her poetry and writings have appeared in numerous publications. Staajabu and her daughter V.S. Chochezi co-authored and published six books of poetry: *Crucial Comments and Vicious Verses, BAMM!!, This Queendome Come, Taking Names and Pointing Fingers, African Reflections and Scribes Rising*. They've also co-produced two spoken word CDs, *Mind Quake* and *Priorities*. Staajabu uses poetry as a tool for consciousness raising. As an environmentalist, a feminist, and a naturalist, she is an open-minded, non-sexist, non-racist pacifist, whose work shows that "levity will lighten the darkest subjects; that truth is the force that binds us all together and that desire for harmony is the universal beacon that can never be extinguished." Kindergarten © 2008 Staajabu. Used by permission. All rights reserved.

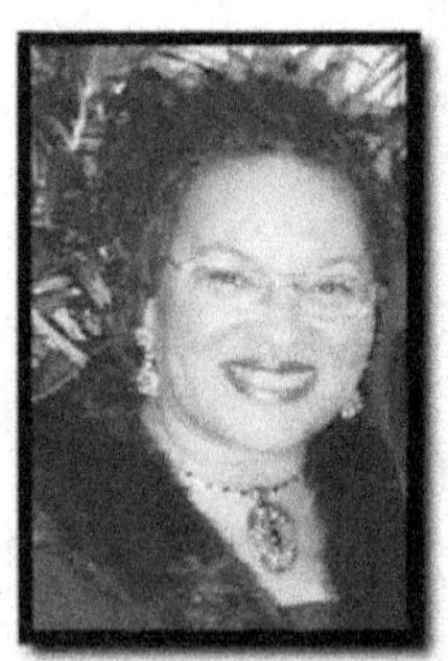

Cloteal Thrower Herron
A True Man After God's Heart

Cloteal Thrower Herron holds a M.A. in Educational Administration and a B.A. in Ethnic Studies. She recently retired as an outreach admission counselor and seminar instructor from Sacramento State University after 34 years of reaching, teaching, motivating and empowering students. Cloteal is the owner and principal consultant of the **TEAL Group** *(Train*Educate*Advocate*Link)*, which specializes in teen and family mentoring and empowerment training to *"help people, help themselves."* Cloteal has created and conducts her motivational empowerment series: *GIRL* Power and Boyz-2-*KINGZ* to foster youth, and students. A dynamic motivational speaker, she "connects in the spirit," with her audience. Called, *"Ms. Teal—"keeping-it-real,"* her desire and personal ministry is to help everyone improve, in order to live the life God has called and ordained for them –thereby blessing our Father. Currently, she serves on several community advisory boards and enjoys traveling with her husband, Minister Rhoecus Herron to visit their children and grandchildren. Ms. Herron can be reached at (916)364-0778 which is her business and fax number. Or you can email her at ctealgroup@aol.com or visit her website www.Tealgroup.org. A True Man After God's Heart © 2008 Cloteal Thrower Herron. Used by permission. All rights reserved.

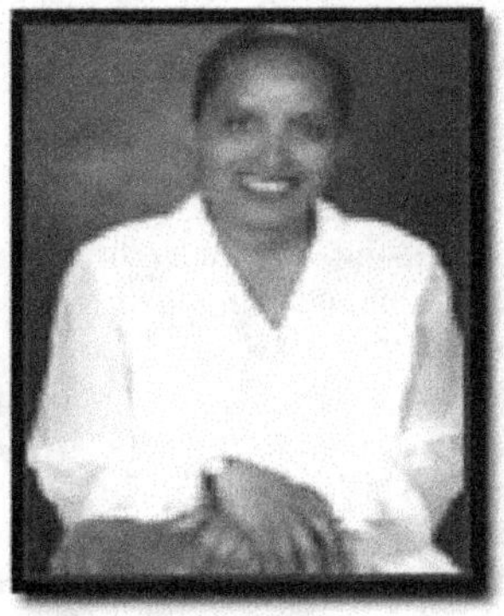

Denise Turney
Destiny Driven: A Legacy of Belief and Courage

Denise Turney is the author of the books, *Portia, Love has Many Faces, Spiral* and *Long Walk Up* (her new release). Denise has more than thirty-four years of book, newspaper, magazine, radio and business writing experience. She is an internationally celebrated author who is listed in various entertainment and business periodicals including industry leaders such as *Who's Who, 100 Most Admired African American Women* and *Crosswalk*. Denise Turney's works have appeared in *Parade, Essence, Ebony, the Pittsburg Quarterly* and *Obsidian II*. Denise would "love it" if you visited her online at **www.chistell.com**. Destiny Driven: A Legacy of Courage and Belief © 2008 Denise Turney. Used by permission. All rights reserved.

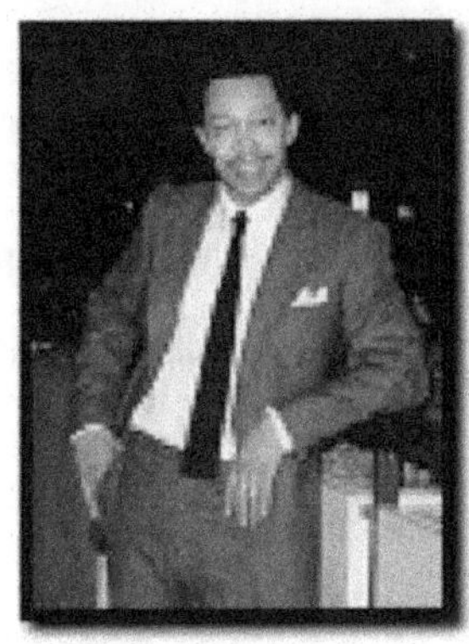

Peter S.Vanderpool
Finally a Father, Man of the Sea was Simply Dad to Me!

Peter Vanderpool is a father, and husband who enjoys family life. He has worked as a radio host on KDVS 90.3 in Davis, CA and played the voice of God in a local play. In addition, he is a voiceover artist with Cast Images Talent Agency. He has a keen interest in architecture and studied in the field for several years. He is grateful for his parents' decision to give him and his siblings a better life, though they never will forget the simple pleasures of their beautiful Guyana. If you're interested in his services for doing voiceover work, Peter can be contacted at (916)346-6086. Man of the Sea was Simply Dad to Me! Finally a Father © 2008 Peter S. Vanderpool. Used by permission. All rights reserved.

Francene G. Weatherspoon
April Love

Mrs. Francene Weatherspoon (M.Ed) is the proud mother of Mac Arthur II, a graduate of Tuskegee University, and Adrian Ja Rell, an undergraduate attending Sacramento City College. She has been happily married for 29 years to Mac Arthur Sr., the Pastor of New Hearts Baptist Church in Rancho Cordova, California. Although a native of Georgia, Mrs. Weatherspoon and family have made Sacramento their home. April Love © 2008 by Francene G. Weatherspoon. Used by permission. All rights reserved.

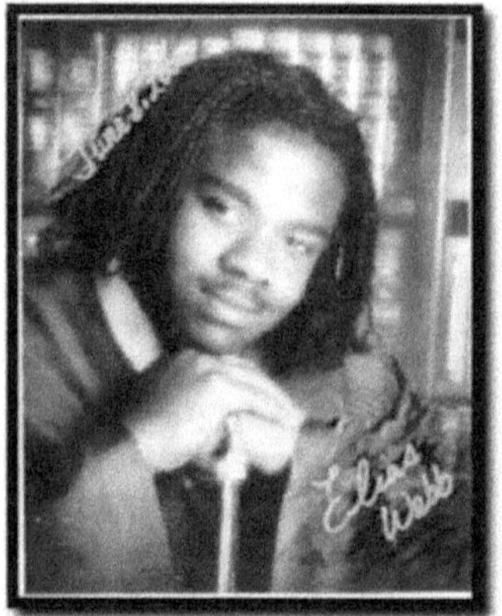

Elias Webb
A Blueprint for Fatherhood

Elias Jackson Webb is the youngest of three sons. He grew up looking up to his two older brothers who worked hard to set a shining example of what a young Black male should be. Elias is a young man with tons of determination who is currently a sophomore at Sacramento State University where he's majoring in Business. On June 12, 2007 his life changed. Once he became a father his determination to succeed and provide for his child more than doubled. Elias desires to be *the man, (bold, black and strong) that his daughter deserves in her life*. A Blueprint for Fatherhood © 2008 Elias Webb. Used by permission. All rights reserved.

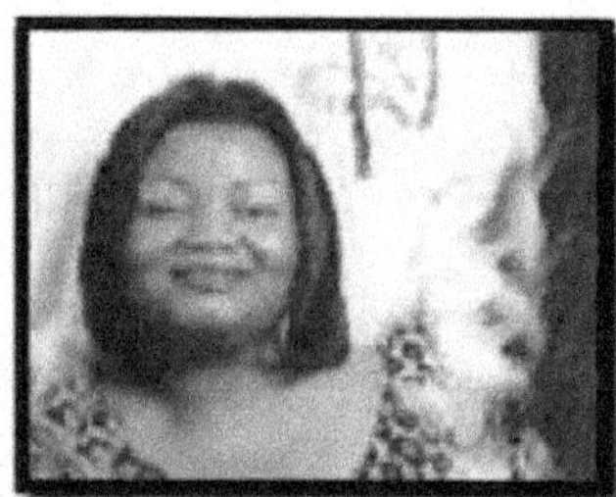

Jacqueline Webb
To Know Him is to Love Him

Jacqueline Webb is a high school teacher and a mother of three. Her passion is writing African American romance stories. In the coming months her debut novel: Greenwood Archer will be released. Ms. Webb also loves singing and nurturing her pride and joy, granddaughter Taylor. To Know Him is to Love Him © 2008 Jacqueline Webb. Used by permission. All rights reserved.

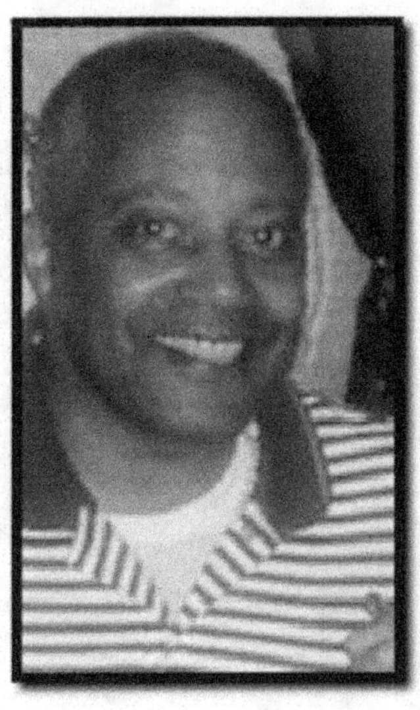

Theodore R. White
Necessity to Nurture

Theodore R. White, known by most as "Teddy," was born November 14, 1951 in New York City. He is the proud father of five children; and four grandchildren. Mr. White is an artist whose talent was noted at age three, and has served the NYC Human Resources Administration in various capacities for 30 years, including six years as a graphics unit director. He hopes to join HRA graphics one day and serve 20 more years. Necessity to Nurture © 2008 Theodore R. White. Used by permission. All rights reserved.

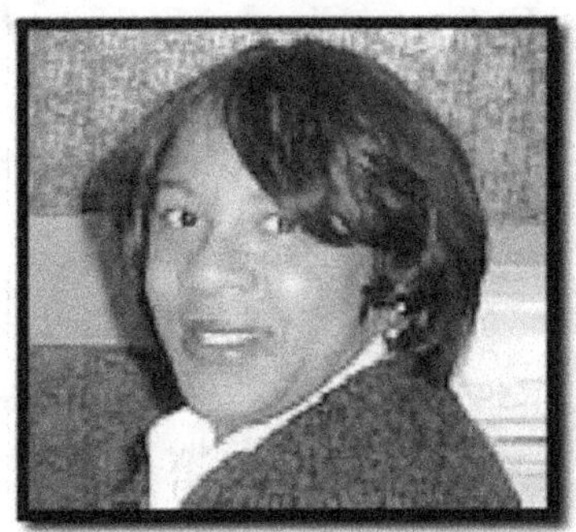

Dera R. Williams
Hope for Dad's First Born

Dera R. Williams has lived, worked and played in the San Francisco/Oakland Bay Area for most of her life. A native of Arkansas, she is the family genealogist and keeper of stories. Rooted in the tales of the ancestors, her stories have been published in a number of anthologies including *Life Spices from Seasoned Sistahs! Help! I've Turned into My Mother* and *A Cup of Comfort for Women*. Her academic contributions have been to Greenwood Publishing Group in the *Encyclopedia of African American Literature* and *The Encyclopedia of Slave Resistance and Rebellions*. A long time book reviewer and interviewer with *Affaire de Coeur* magazine, Dera is also an editor with the online review team, *A Place of Our Own*. She is completing a coming-of-age novel set in the South and has a number of other projects she's working on. Currently, Ms. Williams works in curriculum development at Merritt College in Oakland, California. Hope's for Dad's First Born © 2008 Dera R. Williams. Used by permission. All rights reserved.

Rod Williams

A Love Letter to My Dad

 Rod Williams is a single African-American father of three. He was born and raised in South Central Los Angeles during the politically charged, expressive and vibrant times of the '70s and '80s. An extensive background in sales and marketing consume the majority of Rod's daytime hours. But it also provides freedom and flexibility to pursue his passion for writing - specifically writing about the warmth and intrigue of relationships and exploring the powerful and long-lasting impact they have on our daily lives. A Love Letter to My Father © 2008 Rod Williams. Used by permission. All rights reserved.

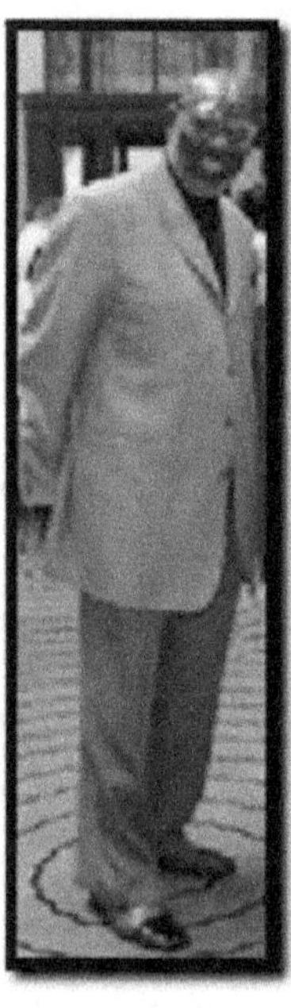

Frank Withrow

He Taught Me, Ebony King, Men of Excellence, Tribute to Father, Father to Son

Frank Withrow is a poet, retired educator and an inspirational motivator. Known as "The Middle Aged Rapper," he empowers youth to reach their potential. He was born and raised in Washington, DC and has taught for 25 years in schools in the District of Columbia and in California. Mr. Withrow has received numerous awards and in 1997 was inducted into the International Educational Hall of Fame. "Your responsibility is to secure knowledge and to develop a technique in which you use that knowledge wisely," is his signature phrase to all he meets. Frank's company is Reasons for Rhyme which markets posters, caps, and books (see resource section for information). Father to Son, Men of Excellence, Ebony Kings, He Taught Me, A Tribute to Father © 2008 Frank Withrow. Used by permission. All rights reserved.

Trinica Woodley

Born Leader

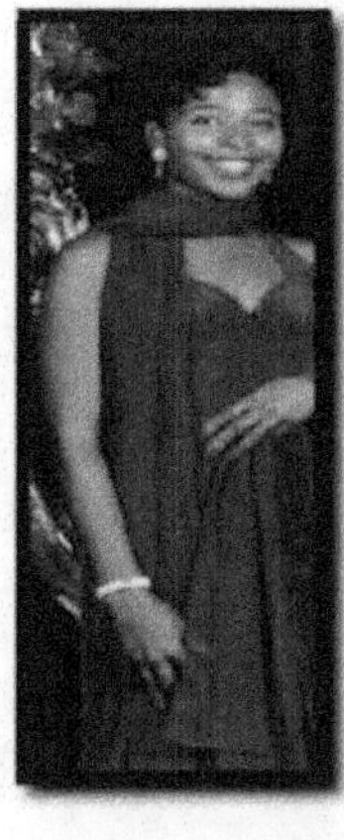

Trinicia M. Woodley was born and raised in Sacramento, California. She is the eldest daughter of Alfred Walker Jr., the loving wife of Michael A. Woodley, and the blessed mother of five children. Ms. Woodley is joyous most of the time because of "My Lord & Savior Jesus Christ. His joy gives me strength and his strength is what I need to get through the tough times and sail through the smooth times." Trinicia loves teaching at her community church, and cooking with her family. Her life long dream is a career in Architecture. She is currently attending Kaplan University and plans to receive a M.A. in Urban Development from UC Berkeley so that she can develop a community for transients, low income individuals and multiple families. Born Leader © 2008 Trinicia M. Woodley. Used by permission. All rights reserved.

Joean Wright
A Portrait of Perseverance

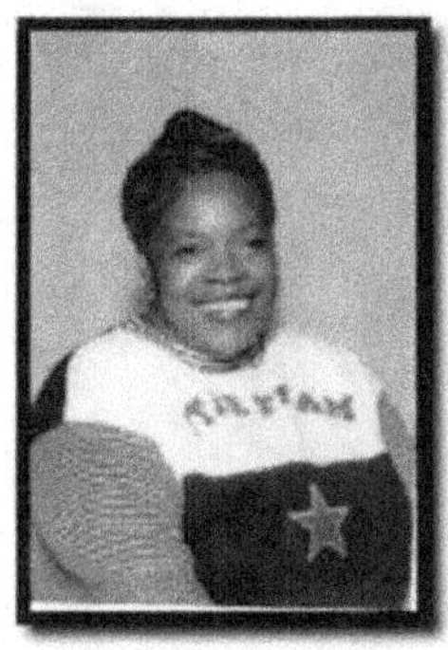

Joean Wright currently lives in Sacramento, California and has two children, Davinia and Kareem and eight grandchildren. She is retired from the city and county of San Francisco where she created *a problem reporting system* and won the top web award in 2004 from the Public Utilities Commission. Before accomplishing that feat, she was one of the first women union representatives for Muni Railways in the '80s. Joean loves reading, walking, and helping others. She draws closer to God in these trying times and is enjoying living her life, being with family and friends and helping others. A Portrait of Perseverance © 2008 Joean Wright. Used by permission. All rights reserved.

Special Thanks and Permissions

Lee E. Downing

A Forgotten Horseman: A Son's Weekend Memoir © 2006 by Lee E. Downing. Used by permission. All rights reserved.

Alan Govenar/Osceola Mays

By permission: The Black Man's Plea for Justice is excerpted from "Osceola: Memories of a Sharecropper's Daughter." Collected and edited by Alan Govenar. Copyright © 2000 by Alan Govenar and Osceola Mays.

Resources

The organizations, agencies, individuals and resources listed are provided for informational purposes. At press time we did our best to ensure the following information was correct. Please notify us at www.5sisterspublishing.com if the information is different for future editions.

100 Black Men of America, Inc. -- With several chapters across the country, the United Kingdom and other regions of the world, 100 Black Men provides educational opportunities to "overcome economic and social disadvantages." Contact information: 100 Black Men of America, Inc. 141 Auburn Avenue, Atlanta, GA 30303. Phone: (404)688-5100. Email: www.100blackmen.org

African American Dad Project – Fatherdad.com is weblog that was created to dispel some of the negative perpetuating myths about black fatherhood. The site offers peer developed parenting strategies and advice on successful co-parenting through interactive posts and podcasts. What's more, it is the first blog in the "daddy blog" genre to identify itself openly as being written by an African American Dad. Website: www.fatherdad.com

African American Male Leadership Institute – The Foundation of African American Male Leadership Institute is to "reaffirm the essence and courage to Black Male Leadership." Contact Information: Mr. Richard Rowe, AAMLI, P.O. Box 32025 Baltimore, MD 21208. Phone: (410)637-5564. Website: www.aamli.org

Alive and Free -- The mission of A&F is to encourage and empower people to success in all endeavors. Each workshop seminar and/or lecture allows individuals to choose a course of action that can help to develop and enhance leadership, social skills, self-esteem, resolution abilities and academic skills. Contact: Jeri Marshall for further information at (916)768-3987 or (916)967-5339.

American Coalition for Fathers and Children – Promotes legislation that considers "all parties" in cases of divorce, and equitable solutions. Website: **www.acfc.org**

Black Fatherhelp -- Working from the belief that giving and receiving love is a human right, *Black Fatherhelp* seeks to remedy obstacles to healthy father-child relationships through outreach, programs, research and advocacy. Please call Jackie Booth at (410)321-7994 for information.

Blackfatherhood.com -- Excellent source of information pertaining to fathers. Website: **www.blackfatherhood.com**

Black Men Raising Girls Alone -- "Dedicated to strengthening the moral and spiritual fiber of the young black woman that is parented only (or primarily) by her father." Website: **www.bmrga.com**

Blackrefer.com – Several links to Black parenting information. Website: www.blackrefer.com

Brave, Bold and Beautiful Book Series -- Dedicated to providing powerful, poignant, inspiring true stories about and from the unacknowledged, forgotten, little known and well-known, in order to preserve legacies and recall the beauty, greatness and humanity that exists in all of us. Contact: joslyngaines@comcast.net and anitaroystonca@gmail.com. Please visit **5sisterspublishing.com** or call **1-800-277-2330** to order books that will engage and inspire, specialty gifts that will empower, and African American Heritage book markers that will enlighten. All products celebrate the legacies of strong, brave and beautiful people with ancestries, stories and lives that must never be forgotten.

Center for Fathers and Families – "The Center for Fathers and Families was established to provide enrichment and educational resources to fathers and fatherless families." Contact: 916-568-DADS (3237). Website: www.fathersandfamilies.com

Center for Urban Families – CFUF "Changes lives by helping their clients build the skills and the confidence to find their personal power to change." Contact: Joe Jones, President/CEO, Center for Urban Families, 3002 Druid Park Drive, Baltimore, MD 21215. Phone: (410)367-5691. Website: www.cfuf.org

Casey Families Services – "CFS offers a wide range of services for foster youth." Contact: Darryl Green, Director, Young Fathers Programs, 25 North Caroline St. Baltimore, MD 21231. Phone: (410) 342-7554 or (800) 992-2802. Website: www.caseyfamilyservices.org

Concerned Black Men -- "Supports youth and strengthens families." Contact information: The Thurgood Marshall Center, 1816 12th Street, NW Ste. 204, Washington, DC 20009. Phone: (202)783-6119 or toll free (888)395-7816. Website: www.cbmnational.org/contact

Daddy's Here – Men's support group for fathers who would like to be more involved or improve their involvement in the lives of their children. Guests speakers range from attorneys to relationship experts. Contact: Terry Moore, Coordinator, (916)568-DADS ext. 205 or email: terry@fathersandfamilies.com

Daddy Hunger – Powerful, award winning documentary with a message of "Redemption, Hope & Love!" Ray Upchurch's documentary *Daddy Hunger* can be ordered via his website at www.daddyhunger.com or by calling (916)333-1606.

(The) Fathers Network -- Information provided to help fathers, families, care providers who work with children with special needs. Website: **www.fathersnetwork.org**

Fathers Rights Help -- Parental rights advocates. Website: **www.parentaladvocates.info**

Fathers Who Care – Established to help non-custodial fathers and custodial fathers who are indigent and want to be engaged in the lives of their children. 3333 West Arthington St., Ste 1051, Chicago, IL 60624 Phone: (773) 638-2052 Website: www.fatherswhocare.us

Frank Withrow -- is powerful poet, educator and motivational speaker. For information about Frank's products, please visit reasonsforrhyme.com. Frank can also be reached at for public engagements. Reasons For Rhyme, 8660 Red Clover Way, Elk Grove, CA 95624. (916)681-1179.

jBanta, Inc. Resource & Support for Fathers, 2831 Fruitridge Road, Ste. M, Sacramento, CA, 95820. Phone: (916) 739-0894 *Fax:* (916) 739-0895. Provides numerous programs to aid fathers. *Email:* info@jbanta.com. Web: www.jbanta.com

The Men's Center -- Large database of information and resources for men. Website: www.themenscenter.com

National Fatherhood Initiative – National Fatherhood Initiative's **mission** "is to improve the well being of children by increasing the proportion of children growing up with involved, responsible, and committed fathers." Contact: www.fatherhood.org

Non-custodial Mothers & Fathers and Non-custodial Parents Meet Ups – Groups around the country that meet and discuss parental issues. Website: noncustodial.meetup.com/

The TEAL Group *(Train*Educate*Advocate*Link)* specializes in teen and family mentoring and empowerment training to *"help people, help themselves." GIRL* Power and Boyz-2-*KINGZ* **is designed to empower** youth. Contact: Cloteal Thrower Herron at (916)364-0778. Email ctealgroup@aol.com or visit her website www.Tealgroup.org

Urban Leadership Institute – Organization that utilizes innovative and "non-traditional approaches" and programs such as *Dare to Be King* to address issues and challenges that youth face. Contact: David E. Miller, Chief Visionary Officer, ULI, 2437 Maryland Avenue, Baltimore, MD 21218. Phone: 1(877)339-4300 toll free or (410)467-1605. Website: www.urbanleadershipinstitute.com/